Complementary and Integrative Therapies for ENT Disorders

Editors

JOHN MADDALOZZO
EDMUND A. PRIBITKIN
MICHAEL D. SEIDMAN

OTOLARYNGOLOGIC CLINICS OF NORTH AMERICA

www.oto.theclinics.com

June 2013 • Volume 46 • Number 3

ELSEVIER

1600 John F. Kennedy Boulevard • Suite 1800 • Philadelphia, Pennsylvania, 19103-2899

http://www.theclinics.com

OTOLARYNGOLOGIC CLINICS OF NORTH AMERICA Volume 46, Number 3
June 2013 ISSN 0030-6665, ISBN-13: 978-1-4557-7154-7

Editor: Joanne Husovski
Development Editor: Gretchen Spencer

Otolaryngologic Clinics of North America (ISSN 0030-6665) is published bimonthly by Elsevier, Inc., 360 Park Avenue South, New York, NY 10010-1710. Months of issue are February, April, June, August, October, and December. Business and Editorial Offices: 1600 John F. Kennedy Blvd., Suite 1800, Philadelphia, PA 19103-2899. Customer Service Office: 6277 Sea Harbor Drive, Orlando, FL 32887-4800. Periodicals postage paid at New York, NY and additional mailing offices. Subscription prices is $348.00 per year (US individuals), $653.00 per year (US institutions), $167.00 per year (US student/resident), $460.00 per year (Canadian individuals), $819.00 per year (Canadian institutions), $516.00 per year (international individuals), $819.00 per year (international institutions), $258.00 per year (international & Canadian student/resident). Foreign air speed delivery is included in all *Clinics'* subscription prices. All prices are subject to change without notice. **POSTMASTER:** Send address changes to *Otolaryngologic Clinics of North America*, Elsevier Health Sciences Division, Subscription Customer Service, 3251 Riverport Lane, Maryland Heights, MO 63043. **Telephone: 1-800-654-2452 (U.S. and Canada); 314-447-8871 (outside U.S. and Canada). Fax: 314-447-8029. E-mail: journalscustomerservice-usa@elsevier.com (for print support); journalsonlinesupport-usa@elsevier.com (for online support).**

Reprints. For copies of 100 or more of articles in this publication, please contact the Commercial Reprints Department, Elsevier Inc., 360 Park Avenue South, New York, NY 10010-1710. Tel.: 212-633-3812; Fax: 212-462-1935; E-mail: reprints@elsevier.com.

Otolaryngologic Clinics of North America is also published in Spanish by McGraw-Hill Interamericana Editores S.A., P.O. Box 5-237, 06500 Mexico D.F., Mexico.

Otolaryngologic Clinics of North America is covered in *MEDLINE/PubMed (Index Medicus), Current Contents/Clinical Medicine, Excerpta Medica, BIOSIS, Science Citation Index,* and *ISI/BIOMED.*

Printed and bound by CPI Group (UK) Ltd, Croydon, CR0 4YY

Transferred to digital print 2012

Contributors

EDITORS

JOHN MADDALOZZO, MD
Attending Physician, Ann & Robert H. Lurie Children's Hospital of Chicago; Professor, Department of Otolaryngology, Feinberg School of Medicine, Northwestern University, Chicago, Illinois

EDMUND A. PRIBITKIN, MD
Professor, Academic Vice Chairman, Department of Otolaryngology-Head & Neck Surgery, Thomas Jefferson University, Philadelphia, Pennsylvania

MICHAEL D. SEIDMAN, MD, FACS
Director, Division Otologic/Neurotologic Surgery, Medical Director for Wellness, Henry Ford Hospital, Medical Director, Center for Integrative Medicine, Henry Ford Health System, West Bloomfield, Michigan; Professor of Otolaryngology-Head and Neck Surgery, Wayne State University, Detroit, Michigan

AUTHORS

GREGORY J. ARTZ, MD
Department of Otolaryngology–Head and Neck Surgery, Thomas Jefferson University Hospitals, Philadelphia, Pennsylvania

BENJAMIN F. ASHER, MD, FACS
Private Practice, Asher Integrative Ear, Nose, and Throat, New York, New York

KATHLEEN R. BILLINGS, MD
Assistant Professor, Division of Pediatric Otolaryngology, Department of Surgery, Children's Memorial Hospital; Assistant Professor, Division of Otolaryngology–Head and Neck Surgery, Department of Surgery, Ann & Robert H. Lurie Children's Hospital of Chicago, and the Northwestern University Feinberg School of Medicine, Chicago, Illinois

SETH M. BROWN, MD, MBA, FACS
Assistant Clinical Professor, Connecticut Sinus Institute, University of Connecticut School of Medicine, Farmington, Connecticut

KYRRAS CONRAD, RN, MA
Certified St John's Neuromuscular Therapist, Center for Integrative Medicine, Conrad Neuromuscular Therapy Center, LLC, Henry Ford Health System, West Bloomfield, Michigan

GRANT GARBO, MD
Resident in Otolaryngology, University of Connecticut School of Medicine, West Hartford, Connecticut

PAULA GARDINER, MD, MPH
Assistant Professor of Family Medicine, Department of Family Medicine, Boston
University Medical Center, Boston University, Boston, Massachusetts

ELIZABETH GRAY-KARAGRIGORIOU, Au.D
Department of Otolaryngology–Head and Neck Surgery, Thomas Jefferson University
Hospitals, Philadelphia, Pennsylvania

JAMES M. HAMILTON, MD
Department of Otolaryngology-Head and Neck Surgery, Thomas Jefferson University,
Philadelphia, Pennsylvania

JENNIFER M. LAVIN, MD
Department of Otolaryngology-Head and Neck Surgery, Northwestern University
Feinberg School of Medicine, Chicago, Illinois

STEPHANIE L. LEE, MD, PhD
Associate Professor of Medicine, Section of Endocrinology, Diabetes, and Nutrition,
Department of Medicine, Boston Medical Center, Boston University School of Medicine,
Boston, Massachusetts

JESSICA R. LEVI, MD
Assistant Professor, Department of Otolaryngology Head and Neck Surgery; Assistant
Professor, Department of Pediatrics, Boston Medical Center, Boston University, Boston,
Massachusetts

JOHN MADDALOZZO, MD
Department of Otolaryngology-Head and Neck Surgery, Northwestern University
Feinberg School of Medicine; Division of Otolaryngology; Professor, Division of
Otolaryngology-Head and Neck Surgery; Professor, Division of Pediatric Otolaryngology,
Department of Surgery, Children's Memorial Hospital, Ann & Robert H. Lurie Children's
Hospital of Chicago, and the Northwestern University Feinberg School of Medicine,
Chicago, Illinois

MATTHEW C. MILLER, MD
Assistant Professor of Otolaryngology and Neurosurgery, Department of
Otolaryngology-Head and Neck Surgery, University of Rochester Medical Center,
Rochester, New York

CHAU T. NGUYEN, MD, FACS
Director, Division of Otolaryngology-Head and Neck Surgery, Department of Surgery,
Ventura County Medical Center, Ventura, California; Assistant Clinical Professor, UCLA
Department of Head and Neck Surgery, Los Angeles, California

ROBERT O'REILLY, MD
Division of Otolaryngology, Department of Surgery, Alfred I. duPont Hospital for Children,
Nemours Children's Clinic, Wilmington, Delaware

EDMUND A. PRIBITKIN, MD
Professor, Academic Vice Chairman, Department of Otolaryngology-Head and Neck
Surgery, Thomas Jefferson University, Philadelphia, Pennsylvania

MASSI ROMANELLI-GOBBI, BM
Jefferson Medical College of Thomas Jefferson University, Philadelphia, Pennsylvania

JENNIFER E. ROSEN, MD, FACS
Assistant Professor of Surgery, Section of Surgical Oncology, Department of Surgery, Boston University, Boston, Massachusetts

MICHAEL D. SEIDMAN, MD, FACS
Director, Division Otologic/Neurotologic Surgery, Medical Director for Wellness, Henry Ford Hospital, Medical Director, Center for Integrative Medicine, Henry Ford Health System, West Bloomfield, Michigan; Professor of Otolaryngology-Head and Neck Surgery, Wayne State University, Detroit, Michigan

GREGORY S. SMITH, MD
Department of Otolaryngology–Head and Neck Surgery, Thomas Jefferson University Hospitals, Philadelphia, Pennsylvania

MICHAEL SPANO, MS, R.Ac
Center for Integrative Medicine, Henry Ford Health System, Northville, Michigan

MALCOLM B. TAW, MD
Assistant Clinical Professor, UCLA Center for East-West Medicine, Santa Monica, California

BELACHEW TESSEMA, MD, FACS
Assistant Clinical Professor, Connecticut Sinus Institute, University of Connecticut School of Medicine, Farmington, Connecticut

DAVID TIEU, MD
Department of Otolaryngology-Head and Neck Surgery, Kaiser Foundation Hospital, Los Angeles, California

GERARD VAN GRINSVEN
President and CEO, Henry Ford West Bloomfield Hospital, West Bloomfield, Michigan

MARILENE B. WANG, MD, FACS
Professor, Department of Head and Neck Surgery, David Geffen School of Medicine at UCLA, Los Angeles, California; Professor, UCLA Department of Head and Neck Surgery, Los Angeles, California

JESSICA R. WEISS, MD
Resident in Otolaryngology–Head and Neck Surgery, University of Connecticut School of Medicine, Farmington, Connecticut

Contents

The authors discuss current medical and surgical regimens, and then provide a review of the current literature on integrative and complementary approaches for treatment of this disorder.

This article discusses the use of an integrative approach to treating tinnitus. The authors begin with a discussion of their approach to tinnitus patients, followed by a detailed look at the physiology of tinnitus and several theories of its mechanism. The many viable options for tinnitus relief are discussed, including sound therapies, Western medical approaches, and herbal and traditional medicines that can be used as integrative and complementary treatments. It concludes with a reminder that a variety of treatment options are available to tinnitus patients to help them take control of their symptoms.

This article presents an overview of balance disorders for the practicing otolaryngologist. The demographics of balance disorders, anatomy and physiology of human balance, clinical features, differential diagnosis, and treatment, within the framework of an holistic approach, are discussed.

Complementary and integrative medicine (CIM) is defined by the National Institutes of Health as a group of diverse medical and health care systems, practices, and products not generally considered part of conventional medicine. CIM practices are grouped into 4 categories: natural products, mind and body medicine practices, manipulative practices, and body-based practices. CIM use in patients is common and a working knowledge is relevant to practicing physicians. This article presents an overview of common forms of CIM and their theoretic framework to review the data regarding CIM use in thyroid disease. The intent is to facilitate communication between patients and physicians regarding CIM.

This article discusses the use of an integrative approach in the evaluation and management of the voice. The article begins with a look at the larynx and antioxidant therapy, followed by methods to relieve the pain associated with myofacial trigger points, and the herbs and supplements that can be used by vocalists to replace conventional medications in allergies and reflux. The article concludes with a reminder of the reasons why many vocalists turn to complementary and integrative treatments.

OTOLARYNGOLOGIC CLINICS OF NORTH AMERICA

**DOWNLOAD
Free App!**

Review Articles
THE CLINICS

NOW AVAILABLE FOR YOUR iPhone and iPad

Complementary and Integrative Treatments
Expanding the Continuum of Care

Matthew C. Miller, MD

KEYWORDS

- Complementary and alternative medicine • CAM • Integrative medicine • CIM
- Otolaryngology • Traditional medicine • Acupuncture
- Homeopathy natural products • Supplements

KEY POINTS

- For a variety of reasons, increasing numbers of patients are using complementary and integrative medicines.
- The list of treatments considered to be complementary and/or integrative is constantly growing and evolving.
- Most patients do not disclose use of complementary and integrative therapies unless specifically asked by their physician.
- Education and communication are paramount to the integration of evidence-based complementary and integrative therapies into Western medicine.
- Complementary and integrative medicines have the potential to be harmful to patients, but they also have the potential to be helpful.

OVERVIEW OF COMPLEMENTARY AND INTEGRATIVE MEDICINE

In the United States, "conventional medicine" is a term that has come to be synonymous with Western (ie, allopathic and osteopathic) medicine and surgery. In practical terms, all other medical systems and practices have been considered to be "complementary" or "alternative." Being outside of what is considered mainstream medicine in the Western world, complementary and integrative medicine (CIM) is often viewed as a single entity and is in many cases marginalized. However, not unlike Western medicine, CIM represents a heterogeneous group of therapies, practices, and philosophies. As such, each has a unique set of distinguishing features, purported benefits, and potential risks. Likewise, there are varying levels of scientific evidence to support or refute their use.

Disclosures/conflicts of interest: none.
Department of Otolaryngology-Head and Neck Surgery, Box 629, 601 Elmwood Avenue, Rochester, NY 14642, USA
E-mail address: Matthew_miller@urmc.rochester.edu

Otolaryngol Clin N Am 46 (2013) 261–276
http://dx.doi.org/10.1016/j.otc.2012.12.003
0030-6665/13/$ – see front matter © 2013 Elsevier Inc. All rights reserved.

oto.theclinics.com

What Constitutes CIM

CIM encompasses a broad array of preventive, therapeutic, and palliative modalities, and the list of what constitutes CIM is ever-evolving. According to the National Center for Complementary and Alternative Medicine (NCCAM), complementary medicines are used concurrently with traditional medical and surgical interventions. They may be used for alleviation of symptoms, reduction of disability, improvement of overall quality of life, or promoting general wellness during treatment. Alternative therapies are used in lieu of traditional Western medicines. The practice of integrative medicine, on the other hand, involves combining allopathic medicine with complementary therapies for which there is scientific evidence of safety and efficacy.[1] In response to the increased awareness of integrative medicine and its relevance to modern medical practice, the term "complementary and integrative medicine," or CIM, has been used interchangeably with complementary and alternative medicine (CAM) in recent years. Although the distinction between these two is subtle, its importance should not be minimized. Although "CAM" continues to be the predominant abbreviation used throughout the medical literature, this review seeks to highlight the integrative nature of the therapies, and hence CIM is used throughout (**Table 1** gives a full list of CIM abbreviations).

CIM Usage

Although CIM is not typically taught in US and European medical schools, it has made significant gains in popularity among patients and practitioners in recent years. Indeed, approximately 38% of the general US population admitted to CIM use in a 2007 survey of more than 23,000 adults conducted by the Centers for Disease Control. The prevalence of CIM use is up nearly 10% when compared with 1991 data.[2,3] This translates to roughly $34 billion in out-of-pocket CIM purchases.[4] When patients visiting general otolaryngology clinics are evaluated as a separate group, more than 60% have been found to be CIM users in some series.[5] Pediatric otolaryngology patients may also use CIM frequently, as evidenced by a recent study by Shakeel and colleagues.[6] They report that nearly 30% of patients presenting to a pediatric otolaryngology clinic

Table 1 Abbreviations: overview of CIM terms	
CAM	Complementary and alternative medicine
CIM	Complementary and integrative medicine
DC	Doctors of Chiropractic
DO	Doctors of Osteopathic Medicine
DSHEA	Dietary Supplement Health and Education Act
NCCAM	National Center for Complementary and Alternative Medicine
NIH	National Institutes of Health
OMM	Osteopathic manipulative medicine
ppm	Parts per million
TCM	Traditional Chinese medicine
TM	Traditional medicine
TT	Therapeutic touch
USP	United States Pharmacopeial
WHO	World Health Organization

have used CIM. Oncology patients may be particularly amenable to CIM use. In large series, prevalence of CIM use ranges from 17% to 91% among this population.[7–11] When patients with head and neck cancer are considered as a separate group, CIM usage prevalence ranges from 6% to 92%.[7,10,12–16]

In response to the growing interest in, use of, and acceptance of complementary and alternative therapies, the US Congress established the NCCAM in 1998. As one of 27 centers within the National Institutes of Health (NIH), NCCAM funds and supports CIM-related research, disseminates CIM-related information, and assists with the integration of proved CIM therapies into medical practice. With an annual operating budget of nearly $128 million, NCCAM's stated mission is "To define, through rigorous scientific investigation, the usefulness and safety of complementary and alternative medicine interventions and their roles in improving health and health care." As such, NCCAM serves as the NIH's liaison to the public and the medical profession with regard to complementary and alternative therapies. They are a repository for CIM-related grant money and a resource for numerous clinical trials.[1]

This review introduces otolaryngologists to several commonly encountered CIM modalities. The goal is to classify and define these entities as well as to provide a historical, cultural, philosophic, and physiologic background for them. The in-depth discussion of individual treatments and their applicability to specific otolaryngologic problems are discussed elsewhere in this issue.

CLASSIFICATION OF CIM MODALITIES

The list of what constitutes CIM is fluid. NCCAM loosely categorizes CIM into several broad domains[1]:

- Traditional medicine and whole medical systems
- Mind-body interventions
- Manipulative and body-based practices
- Movement therapies
- Natural products
- Energy therapies

There is often overlap between the subgroups, and individual treatments are continuously being added to the list. Examples of CIM that fall within each of these categories can be seen in **Box 1**.

TRADITIONAL MEDICINE AND WHOLE MEDICAL SYSTEMS

The World Health Organization (WHO) estimates that less than 40% of the world's population practices conventional Western medicine[1] (ie, medical practice founded on the biochemical and pathophysiologic basis for disease). The remainder of the world's population practices what is referred to as traditional or "folk medicine." In their 2002 report on the state of traditional medicine (TM), the WHO defines TM as a group of "diverse health practices, approaches, knowledge and beliefs incorporating plant, animal, and/or mineral based medicines, spiritual therapies, manual techniques and exercises applied singularly or in combination to maintain well-being, as well as to treat, diagnose or prevent illness."[17]

In developing nations, up to 90% of the population receive their primary medical care from practitioners of TM.[17] In developed countries, particularly those in Asia and Latin America, the practice of TM is also widespread, despite the availability of conventional Western medicine.[17] Moreover, it has been demonstrated that large proportions of Asian

Box 1
Categories and examples of CIM

Traditional healers

    Native American Shaman

Whole medical systems

    Traditional Chinese medicine

    Ayurveda

    Homeopathy

    Naturopathy

Mind-body medicine

    Meditation

    Yoga

    Prayer and intercessory prayer

    Music and art therapy

    Guided imagery

    Aromatherapy

    Deep breathing exercises

    Hypnotherapy

Manipulative and body-based practices

    Acupuncture

    Moxibustion

    Chiropractic and osteopathic manipulation

    Biofeedback

Movement therapies

    Pilates

    Tai Chi

Natural products

    Herbal remedies

    Megadose vitamins

    Animal-derived extracts (eg, shark-fin cartilage and rhinoceros horn)

    Plant extracts

    Enzymes and enzyme derivatives

    Special diets

Energy therapies

    Reiki

    Therapeutic touch

    Qigong

Indian and Chinese immigrants continue to use TM after emigrating to the United States and that the phenomenon of acculturation often does not apply in this context.[18–20]

The cultural, spiritual, and geopolitical contexts within which a given form of TM exists has a tremendous influence on the philosophies and treatment modalities that are practiced. In some cases, these have evolved into well-defined medical systems. These so-called alternative medical systems are complete systems of theory and practice. They are philosophically rather than scientifically rooted. Practitioners and supporters of these systems cite the importance of balance and harmony between the physical, mental, and spiritual self. Interventions and therapies in these systems are aimed at reestablishing such a balance to facilitate the body's innate capacity for healing.[1,21] Traditional Chinese medicine (TCM) and Eastern medical philosophies have been practiced for centuries, as has the Indian system of Ayurveda. Over time, many of the teachings and practices of these and other systems have been imported to and adopted by Western societies. In some cases, entirely new systems have developed based on the Eastern principles of restoring inner harmony to promote the body's self-healing capacity. Examples of alternative medical systems that have developed in Western cultures include homeopathic and naturopathic medicine. Although complete reliance on an alternative medical system is uncommon in the United States today, many individual CIM therapies currently practiced either directly or indirectly trace their roots to one of these systems.

There are few articles in the literature that specifically discuss the applications of alternative medical systems to otolaryngology. However, an understanding of the philosophic undertones of these systems can allow for a better understanding of the decision-making process of patients who subscribe to them. A brief overview of 4 common alternative medical systems, TCM, Ayurveda (traditional Indian medicine), homeopathy, and naturopathy, is provided herein.

Traditional Chinese Medicine

TCM is an ancient practice and considers humans to be at the center of the universe and an essential link between the celestial and the earthly worlds.[22] The world and the individual exist in a zero net gain state of homeostasis between *yin* and *yang*, or positive and negative energies. Disruptions in this equilibrium are thought to affect health and well-being. To restore harmony between yin and yang, the flow of 4 vital humors (blood, moisture, essence, and *qi*, or "life energy") must be manipulated. Multiple different modalities are used by practitioners of TCM to balance yin and yang. Principal among these are meditation, acupuncture, and a large number of biologically based therapies.[1,21,22] Despite the vast number of TCM modalities practiced for a myriad of diseases and conditions, there continues to be insufficient scientific evidence to support their widespread use, which is perhaps best evidenced by the work of Manheimer and colleagues[23] in their 2008 query of the Cochrane database for systematic reviews of TCM. They found that most trials evaluating TCM modalities suffered from methodological flaws and heterogeneity, ultimately leading them to conclude that further rigorous investigation is warranted before definitive recommendations regarding TCM can be made.

Ayurveda

Ayurveda is perhaps the oldest medical system still in practice in the world today. It began in India several millennia ago and is still practiced by nearly 50% of India's population. The name comes from the Sanskrit words *ayur* (life) and *veda* (knowledge). The principal tenets are that humans and their universe are interconnected and that all of material creation comprises 5 elements: space, air, fire, water, and earth. Each person possesses a unique proportion of these elements at birth—a ratio that is in turn the foundation for 3 governing life forces or *doshas*. It is the relationship between the 3 doshas that dictates each person's biologic makeup and hence, their physical makeup, physiologic functioning, and psychological characteristics.[1,21,22,24,25]

Each person has a predominant dosha, and the doshas must exist in their native state of balance for the maintenance of health. Exposure to anything that alters this delicate interplay manifests itself by disease. To restore balance, several different therapies are used. These have traditionally included biologically based modalities such as herbals and special diets. Purging treatments play a prominent role as well—with vomiting, nasal irrigation, enemas, and bloodletting used to "detoxify" in an attempt to restore balance. There is a strong mind-body component as well, with an emphasis on visualization techniques, oil massage, and yoga.[1,24,25]

Homeopathy

Homeopathy was founded in the late 1700s by Samuel Hahnemann. It holds as its most basic tenet the notion that "Like cures like." Homeopaths contend that the body may be stimulated to heal itself by being exposed to small doses of substances that would in larger doses cause symptoms akin to their disease.[1,21,26] Homeopathic remedies are generated by performing serial dilutions while agitating the mixture to extract the "vital essences" of the offending substance. The most common denotation of a homeopathic preparation is $\_\times$, which refers to the number of 1:10 dilutions performed. A $6\times$ would be a concentration of $1:10^6$ or 1 part per million (ppm). So miniscule is the dose delivered in most homeopathic remedies that they are exempt from much of the US Food and Drug Administration (FDA) oversight that is characteristic of other medications. However, the FDA does regulate that package inserts for homeopathic medicines include an ingredients list, instructions for safe use, at least one major indication, and the dilution. At present, 3 states offer licensure to practice homeopathy. Only one (Nevada) requires formal training before license application.[27]

Despite the apparent lack of a measurable pharmacologic effect, a limited amount of evidence does support the efficacy of homeopathy in certain conditions treated by otolaryngologists. For instance, a systematic review suggests that it is effective in the treatment of chemotherapy-induced stomatitis, radiodermatitis, and general adverse events from radiotherapy.[28] In a randomized double-blinded trial comparing the homeopathic remedy VertigoHeel, there was an observed reduction in the frequency, duration, and intensity of vertigo attacks that was equivalent to standard therapy with betahistadine.[29] It has been argued that the placebo effect may be entirely responsible for the observed effects of homeopathy.[30] However, other factors such as patient expectations and openness to the mind-body connection and practitioner empathy may also play a role in the observed benefits of these remedies.[31]

Naturopathy

Naturopathy is a medical system that originated in the Western world. As a consequence, its practitioners do concern themselves with the pathophysiologic nature of disease and scientific method. However, at its core, naturopathy shares many of the philosophies and traditions of Eastern practices such as Ayurveda and TCM. Naturopathy emphasizes prevention and self-care to restore a "healthy internal environment." Naturopathic practitioners believe that this in turn promotes the body's innate self-healing mechanisms.[1,32,33] Most treatment strategies rely on natural healing methods. Today, these consist primarily of herbal remedies, supplements, and special diets.[1,32] Naturopathy is unique among the alternative medical systems in that the education and professional licensure criteria are stringent. A total of 17 states and 2 US territories now offer professional licenses to naturopathic physicians. There are numerous postbaccalaureate programs offering Naturopathic Doctor (ND) degrees. These programs are accredited by the US Department of Education and feature training in naturopathy as well as basic and clinical sciences traditionally taught in allopathic medical curricula.[27,32,33]

MIND-BODY MEDICINE

The mind-body interventions are a diverse group of techniques designed to enhance the mind's capacity to affect bodily function and symptoms. Some techniques that were thought to be alternative in the past have become mainstream (eg, patient support groups and cognitive-behavioral therapy).[1] Other mind-body interventions are still considered CIM by most. These include, but are not limited to, meditation, prayer, mental healing, yoga, aromatherapy, and therapies that use creative outlets such as art, music, or dance. Mind-body techniques are among the most common forms of CIM used in the United States, and their use seems to be on the rise. According to the 2007 National Health Information Survey (NHIS) data, mind-body techniques experienced the greatest increase in use during the period between 2002 and 2007.[3] Another survey of more than 2000 American households found that nearly 19% of all respondents had used at least one form of mind-body intervention within the previous 12 months.[34] When prayer for self or others is included in the analysis, the prevalence of mind-body therapy use can approach 90%.[7–9]

Mind-body interventions tend to be low-risk forms of CIM, as they typically pose little to no physical or emotional danger to patients. Several validated patient surveys have shown that they are also considered to be among the most efficacious group CIM in terms of promoting overall wellness. There seems to be clear evidence to support the use of these techniques for the reduction of anxiety and emotional distress, improvement of the patient's perceived social support, sleep quality, and overall sense of well-being.[21,35,36]

Physiologic and biochemical measures of the mind-body connection have also been reported. Yoga and guided meditation have been shown to reduce blood pressure, improve cardiovascular risk profiles, and promote better vascular endothelial function among patients with coronary artery disease.[37–39] Among patients with breast and prostate cancer, mind-body interventions have also demonstrated the ability to shift serum cytokine and T-cell profiles toward normal levels.[35,36] Solberg and colleagues[40] found that baseline melatonin levels were significantly higher in meditators than in nonmeditators and that serotonin levels decrease precipitously after an hour of meditation.

MANIPULATIVE AND BODY-BASED TECHNIQUES

Members of this subgroup share in common with one another the use of physical force to move and/or manipulate a particular body part, the principle that the human body is self-regulating and has the ability to heal itself, and the notion that all parts of the human body are interconnected and interdependent.[1] The general goal of manipulative techniques is to alter function through the alteration of form. Common examples of these interventions include acupuncture, chiropractic and osteopathic manipulation, massage, and reflexology.

Acupuncture

Acupuncture has been practiced for several millennia and is a central feature of TCM. In the United States, there are more than 3000 physicians and more than 14,000 licensed acupuncturists in practice. Licensure is available in 42 states to individuals who have completed a 3-year training program. In several states, the practice of acupuncture is actually incorporated into physician licensure.[27]

There are numerous different techniques and descriptions of acupuncture, although the most commonly described method uses thin metal needles that pierce the skin at various points across the body's surface.[1,41] According to TCM teachings, these points are chosen for their relationship to the flow of qi along conduits known as meridians.[21,41] Stimulation along the meridians is thought to alter this flow and promote balance of qi and the overall restoration of health. A more physiologic basis has been ascribed to the stimulation of afferent neurons (primarily group I and II afferents) by acupuncture needles,[42] which results in several neurophysiologic responses. Pain relief comes as a result of an increase in the release of enkephalins and endorphins, which in turn inhibit nociceptive fibers.[43] Levels of cortisol, interferons, interleukins, and natural killer cell activity have also been shown to increase with acupuncture,[44,45] suggesting a role in immune activation and responsiveness.

Acupuncture has numerous potential applications in otolaryngology, particularly with respect to the management of head and neck cancer symptoms. Its efficacy in pain control has been well established.[10] Acupuncture has also been suggested as a treatment of chemotherapy-induced nausea. Dundee and colleagues[46] demonstrated a reduction in chemotherapy-associated emesis in 97% of patients. A 2006 Cochrane review concluded that acupuncture was beneficial for acute nausea but argued that head-to-head comparison with the newest antiemetic medications was needed to further elucidate acupuncture's role in this context.[47] There have been several reports that acupuncture or acupuncture-like stimulation improves salivary flow in patients with radiation-induced xerostomia. This improvement has been noted for subjective symptom scores as well as baseline and stimulated salivary flow rates.[48-50] Adverse effects of acupuncture are rare and typically mild.[41] Although there are apparently no absolute contraindications, care should be taken in any patient who is concurrently receiving anticoagulant therapy or who has an innate coagulopathy.

Chiropractic Manipulation and Osteopathic Manipulative Medicine

Musculoskeletal manipulative therapies have been present since the time of Hippocrates and have been prominent features of several traditional medical practices. Today, these techniques are most commonly associated with chiropractic and osteopathy. Chiropractic and osteopathic manipulations are the second and fourth most common types of CIM used by children and adults in the United States, respectively.[3] This amounts to more than 20 million visits annually with total out-of-pocket costs approaching $4 billion.[4] Both Doctors of Chiropractic (DC) and Doctors of Osteopathic Medicine (DO) are required to undergo 4 years of postbaccalaureate training. Licensure is available in all 50 states.

Conceived at the turn of the twentieth century, chiropractic developed out of a belief that spinal misalignment results in aberrant flow of energy between the brain and the body's organ systems, thus resulting in disease processes. Adjustments of the vertebrae are thought to allow for the body to heal itself through the reestablishment of the natural communication between the body and the central nervous system.[1,51] Chiropractic manipulation has been promoted as a treatment of both somatic and visceral conditions. However, the scientific basis for its efficacy in treating nonmusculoskeletal disorders is lacking. Indeed, a 1995 paper by 2 chiropractors concluded that "no appropriately controlled studies that establish that spinal manipulation or any other form of somatic therapy represents a valid curative strategy for the treatment of any internal organ disease." The investigators concluded that the benefit of spinal manipulation (and other manipulative therapies) in these instances was likely due to somatic-visceral mimicry.[52]

Osteopathic medicine was founded in the mid-1800s by an allopathic physician (Andrew Taylor Still, MD). Still was discouraged by the ineffectual and often harmful nature of medicine at the time. He believed that the body possessed an innate capacity to heal itself and eventually came to the conclusion that alterations in structure could have profound effects on function. It was and continues to be postulated that manipulative techniques can facilitate the body's self-healing powers.[53] Similar to chiropractors, osteopathic physicians perform several different spinal manipulations that at are directed at both somatic and visceral disorders, although subtle variations in technique do distinguish the two. The principal difference between osteopathy and chiropractic resides in the fact that osteopathic practitioners in the United States are physicians, whereas chiropractors are not. Indeed, osteopathic medical education is actually similar in content and rigor to allopathic medical school. Graduates of osteopathic medical schools may become licensed physicians and practice within any of the medical or surgical disciplines. Although osteopathic manipulative medicine (OMM) continues to be featured prominently during education and training, its role in the day-to-day practices of DOs seems to be diminishing. Results from a survey of 955 osteopathic physicians revealed that most DOs (86%) use OMM infrequently (ie, for less than 25% of their patients).[54]

Although the benefits for visceral disorders are somewhat suspect, spinal manipulative therapies do seem to have efficacy in the management of acute and chronic musculoskeletal pain.[55–57] However, spinal manipulation is not without risk. Complications of these therapies are thought to be widely underreported.[58] Although the incidence of adverse events among patients undergoing spinal manipulation is largely unknown, a recent systematic review suggested that complications occurred in 33% to 61% of these procedures.[59] Although most of these were minor and short-lived, serious events including stroke, myelopathy, arterial dissection, vertebral disk displacement, epidural hematoma, and death have been reported. These are estimated to occur at a rate of approximately 1.5 per 100,000 manipulations.[59]

NATURAL PRODUCTS

The collective group of natural products is perhaps the largest, most diverse, and most rapidly evolving class of CIM.[1,2] According to the National Health Interview Survey, non-vitamin, nonmineral natural products are the most commonly used forms of CIM in the United States today.[3] This category encompasses a variety of treatments including simple dietary modifications, vitamins and minerals, herbals, animal-derived products, and other substances. That they are largely unprocessed and scientifically unproven renders them complementary or alternative. However, a great number of these products have true pharmacologic, physiologic, and toxicologic effects. Numerous medicines now considered to be mainstream were developed only after the medicinal properties of their raw or unprocessed forms were recognized. Examples include

- Willow bark (aspirin)
- Foxglove (digoxin)
- Belladonna (atropine)
- Opium poppy (morphine)
- Pacific yew berry (taxane antineoplastics)

For the most part, biologically based CIM therapies are now designated by the FDA and available to the consumer as dietary supplements. The 1990s saw a dramatic increase in the use of these so-called natural supplements.[2] The growth of the Internet and the dawn of the information age may be partially responsible, but the boon has most certainly been hastened by the passage of the Dietary Supplement Health and Education Act (DSHEA) of 1994. Under this act, Congress defined a new nonfood, nondrug category of ingestibles known as dietary supplements. According to DSHEA, a dietary supplement[60]

- Is a product (other than tobacco) that is intended to supplement the diet that bears or contains one or more of the following dietary ingredients: a vitamin, a mineral, an herb or other botanic, an amino acid, a dietary substance for use by man to supplement the diet by increasing the total daily intake, or a concentrate, metabolite, constituent, extract, or combinations of these ingredients.
- Is intended for ingestion in pill, capsule, tablet, or liquid form.
- Is not represented for use as a conventional food or as the sole item of a meal or diet.
- Is labeled as a "dietary supplement."
- May not claim to diagnose, prevent, mitigate, treat, or cure a specific disease.
- Must bear the statement "This statement has not been evaluated by the Food and Drug Administration. This product is not intended to diagnose, treat, cure, or prevent any disease."

Before the passage of the DSHEA, most substances that are now considered supplements were subject to premarketing scrutiny by the FDA and held to the standards of foods and/or drugs. Since DSHEA was passed, the task of ensuring truth in labeling and safety of a supplement before sale lies with the manufacturer. The FDA does engage in postmarketing surveillance and sanctioning in the event of a reported safety hazard.[60,61] Due to the lack of oversight and relative ease of bringing new products to the consumer, the supplement market exploded following the passage of DSHEA.

To keep up with the growing numbers of adulterated products, safety risks, and illicit claims of efficacy, the US Pharmacopeial Convention, Inc. (USP) launched a verification program for dietary supplements in 2001. This program was designed to provide assurance to consumers that the products they purchase contain the ingredients listed on the label at the stated levels. In addition, the program evaluates and verifies supplements according to stringent standards for product purity, accuracy of ingredient labeling, and proper manufacturing practices.[62] Supplements meeting these standards may display the USP label on their package. Patients choosing such therapies should be advised to seek products with the USP label as it represents the most rigorous oversight of supplements in the United States today.

An exhaustive list of these biologically based CIM modalities is beyond the scope of even the most comprehensive review. However, the 10 most commonly used natural products (as determined by the 2007 NHIS survey) are listed in **Box 2**.[2]

ENERGY THERAPIES

Energy therapy is the least common and perhaps the most controversial category of CIM. It involves the harnessing and manipulation of the body's energy fields. NCCAM defines energy therapy into 2 categories:

1. Those involving veritable energy
2. Those involving putative energy

Veritable energies are those energies that can be quantified as having a specific wavelength and frequency within the electromagnetic spectrum. Theoretically,

Box 2
Most commonly used natural products
Fish oil/omega 3
Glucosamine
Echinacea
Flaxseed oil
Ginseng
Combination herb pills
Ginkgo biloba
Chondroitin
Garlic supplements
Coenzyme Q10

physical and electrochemical changes may be induced by placing the body or body parts into contact with these forces.

Putative energies, on the other hand, are energies that have never been objectively demonstrated by scientific measures. These exist as "vital fields" that purportedly infuse and surround the human body. Practitioners of energy medicine believe that they can restore or reset the balance of an individual's energy fields.[1,21] Once the proper energy flow is achieved, it is believed that disease states may be resolved.

Veritable energy as CIM is best exemplified by magnet therapy. Patients may use magnets because they have long been touted in anecdotal reports for their ability to reduce pain. However, well-controlled trials have failed to demonstrate their effectiveness in this capacity.[63,64] Magnet therapy has also been reported to be effective in the management of nausea.[65] Although magnet therapy seems to be safe, further research into their analgesic and antiemetic properties must be conducted before conclusions regarding their efficacy can be made.

Putative energy therapies each involve restoring balance and flow of a vital energy force. Examples of this force are the doshas of Ayurvedic medicine or the qi of TCM. Practitioners of energy therapy attempt to manipulate these so-called biofields. Several ailments (including death) are reportedly amenable to cure by realignment of biofields.[66]

Qigong is a component of TCM that teaches deep breathing and meditation techniques to bring the flow of qi back into harmony, thereby facilitating self-healing.[1] Reiki (a Japanese energy therapy) and therapeutic touch (TT) are modalities that rely on a practitioner to detect and remove blockages to biofield flow, again facilitating balance of vital energies and promoting health.[1,21] However, a 1998 study demonstrated that practitioners of TT were no better than chance alone at detecting a patient's putative energy field.[66]

BARRIERS TO INTEGRATION OF CIM

Despite its growing popularity and NIH endorsement, CIM has not yet been fully incorporated into allopathic medical practice, and true integrative medicine remains elusive; this is perhaps best reflected by the fact that CIM is not routinely discussed during medical visits. In most large series, only about 30% to 60% of CIM users disclose the use of CIM to their health care provider.[3,5,16,67,68] When patients and physicians do speak about CIM, the discussion is initiated by the patient twice as often as it is by the physician.[3] The most common reason that CIM users have cited for not disclosing CIM with health care providers is that the provider simply never asked. Approximately one-third also expressed concern that their provider either did not know enough about CIM or would be dismissive.[3] That many physicians avoid discussing CIM might give the impression that the latter is true. However, survey data suggest otherwise. A recent Mayo Clinic report queried 233 physicians regarding their knowledge base and attitudes toward CIM. Most believed that physicians should have an understanding of common CIM treatments and that incorporating CIM into their practice would have a positive effect on patient satisfaction. Most respondents also believed that they lacked sufficient knowledge to appropriately counsel patients about CIM.[69] Physicians polled in this and other studies have repeatedly indicated that they would like to receive more training with respect to CIM.[69–71]

The major limitation to educating doctors about unconventional therapies is the paucity of evidence with regard to their efficacy and safety. The challenges of CIM research are multifactorial. It has been argued that the lack of standardization and uniformity of certain therapies makes direct comparisons and reproducible data difficult to come by; that it is difficult to find adequate placebos for some CIM interventions, making a controlled and blinded trial impossible; that the subject is emotionally charged and renders patient recruitment extremely difficult; that funding for CIM research is scarce and is of low priority, and that CIM providers have little to no incentive to submit their methods to the scrutiny of science.[72] However, the continued growth in CIM's popularity and a desire to meet patient needs and desires will likely be the impetus for improved quality and scope of research.

In the meantime, patients continue to be inundated with CIM-related materials through the popular media and Internet. This information is widely available but is of variable quality.[73,74] Misleading and unsubstantiated claims abound on the World Wide Web and patients not savvy to the lack of scientific methodology might be convinced to undergo useless or even harmful treatments. The means to counteract this risk rests in physicians' ability to initiate an open and fact-based discussion about CIM with their patients. Several investigators have outlined techniques for bridging the CIM communication gap.[2,7,15,21,75,76] Central to each of their approaches is the notion that physicians are obligated to first educate themselves about CIM. Doing so allows physicians to fulfill what has been described as "an obligation to provide evidence-based advice in a manner that shows respect for the patient's beliefs and choices."[76] Only after physicians are educated and open minded can they begin to attempt to meet the needs of patients with respect to CIM.

SUMMARY

CIM is a rapidly growing and evolving phenomenon. The list of complementary, alternative, and integrative therapies is ever-changing, and the line between these treatments and Western medicine is often blurred. Consequently, it is a daunting task for otolaryngologists and other physicians to be well-versed in all facets of CIM. It is hoped that through this review, the reader will develop an understanding of what types of treatments constitute CIM and a framework for counseling patients who wish to pursue specific complementary or integrative therapies.

Today's physicians are tasked with providing evidenced-based care to a patient population with seemingly limitless access to medical information via the World Wide Web and other sources. At the same time, a greater emphasis has been placed on patient autonomy in medical decision making. Under this construct, it behooves practitioners to educate themselves about complementary and integrative therapies, to engage their patients in frank discussions about the topic, to abandon preconceived notions and biases that they may harbor, to critically evaluate the scientific literature, and to champion the concept of integrative medicine as it pertains to their patient population.

REFERENCES

1. The National Center for Complementary and Alternative Medicine (NCCAM) Web site. Available at: http://nccam.nih.gov. Accessed January 6, 2012.
2. Eisenberg DM, Davis RB, Ettner SL, et al. Trends in alternative medicine use in the United States, 1990-1997: results of a follow-up national survey. JAMA 1998;280(18):1569–75.
3. Barnes PM, Bloom B, Nahin RL. Complementary and alternative medicine use among adults and children: United States, 2007. Natl Health Stat Report 2008;(12):1–23.
4. Nahin RL, Barnes PM, Stussman BJ, et al. Costs of complementary and alternative medicine (CAM) and frequency of visits to CAM practitioners: United States, 2007. Natl Health Stat Report 2009;(18):1–14.
5. Shakeel M, Trinidade A, Jehan S, et al. The use of complementary and alternative medicine by patients attending a general otolaryngology clinic: can we afford to ignore it? Am J Otolaryngol 2010;31(4):252–60.
6. Shakeel M, Little SA, Bruce J, et al. Use of complementary and alternative medicine in pediatric otolaryngology patients attending a tertiary hospital in the UK. Int J Pediatr Otorhinolaryngol 2007;71(11):1725–30.
7. Yates JS, Mustain KM, Morrow GR, et al. Prevalence of complementary and alternative medicine use in cancer patients during treatment. Support Care Cancer 2005;13:806–11.
8. van der Weg F, Streuli RA. Use of alternative medicine by patients with cancer in a rural area of Switzerland. Swiss Med Wkly 2003;133:233–40.
9. Dy GK, Bekele L, Hanson LJ, et al. Complementary and alternative medicine use by patients enrolled onto phase I clinical trials. J Clin Oncol 2004;22:4810–5.
10. Hyodo I, Amano N, Eguchi K, et al. Nationwide survey on complementary and alternative medicine in cancer patients in Japan. J Clin Oncol 2005;23:2645–54.
11. Lafferty WE, Bellas A, Corage Baden A, et al. The use of complementary and alternative medical providers by insured cancer patients in Washington State. Cancer 2004;100:1522–30.
12. Davis GE, Bryson CL, Yueh B, et al. Treatment delay associated with alternative medicine use among veterans with head and neck cancer. Head Neck 2006; 28(10):926–31.
13. Molassiotis A, Ozden G, Platin N, et al. Complementary and alternative medicine use in patients with head and neck cancers in Europe. Eur J Cancer Care 2005; 15:19–24.
14. Talmi YP, Yakirevich A, Migirov L, et al. Limited use of complementary and alternative medicine in Israeli head and neck cancer patients. Laryngoscope 2005; 115:1505–8.
15. Warrick PD, Irish JC, Morningstar M, et al. Use of alternative medicine among patients with head and neck cancer. Arch Otolaryngol Head Neck Surg 1999; 125:573–9.
16. Miller MC, Pribitkin EA, Difabio T, et al. Prevalence of complementary and alternative medicine use among a population of head and neck cancer patients: a survey-based study. Ear Nose Throat J 2010;89(10):E23–7.

17. The World Health Organization. WHO traditional medicine strategy 2002–2005. Geneva (Switzerland): World Health Organization; 2002. Available at: http://apps.who.int/medicinedocs/en/d/Js2297e/. Accessed December 22, 2011.
18. Wu AP, Burke A, LeBaron S. Use of traditional medicine by immigrant Chinese patients. Fam Med 2007;39(3):195–200.
19. Misra R, Balagopal P, Klatt M, et al. Complementary and alternative medicine use among Asian Indians in the United States: a national study. J Altern Complement Med 2010;16(8):843–52.
20. Hsiao AF, Wong MD, Goldstein MS, et al. Complementary and alternative medicine use among Asian-American subgroups: prevalence, predictors, and lack of relationship to acculturation and access to conventional health care. J Altern Complement Med 2006;12(10):1003–10.
21. Cassileth BR, Deng G. Complementary and alternative therapies for cancer. Oncologist 2004;9:80–9.
22. Patwardhan B, Warude D, Pushpangadan P, et al. Ayurveda and traditional Chinese medicine: a comparative overview. Evid Based Complement Alternat Med 2005;2(4):465–73.
23. Manheimer E, Wieland S, Kimbrough E, et al. Evidence from the Cochrane collaboration for traditional Chinese medicine therapies. J Altern Complement Med 2009;15(9):1001–14.
24. National Institute for Ayurvedic Medicine Web site. Available at: http://niam.com/corp-web/index.htm. Accessed January 20, 2012.
25. Chopra A, Doiphode VV. Ayurvedic medicine. Core concept, therapeutic principles, and current relevance. Med Clin North Am 2002;86(1):75–89, vii.
26. Stehlin I. Homeopathy: real medicine or empty promises? FDA Consumer – On Line Edition. 1996;30(10). Available at: http://www.fda.gov/fdac/features/096_home.html. Accessed January 10, 2012.
27. Eisenberg DM, Cohen MH, Hrbek A, et al. Credentialing complementary and alternative medical providers. Ann Intern Med 2002;137:965–73.
28. Milazzo S, Russell N, Ernst E. Efficacy of homeopathic therapy in cancer treatment. Eur J Cancer 2006;42:282–9.
29. Linde K, Clausius N, Ramirez G, et al. Are the clinical effects of homoeopathy placebo effect? A meta-analysis of placebo-controlled trials. Lancet 1998;350:834–43.
30. Ernst E. A systematic review of systematic reviews of homeopathy. Br J Clin Pharmacol 2002;54(6):577–82.
31. Thompson TD, Weiss M. Homeopathy–what are the active ingredients? An exploratory study using the UK Medical Research Council's framework for the evaluation of complex interventions. BMC Complement Altern Med 2006; 6:37.
32. Smith MJ, Logan AC. Naturopathy. Med Clin North Am 2002;86(1):173–84.
33. American Association of Naturopathic Physicians Web site. Available at: www.naturopathic.org. Accessed January 6, 2012.
34. Wolsko PM, Eisenberg DM, Davis RB, et al. Use of mind–body medical therapies: results of a national survey. J Gen Intern Med 2004;19:43–50.
35. Anderson BL, Farrar WB, Golden-Kreutz DM, et al. Psychological, behavioral, and immune changes after a psychological intervention: a clinical trial. J Clin Oncol 2004;22:3570–80.
36. Carlson LE, Speca M, Patel KD, et al. Mindfulness-based stress reduction in relation to quality of life, mood, symptoms of stress, and immune parameters in breast and prostate cancer outpatients. Psychosom Med 2003;65:571–81.

37. Nidich SI, Rainforth MV, Haaga DA, et al. A randomized controlled trial on effects of the Transcendental Meditation program on blood pressure, psychological distress, and coping in young adults. Am J Hypertens 2009;22(12):1326–31.

38. Sivasankaran S, Pollard-Quintner S, Sachdeva R, et al. The effect of a six-week program of yoga and meditation on brachial artery reactivity: do psychosocial interventions affect vascular tone? Clin Cardiol 2006;29(9):393–8.

39. Khatri D, Mathur KC, Gahlot S, et al. Effects of yoga and meditation on clinical and biochemical parameters of metabolic syndrome. Diabetes Res Clin Pract 2007;78(3):e9–10.

40. Solberg EE, Holen A, Ekeberg Ø, et al. The effects of long meditation on plasma melatonin and blood serotonin. Med Sci Monit 2004;10(3):CR96–101.

41. Cohen AJ, Menter A, Hale L. Acupuncture: role in comprehensive cancer care – a primer for the oncologist and review of the literature. Integr Cancer Ther 2005; 4(2):131–43.

42. Kawakita K, Shinbara H, Imai K, et al. How do acupuncture and moxibustion act? Focusing on the progress in Japanese acupuncture research. J Pharmacol Sci 2006;100:443–59.

43. Han JS. Acupuncture and endorphins. Neurosci Lett 2004;36:258–61.

44. Yu Y, Kasahara T, Sato T, et al. Enhancement of splenic interferon gamma, interleukin 2, and NK cytotoxicity by S36 acupoint acupuncture in F344 rats. Jpn J Physiol 1997;47:173–8.

45. Cheng R, McKibbin L, Roy B, et al. Electroacupuncture elevates blood cortisol levels in naive horses, sham treatment has no effect. Int J Neurosci 1980;10:95–7.

46. Dundee JW, Ghaly RG, Fitzpatrick KT, et al. Acupuncture prophylaxis of cancer chemotherapy-induced sickness. J R Soc Med 1989;82(5):268–71.

47. Ezzo JM, Richardson MA, Vickers A, et al. Acupuncture-point stimulation for chemotherapy-induced nausea or vomiting. Cochrane Database Syst Rev 2006;(2):CD002285.

48. Blom M, Dawidson I, Fernberg JO, et al. Acupuncture treatment of patients with radiation-induced xerostomia. Eur J Cancer B Oral Oncol 1996;32B(3):182–90.

49. Johnstone PA, Peng YP, May BC, et al. Acupuncture for pilocarpine-resistant xerostomia following radiotherapy for head and neck malignancies. Int J Radiat Oncol Biol Phys 2001;50(2):353–7.

50. Raimond K, Jones GW, Sagar SM, et al. A phase I-II study in the use of acupuncture-like transuctaneous nerve stimulation in the treatment of radiation-induced xerostomia in head and neck cancer patients treated with radical radiotherapy. Int J Radiat Oncol Biol Phys 2003;57(2):472–80.

51. Homola S. Chiropractic: history and overview of theories and methods. Clin Orthop Relat Res 2006;444:236–42.

52. Nansel D, Szlazak M. Somatic dysfunction and the phenomenon of visceral disease simulation: a probable explanation for the apparent effectiveness of somatic therapy in patients presumed to be suffering from true visceral disease. J Manipulative Physiol Ther 1995;18(6):379–97.

53. A history of osteopathic medicine. American Association of Colleges of Osteopathic Medicine Web site. Available at: http://www.aacom.org/. Accessed December 31, 2011.

54. Johnson SM, Kurtz ME. Diminished use of osteopathic manipulative treatment and its impact on the uniqueness of the osteopathic profession. Acad Med 2001;76(8):821–8.

55. Swenson R, Haldeman S. Spinal manipulative therapy for low back pain. J Am Acad Orthop Surg 2003;11(4):228–37.

56. Rubinstein SM, van Middelkoop M, Assendelft WJ, et al. Spinal manipulative therapy for chronic low-back pain: an update of a Cochrane review. Spine (Phila Pa 1976) 2011;36(13):E825–46.

57. Bronfort G, Haas M, Evans RL, et al. Efficacy of spinal manipulation and mobilization for low back pain and neck pain: a systematic review and best evidence synthesis. Spine J 2004;4(3):335–56.

58. Ernst E. Adverse effects of spinal manipulation: a systematic review. J R Soc Med 2007;100(7):330–8.

59. Gouveia LO, Castanho P, Ferreira JJ. Safety of chiropractic interventions: a systematic review. Spine (Phila Pa 1976) 2009;34(11):E405–13.

60. Dietary Supplement Health and Education Act of 1994. U.S. Food and Drug Administration Center for Food Safety and Applied Nutrition Web site. Available at: http://ods.od.nih.gov/about/dshea_wording.aspx. Accessed January 5, 2012.

61. Regulatory strategy for the further implementation and enforcement of the Dietary Supplement Health and Education Act of 1994. U.S. Food and Drug Administration Center for Food Safety and Applied Nutrition Web site. Available at: http://www.fda.gov/Food/DietarySupplements/Alerts/ucm111110.htm. Accessed January 8, 2012.

62. USP-verified dietary supplements. US Pharmacopeia Web site. Available at: http://www.usp.org/USPVerified/dietarySupplements/. Accessed January 10, 2012.

63. Collacott EA, Zimmerman JT, White DW, et al. Bipolar permanent magnets for the treatment of chronic low back pain: a pilot study. JAMA 2000;283:1322–5.

64. Borsa PA, Liggett CL. Flexible magnets are not effective in decreasing pain perception and recovery time after muscle microinjury. J Athl Train 1998;33(2):150–5.

65. Riddle GE. Treating nausea and vomiting with magnets. Can Fam Physician 2004; 50:871–2.

66. Rosa L, Rosa E, Sarner L, et al. A close look at therapeutic touch. JAMA 1998; 279:1005–10.

67. Kennedy J, Wang CC, Wu CH. Patient disclosure about herb and supplement use among adults in the US. Evid Based Complement Alternat Med 2008;5(4):451–6.

68. Eisenberg DM, Kessler RC, Foster C, et al. Unconventional medicine in the United States: prevalence, costs, and patterns of use. N Engl J Med 1993;328:246–52.

69. Wahner-Roedler DL, Vincent A, Elkin PL, et al. Physicians' attitudes toward complementary and alternative medicine and their knowledge of specific therapies: a survey at an academic medical center. Evid Based Complement Alternat Med 2006;3(4):495–501.

70. Milden SP, Stokols D. Physicians' attitudes and practices regarding complementary and alternative medicine. Behav Med 2004;30(2):73–82.

71. Waterbrook AL, Southall JC, Strout TD, et al. The knowledge and usage of complementary and alternative medicine by emergency department patients and physicians. J Emerg Med 2010;39(5):569–75.

72. Ernst E. The current position of complementary/alternative medicine in cancer. Eur J Cancer 2003;39:2273–7.

73. Schmidt K, Ernst E. Assessing websites on complementary and alternative medicine for cancer. Ann Oncol 2004;15:733–42.

74. Pilkington K, Gamst A, Liu I, et al. The International Collaboration on Complementary Therapy Resources (ICCR): working together to improve online CAM information. J Altern Complement Med 2011;17(7):647–53.

75. Eisenberg DM. Advising patients who seek alternative medical therapies. Ann Intern Med 1997;127:61–9.

76. Weiger WA, Smith M, Boon H, et al. Advising patients who seek complementary and alternative medical therapies for cancer. Ann Intern Med 2002;137:889–903.

Complementary and Integrative Treatments Healthy Living: Strategies to Live Longer

Kyrras Conrad, RN, MA[a,b], Michael Spano, MS, R.Ac[c],
Michael D. Seidman, MD[d],*

KEYWORDS

- Complementary treatments • Integrative treatments • Aging • Health

KEY POINTS

- The 3 leading theories of aging are the telomerase theory of aging, the dysdifferentiation hypothesis of aging, and the membrane hypothesis of aging, also known as the mitochondrial clock theory of aging.
- The best way to practice healthy nutrition is to increase the daily intake of plants and reduce highly processed foods.
- Postural distortion can put patients at risk for a variety of symptoms and diseases. Many of these respond well to soft tissue therapies such as St John integrative neurosomatic therapy, myofascial release, Rolfing, and structural integration.
- The 3 major aspects of traditional Chinese medicine are botanic medicine, tai qi and qi gong, and acupuncture.
- Healthy living can be achieved by making sensible lifestyle choices, such as improving nutrition, exercising, and a judicious choice of nutritional supplements.

OVERVIEW

Aging is a complex process that involves metabolic and physiologic changes that lead to an increasing susceptibility to disease and ultimately death. Scientists, physicians, and con-men have been trying to find the fountain of youth for millennia. No one wants

Disclosure: Michael D Seidman is the founder of Body Language Vitamin Co., which produces nutriceuticals that use such compounds; in addition, he is the Chief Scientific Officer of Visalus Sciences, a company that markets formulations targeting health, wellness, and obesity. Kyrras A Conrad is a LifeVantage/Protandim independent distributor.
[a] Center for Integrative Medicine, Henry Ford Health System, 40000 W. 8 Mile Road, Northville, MI, 48167, USA; [b] Conrad Neuromuscular Therapy Center, LLC, 5600 W. Maple D-408, West Bloomfield, MI 48322, USA; [c] Center for Integrative Medicine, Henry Ford Health System, 40000 W. 8 Mile Road, Northville, MI, 48167, USA; [d] Otologic/Neurotologic Surgery, Center for Integrative Medicine, Henry Ford West Bloomfield Hospital, 6777 W. Maple Road, West Bloomfield, MI, 48322, USA
* Corresponding author.
E-mail address: Mseidma1@hfhs.org

to grow old, and although everyone understands that aging is inevitable, everyone is also fascinated with the possibility that one day science will prevail and it will be possible to greatly slow or even reverse the processes of aging. This article discusses the mechanisms of aging, future areas of exploration, and strategies to achieve successful aging given the current state of medical knowledge.

PHYSIOLOGY AND ANATOMY: THE PROCESSES OF AGING

Discussion of several of the most important mechanisms of aging is relevant to better understand how to address methodology to slow the aging process. There are many theories to explain the aging process. Three leading theories have the greatest scientific support:

1. Telomerase theory of aging
2. Dysdifferentiation hypothesis of aging
3. Membrane hypothesis of aging, also known as the mitochondrial clock theory of aging, which has been the focus of the authors' laboratory for many years.

Telomerase Theory

The end of a chromosome is made up of a structure called the telosome. The tip of the telosome is a region of repeating DNA sequences and proteins called the telomere. The telomerase theory of aging suggests that there is a reduction in telomere length over time.[1] The telosome can be thought of as being similar to the tail of a rattlesnake. There are a finite number of rings on a telosome (or a rattlesnake's tail) and each time the telosome reproduces, 1 ring is lost. When there are only a few rings of the telosome remaining, death is imminent. It is possible to manipulate the activation of the enzyme responsible for making these rings disappear; it is called the telomerase enzyme. What is perhaps more fascinating is that certain cancers work precisely by altering the telomerase enzyme. It is thought that certain genes, called viral oncogenes, may produce immortality of a cell or tissue by activating telomerase, thus preventing telomere shortening and sustaining cellular growth of tumors.[2] Thus, although many aspects of telomerase activity remain undefined, it has been hypothesized that the balance between telomere shortening and telomerase activity may underlie the cellular aging processes. Caution must be exercised when these genes are manipulated because of the potential to trigger cancerous change.

Dysdifferentiation Hypothesis

The dysdifferentiation hypothesis suggests that there is a preprogrammed activation of genes that are deleterious to the cell and that lead to activation of enzymes and reactions that are responsible for age-related changes. This line of reasoning was, in part, brought to the forefront from work elaborating control mechanisms of aging in the earthworm. Two main genes, BAX and BCL2, have essential roles in cellular aging and immortality respectively. Scientists were able to increase the lifespan of the common earthworm by 30% to 40% by increasing the activity of the BCL2 gene. Moderation and ethics enter the picture: the moment a cure or treatment of aging seems imminent, a potential obstacle often looms nearby. In this situation, it is known that several cancers have overwhelmed the body by upregulating the BCL2 gene. The need for caution intervenes once again.[3]

Membrane Hypothesis of Aging

The membrane hypothesis of aging, also called the mitochondrial clock theory of aging, is based on the progressive accumulation of oxidative damage and mitochondrial dysfunction. This damage occurs secondary to the action of reactive oxygen species (ROS), also known as free radicals, which are generated in increasing quantities with age.[4,5] ROS are known to damage DNA in general, and mitochondrial DNA (mtDNA) in particular, as well as cells and tissue. The mtDNA damage leads to reduced capacity for energy generation within the mitochondria and ultimately causes aging and death, which is the premise for the use of powerful antioxidants to perhaps slow the processes of aging. Perhaps more important are compounds that may safely upregulate mitochondrial function.[6] Nuclear factor (erythroid-derived 2) –related 2, also known as Nrf2, is a transcription factor that is a master regulator of the antioxidant response. Recent breakthroughs with nrf2 activator compounds show promise for increasing endogenous antioxidants, resulting in significant reduction of oxidative stress.[7–12] Nrf2 activators are currently available as functional food supplements[7] and are being developed in pharmaceutical form.[13,14]

The mitochondrion is a structure inside a cell and is the primary generator of energy, in the form of adenosine triphosphate (ATP). The mitochondria have their own DNA that determines all the functions of the mitochondria. The mtDNA is made up of 16,569 base pairs that, when intact, efficiently make energy for the body, but, if there are subtle changes in the mtDNA, there can be serious effects on mitochondrial function and energy production. Research in our laboratory as well as several others around the world have identified a specific deletion (or elimination) in mtDNA segments that is known to occur in response to aging. It is called the common aging deletion and consists of the loss of 4977 base pairs. Removal of approximately one-third of the mtDNA would cause significant problems. A primary problem is that mitochondria with this deletion can no longer produce energy efficiently. It has been found that even minor amounts of this deletion severely alter energy production and cellular function. This deletion can be measured with tools that are currently available, and this offers a molecular test for aging; although not yet commercially available, our laboratory has been studying this deletion in mice, rats, and humans since 1988. This deletion can be identified in human cells as early as 25 to 30 years of age, and there are some medical conditions in which this deletion occurs even earlier.

Studies have shown an age-related increase in the presence of the common mitochondrial deletion (mtDNA^{4977}).[15] We identified the common aging deletion in 1 of 15 young rats, whereas 11 of 14 aged rats had the mtDNA deletion. The aged rats also had hearing loss, and the 3 aged rats without the deletion had better hearing compared with the 11 with the deletion. In addition, we were able to study mitochondrial function in aged rats and humans, and it is significantly reduced compared with the young subjects.[3] Human studies have revealed the presence of this mtDNA deletion in white blood cells of patients with age-related hearing loss more often than in control patients.[16] Two other human studies have identified the common aging deletion (mtDNA^{4977}) in patients with age-related hearing loss more than in control subjects.[17,18] Certain tissues are more susceptible to oxidative damage (damage from free radicals) and reduced energy supply; this is especially true for tissues that no longer make new cells. For example, brain, eye, inner ear, and all muscle tissues can accumulate large amounts of these deletions, making them more susceptible to free radical damage than other tissues. Thus, increased oxidative damage that is associated with aging preferentially affects these tissues.

The process of aging is associated with many molecular, biochemical, and physiologic changes including increases in DNA damage, reduction in mitochondrial function, decreases in cellular water concentrations, ionic changes, and decreased elasticity of cellular membranes. One contributing factor to this process is altered vascular characteristics, such as reduced flow and vascular plasticity, as well as increased vascular permeability.[15,19] Atherosclerosis and high lipids and cholesterol adversely affect these situations and reduce the overall blood flow to many tissues in the body. These age-related changes result in reductions in oxygen and nutrient delivery, and also in waste elimination.[20–23] These physiologic inefficiencies favor the production of ROS. Furthermore, there is support in the literature for age-associated reduction in enzymes that protect from ROS damage, including superoxide dismutase, catalase, and glutathione.[24–26] These changes collectively enhance the generation of ROS.

Factors in Healthy Aging

Is there hope? Can death be delayed with the tools available now? Participating in the success or failure of their own health is a clear choice that all individuals must make. Successful aging is a function of genetics, along with lifestyle and environmental factors. It is the responsibility of health care providers to educate themselves and their patients or to aggressively refer them to people who will educate and support them in making healthy choices.

Behavioral choices profoundly affect life span.[27] Nutrition and exercise are two of the most commonly discussed elements because they are of primary importance.[28] Enhancement of healthy aging for clinicians and patients includes identifying and managing stress, having a positive rather than a pessimistic outlook, participating in a meaningful social network, and having a support system.[29,30] Other physical and emotional factors that can have a profound effect on successful longevity include environment, alcohol and/or drug abuse, tobacco use, sun exposure, marital stability, exercise, body mass index, posture, coping mechanisms, and education.[31] Although there is little choice in genetic factors, behavioral choices can strongly affect both genetic expression and the consequences of trauma or surgery.[32–34]

One of the few proven strategies to extend life is caloric restriction. This has been shown in multiple species.[35] The mechanism is thought to relate to reduction in overall oxidative stress and a reduction in bioinflammation. It is thought that a reduction of caloric intake by 30% can lead to a 30% increase in life span.[36] In humans, this practice would require significant reduction in consumed calories and this would mean a diet on the order of no more than 1000 to 1200 calories per day, which is enough caloric intake to maintain basic body functions; weight loss, if any, would occur quickly, a plateau in weight would be reached, and a steady state would ensue. Most people would feel hungry all the time and would not find this strategy acceptable. It has been suggested that resveratrol, the chemical found in red wine, peanuts, and so forth, can to some degree mimic the effects of caloric restriction.[37,38]

This article first identifies common causes of death and then discusses contributing factors over which people have control. According to the US Centers for Disease Control and Prevention's National Vital Statistics Reports for 2009,[39] the most recent year for which there are figures, the 15 most common causes of death, in chronologic order, are:

1. Diseases of the heart
2. Malignant neoplasms
3. Chronic lower respiratory diseases
4. Cerebrovascular diseases
5. Accidents (unintentional injuries)
6. Alzheimer disease
7. Diabetes mellitus
8. Influenza and pneumonia

9. Nephritis, nephrotic syndrome, and nephrosis
10. Intentional self-harm (suicide)
11. Septicemia
12. Chronic liver disease and cirrhosis
13. Essential hypertension and hypertensive renal disease
14. Parkinson disease
15. Assault (homicide)

Nine of the 15 have well-established links to lifestyle choices centering on nutrition and exercise, and all other causes may or may not have links to lifestyle choices for any given individual.[40–53] However, avoiding early death is not enough. The real question is how can aging be successful?

INTEGRATIVE TREATMENT APPROACHES AND OUTCOMES
Nutrition

Physicians receive little education about nutrition outside of interventions for acute illness such as for renal disease, for cardiovascular disease, using total parenteral nutrition, and so forth. There is a large, varying, and conflicting amount of information in the lay press and the Internet on general nutrition. Current research indicates a plant-based diet as optimal[28]:

- A diet of 5 to 10 helpings of fruit and vegetables per day
- Starches only in the form of whole grains and beans
- Animal products severely limited or absent
- Supplementation can be useful but should be an adjunct to a healthy diet, not to replace a healthy diet

There are virtually no nutrients in animal-based foods that are not better provided by plants (**Table 1**).

Table 1 Nutrient composition of plant-based and animal-based foods (per 500 calories of energy)		
Nutrient	Plant-based Foods[a]	Animal-based Foods[b]
Cholesterol (mg)	—	137
Fat (g)	4	36
Protein (g)	33	34
Beta-carotene (μg)	29,919	17
Dietary fiber (g)	31	—
Vitamin C (mg)	293	4
Folate (μg)	1168	19
Vitamin E (mg ATE)	11	0.5
Iron (mg)	20	2
Magnesium (mg)	548	51
Calcium (mg)	545	252

Abbreviation: mg ATE, milligrams of alpha-tocopherol equivalents.
 [a] Equal parts of tomatoes, spinach, lima beans, peas, and potatoes.
 [b] Equal parts of beef, pork, chicken, and whole milk.
 From Campbell TC, Campbell TM. The China Study. Dallas, TX: Benbella Books 2005;230; with permission.

Why have we become so dependent upon drugs, surgery, and other debilitating treatments? The answer, very simply, is this: We are sick because Nature never intended for us to eat the foods we are eating today. When looked at from the perspective of human history, the diet we are eating – loaded with fat, cholesterol, animal protein, processed foods, and artificial ingredients – is a bizarre anomaly. Our blood, arteries, and cells were not designed to live under all that fat and choles- terol that covers them today. Our intestines were not intended to work in the absence of fiber, and clogged with flesh. Our immune system was not meant to function under the burden of a thrice-daily load of fat, without an abundant supply of plant-based nutrients and phytochemicals... With our cells drowning in fat, cholesterol, animal proteins, and artificial chemicals, and our immune systems deprived of what they need to maintain health, it's no wonder so many of us get cancer, heart disease, high blood pressure, adult-onset diabetes, arthritis, osteo- porosis, and other age-related illnesses. In fact, it is a testament to the strengths of the human body that anyone has the slightest semblance of health.[54]

Good nutrition is simple to define, but harder to practice, especially in American culture. Eat plants; that is it. In general, it is not necessary to count nutrients, proteins, or calories (but caloric restriction is an appropriate validated methodology to increase lifespan): if people eat a wide range of plants, they get all the nutrients they need, with the sole exception of vitamin B_{12}, which is needed as an occasional supplement but is easily obtained. Use of other supplements can be beneficial, notably antioxidants and nrf2 activators as mentioned earlier, because many of the plants that are available are grown in soils deficient of a wide range of vitamins or are picked well before ripening (and thus before uptake of available vitamins and minerals is complete). Implementing a plant-based diet within American cultural norms can be challenging; it is easy to go home and throw a steak on the grill and challenging to find low-fat or no-fat-added tasty meals in restaurants. However, there are a plethora of cook books, Web sites, and how-to books available with enough delicious foods and recipes to make people forget about animal products if they wish to move toward a plant-based diet. As with most other things, the most challenging part of changing how people eat is deciding to do so. Switching to plant-based eating can change life so much for the better that many other things that are listed in this article to achieve successful longevity will be easier to do or may no longer be as important.

There are differences among nutritionists and nutritional outlooks that are starting to converge, although traditional nutritionists still insist that people include meat and dairy in their diet, whereas the new/holistic nutritionists advocate getting proteins and calcium from the same place cows do: plants.

Antioxidants: Useful Elements for Successful Aging

Alpha lipoic acid

Alpha lipoic acid (ALA) is a nutrient that is necessary for normal mitochondrial function and energy production. Recent laboratory studies have shown that this vitaminlike substance shows improvement in age-related hearing loss.[6] Dietary supplementation of ALA successfully reduces heart damage induced by reduced blood supply as is seen in myocardial infarction. At present, its primary therapeutic use is for the treat- ment of diabetes-induced nerve dysfunction (neuropathy). The reduced form of lipoic acid is dihydrolipoic acid (DHLA). DHLA prevents lipid peroxidation, which is the end stage of free radical damage. It does this by reducing glutathione, which in turn recy- cles vitamin E. DHLA has also been shown to be an ROS scavenger (an antioxidant); to reduce peroxyl, ascorbyl, and chromanoxyl radicals; and to inhibit singlet oxygen (these are all beneficial effects).

Acetyl L-carnitine

Acetyl L-carnitine (ALCAR), a biologic compound, plays an important role in the transport of fatty acids from inside the cell to the mitochondria for oxidation. This step is crucial for energy production. ALCAR controls the metabolism of sugars, lipids, and amino acids, thus playing a pivotal role in cellular energy and turnover of cell membranes and proteins. Chronic treatment with ALCAR enhances stimulation of antioxidant defenses. It also enhances the age-related effect of glucocorticoid secretion and improves learning and memory, possibly because of its ability to increase the release of acetylcholine. Studies in our laboratory have shown improved hearing in aged subjects compared with controls. In addition, the treated subjects had improved mitochondrial function and energy production, and there was evidence for a reduction in mitochondrial damage.[6] ALCAR has been shown to be capable of restoring the integrity of the cardiac mitochondrial membrane altered by aging (specifically the cardiolipin content), thereby restoring the normal activity of cytochrome oxidase, adenine nucleotide translocase, and phosphate carrier.

Coenzyme Q-10

Coenzyme Q-10 (CoQ-10) is a crucial coenzyme for mitochondrial function and is essential in the generation of energy. It was first recognized in 1957 as a component necessary for oxidative phosphorylation (the process by which the mitochondrion makes energy). Reduced CoQ-10 functions as an antioxidant and can therefore combat the production of free oxygen radicals. In addition, it seems to function by preventing the initiation and propagation of lipid peroxidation (the end stage of free radical damage). There is evidence supporting an age-related decline of CoQ-10 in humans and other species, thus further supporting the membrane hypothesis of aging. CoQ-10 is currently used alone or in combination as a health/nutritional supplement. It has shown promise in enhancing heart function and has been used medicinally in European countries for this purpose. It may also be useful in cognitive and other neurologic disorders (ie, Alzheimer disease and diseases that produce muscle weakness, such as certain muscular dystrophies).

Glutathione

Glutathione (L-K-glutamyl-L-cysteinyl-glycine) detoxifies ROS (it acts as an antioxidant). It is also involved in the metabolism and detoxification of certain drugs. Mitochondrial glutathione is critical to cell viability and the glutathione redox cycle is a primary antioxidant defense system within the mitochondrion. Additional functions include intracellular binding, transport of lipophilic substances, and prostaglandin synthesis.

Many studies have shown that alterations of glutathione levels through excess or reduced production have a beneficial or harmful influence on cellular function, respectively. Glutathione reduces gentamicin-induced cochlear damage and gentamicin ototoxicity may be attenuated using glutathione. The mechanism for toxicity of certain clinically used drugs occurs secondary to reduced glutathione levels with an increase in ROS. Recent studies have shown an age-associated 86% reduction in glutathione levels in the auditory nerve.[55] Thus, hearing loss may occur in part because of reduction in glutathione levels with age. Studies of patients with Alzheimer disease have shown age-dependent decreases of glutathione-peroxidase activities and their cofactors.[56] The senior author (MDS) has been awarded a patent on the combination of the 4 ingredients listed earlier as an antiaging and hearing loss prevention strategy.

Multivitamin and mineral formulas

There are many other compounds that are relevant, including resveratrol, phosphatidyl-choline, phosphatidylserine, nrf2 activators, and ingredients found in multivitamin and mineral formulas.

Resveratrol (trans 3,5,4'-trihydoxystilbene), a compound found mainly in the skin and seeds of grapes and widely accessible in the form of red wine, is recognized for both its antioxidant and antiinflammatory properties and its potential to reduce the risk of cancer and heart disease. It has been touted as a possible explanation for the French paradox: the low incidence of heart disease among French people, who consume a high-fat diet.[57] Resveratrol has many other important biologic activities, including inhibition of lipid peroxidation,[58] chelation of copper, free radical scavenging,[59] alteration of eicosanoid synthesis, inhibition of platelet aggregation,[60] antiinflammatory and anticancer activity,[61] modulation of lipid metabolism, vasorelaxing activity, estrogenic activity, cardioprotective activity, and neuroprotective actions.[62,63]

Oxidative stress in the central nervous system (CNS) may cause oxidation of lipoprotein particles. The oxidized lipoproteins may damage cellular and subcellular membranes, leading to tissue injury and cell death. Draczynska-Lusiak and colleagues[64] showed that antioxidants, such as resveratrol, as well as vitamins E and C, protect neuronal cell damage from oxidative stress in vivo. Zini and colleagues[65] studied the possible effects of resveratrol on the mitochondrial respiratory chain in rat brains. Resveratrol decreased complex III activity in the rat brain by competition with coenzyme Q. By decreasing the activity of complex III, resveratrol not only suppresses the production of ROS but also scavenges them. Virgili and Contestabile[63] reported that chronic administration of resveratrol to young adult rats significantly protects against damage induced by systemic injection of the excitotoxin kainic acid in the olfactory cortex and the hippocampus. Resveratrol also suppresses tumor necrosis factor–induced activation of nuclear transcription factor NF-kappa B, activator protein-1, and apoptosis.[66]

It is generally accepted that at least 2 isoforms of the principal enzyme responsible for prostaglandin (PG) synthesis exist: cyclooxygenase-1 (COX-1) and cyclooxygenase-2 (COX-2). Constitutive COX-1 activity provides prostaglandins involved in physiologic reactions and performs a housekeeping function that regulates normal cell activity. COX-2 is normally either not present or present in very small amounts in the resting cell. However, levels of COX-2 can be strongly induced by various cytokines, growth factors,[67,68] and endotoxins. There is mounting evidence that upregulation of COX-2 expression contributes to ischemic brain damage,[68] Alzheimer disease,[69] inflammatory states,[70] various tumors,[71] and to the aging process.[72] Studies have shown that selective COX-2 inhibitors can attenuate the ischemia or reperfusion-induced brain damage.[73] In a study by Kim and colleagues,[74] COX-2 mRNA, protein levels, and COX-2 activity increased with age in the heart (using, respectively, reverse-transcription polymerase chain reaction, Western blotting, and prostaglandin E2 synthesis), whereas those of COX-1 showed no change.

THE ROLE OF POSTURE

The beginning of the disease process starts with postural distortions.
— Dr Hans Selye, Nobel Laureate, Professor of Endocrinology, McGill University; father of modern stress management.

Postural Distortion: Effect on Health

Postural distortion can interfere with nerve and organ function secondary to mechanical compression or referrals from trigger points. For example, severe scoliosis can cause mechanical compression of the lungs, restricting breathing and reducing oxygen levels, as well as affecting the heart[75,76]; less well known are the effects of lesser postural distortions. Any postural distortion that causes mechanical compression can diminish the function of the affected tissues. Any effect of postural distortion on tissues is not an all-or-nothing event, it is a continuum of slight to severe results. A minor problem such as constipation can stem from mechanical compression of the transverse colon, whereas a more significant problem might be hypertonic anterior cervical musculature causing a kyphotic cervical spine leading to posterior disc bulging. A trigger point is defined as a focus of hyperirritability in a tissue that is symptomatic with respect to pain; it refers a pattern of pain and ischemia when stimulated.[77] Other referred sensations from trigger points can be numbness, itching, paresthesia, or swelling. Severity of symptoms stemming from postural distortions and from related trigger points can range from simple restriction of motion to disabling pain, the continuum of which can profoundly affect quality of life. Postural distortions and uneven hypertonicity are addressed by specific soft tissue therapies such as St John integrative neurosomatic therapy, myofascial release, Rolfing, and structural integration.

Postural Distortion and the Righting Reflex

It is necessary to satisfy the righting reflex. If this is not done, perhaps because of the sequelae of trauma or surgery, repetitive use positions, or genetics, there will then be contraction of any musculature needed to satisfy the righting reflex. This righting effort, with the influence of gravity continually pulling an individual further out of alignment, may cause an early slight postural distortion to become progressively worse over time, which is why many patients have pain symptoms that seem to have no clear antecedent.

Postural distortion is a deviation off the coronal and midsagittal planes. The greater the degrees of distortion off the coronal and midsagittal planes, the more the muscles tighten unevenly in an attempt to bring the body back to optimal posture, thus satisfying the righting reflex. An example is a garden shed that is leaning a small amount. It looks slightly off kilter but the windows and doors open easily; it functions with no problems. A year later, the shed is leaning a bit more and, although it looks the same, the door sticks or a few nails start to pop; it is symptomatic. Gravity has pulled it further out of alignment.

Symptoms Potentially Related to Postural Distortion

Once humans deviate from erect coronal and midsagittal planes, they are at risk for symptoms related to uneven muscle hypertonicity and/or trigger points: pain (back, neck, headache, abdominal), disease resulting from ischemic tissues (eg, hypothyroidism, tinnitus, low sperm count), and symptoms that seem to come out of nowhere as the organism moves further away from optimal posture. How far away from structurally erect a person can get before symptoms develop depends on many factors; some individuals have posture-related symptoms after a brief period of distortion, some individuals take decades to develop them. When long-term postural distortion is the source of the symptom, that symptom is usually not in the same location as the problem (eg, migraines caused by a leg length difference or temporomandibular joint [TMJ] pain caused by an uneven pelvic flexion).

Soft tissue hypertonicity is not detectable by any current laboratory or diagnostic imaging,[77] so it is sometimes the forgotten differential diagnosis, but is easy to assess by someone trained in accurate postural assessment and palpation. Posture-related nerve compression and myofascial problems that are treated by cortisone injections, nerve blocks, or pain medications, and so forth only result in reoccurrences if the perpetuating factors of ongoing concentric contractions, sporadic overload, and repetitive use are not addressed.[78]

Tinnitus, vertigo, TMJ dysfunction, throat and neck pain, among many other pain syndromes of otherwise unidentified origins, whose sufferers have failed traditional medical interventions and physical therapy, often respond well to St John integrative neurosomatic therapy (SJINT), a structurally driven therapy.[79,80] A recent case study of a patient with somatic tinnitus is an example of the use of SJINT: Mr C reports that, on Thanksgiving weekend 2011, he had used a power router and consequently developed mild ringing in the right ear. Three days later he developed loud, high-pitched ringing in the left ear that has been persistent ever since. A day or two later he also had a loud ringing in the right ear, which has since been intermittent at a milder rate. He was evaluated by a Henry Ford ENT physician and the patient described his tinnitus as bilateral (left more than right) ringing with the severity of 7 to 8 out of 10, where 0 is no noise and 10 is so severe he would consider brain surgery. His Tinnitus Reaction Questionnaire (TRQ) score was 58. The patient was then referred to SJINT at the Henry Ford Center for Integrative Medicine and was found to have a right obliquity of the cranium and the pelvis, the right shoulder inferior to the left, and an uneven pelvic flexion with flexion of 10° on the left and 20° on the right; he also had an approximately 10-cm forward head posture. After treatment that day and 4 additional 1-hour sessions over the following 4 weeks treating the neck flexors, cranial musculature, right shoulder depressors, and hip flexors, and assignment of specific stretches, he returned for an audiology evaluation in which the TRQ was again administered: the patient had a score of 2 on January 27, 2012.

ACUPUNCTURE, TRADITIONAL CHINESE MEDICINE, AND HEALTHY AGING

Throughout Chinese history, Emperors and scholars have sought the key to immortality. In 220 BCE, Emperor Qin Shihuang sent his scholars abroad to find the 5 varieties of chi, the mystical plant of immortality, as well as Sheng Anqi, a magician reputed to be more than 1000 years old, in order to find the elixir of immortality.[81,82] The envoys never returned and thus ensued more than 2 millennia of inquiry into the secrets of physical longevity and health.

Traditional Chinese medicine (TCM) has a rich, dynamic history in China dating back more than 2500 years and continues to evolve. Although in Western cultures acupuncture is thought to be the cornerstone of TCM, acupuncture is only 1 of 3 major aspects of TCM. First and foremost is botanic medicine, then tai qi and qi gong, and then acupuncture.

Botanic Medicines

It is estimated that, in the United States, more than 60% of patients with cancer use botanic medicines during or after chemotherapy, compared with 18% of the population at large.[83–86] Quality of life, cancer symptoms, management of treatment side effects, and fear of cancer recurrence are motivating forces that lead patients to take botanicals.[87]

Research is ongoing worldwide to assess the effects of botanicals and their role in healthy aging, and evidence has long shown that many TCM botanicals have specific effects. TCM herbal extracts of several plants possess antioxidant properties and these properties can play an essential role in the biologic activity of those extracts. It has also been shown that the antioxidant activity of extracts is closely related to their polyphenol content, which includes flavonoids and tannins.[88,89] These compounds have an ability to directly scavenge free radicals and chelate metal ions.[90]

TCM herbals have been used in China by the general population not only as a treatment of disease but also for changes in life, seasons, and even the weather. Herbal formulas may have from 2 to more than 30 different herbs and each concoction is prepared to respond to multiple conditions of the individual and to balance the potential side effects of the herbs. Intrinsic to the history of herbal medicine is the belief that herbs have properties germane to the outward expressions of disease: for example, when patients are hot, as with fever or chronic infection, they are treated with herbs that have cooling properties. These herbal properties have been determined through thousands of years of experimentation. The complexities of TCM exist within this framework and, as each individual ages, that person's herbal formula becomes a creative balance between cold and hot, or, in TCM theory, balanced between yin and yang. Herbs high in polyphenol have a traditional TCM designation as cooling herbs. Many diseases of aging in which ROS may have a potential impact, such as cancer and coronary artery disease, are commonly considered in TCM to be heat diseases. To reduce the potential for harm that may occur by introducing solely a cold herb to treat hot diseases, TCM herbal formulas balance the effects of some of the herbs with other herbs to support subsequent effects on other systems within the body. Several studies have shown that combinations of some herbs in traditional formulas may have a greater effect in reducing oxidative stress than their individual components alone.[91,92]

Tai Chi and Qi Gong

Although herbal formulas are essential in TCM support of healthy aging, exercise and movement are the cornerstones of lifestyle choices. Early morning in the parks in China, and increasingly in the United States, it is common to see large groups of senior citizens practicing tai qi and qi gong. "I am in the best shape of my life," relates 81-year-old Qin Meihua of Shanghai. She practices, as does everyone in her peer group of about 40 retired individuals, from 6 to 9 AM, every morning, 7 days a week. Tai qi and qi gong combine self-awareness with self-correction of the posture, movement of the body, flow of breath, and stilling of the mind. All these are thought to comprise a state that activates a natural self-regulatory (self-healing) capacity and a wide array of natural health recovery mechanisms that, when evoked, integrate body and mind.[93] Qi gong and tai qi are similar in application and intent, so they can be viewed from the same perspective as long as each practitioner focuses on the intended movement and breath. Qi gong and tai qi benefit bone health, cardiopulmonary fitness and related biomarkers, physical function, falls prevention and balance, general quality of life (as measured by patient-reported outcomes tools), immunity, and psychological factors such as anxiety and depression.[94]

Acupuncture

Acupuncture, the third TCM application, is intended to restore and maintain health through the stimulation of specific points on the body with fine, sterile, single-use disposable needles. As people age, their bodies slow down: they have less range of motion, lower body temperatures, less ability to heal, and metabolism may decrease. These decreases can adversely affect quality of life. In acupuncture terms, these decreases are known as stagnated flow of vitality, or qi (pronounced chee), and can result in pain conditions, cancers, cardiac and vascular problems, and sensory loss. Acupuncture treatments work toward alleviating symptoms surrounding the injury or condition. Treatments can range from a single 45-minute session to a series of several treatments, depending on the severity and longevity of the condition. The number of needles inserted can range from 4 to more than 50, again, depending on the condition.

Although TCM acupuncturists work under the TCM model of health, several theories as to how acupuncture works within the biochemical model have been investigated. They can range from the concept that acupuncture causes localized stimulation of circulation and lymphatics, leading to more elasticity of cells,[95] the release of pain-relieving endogenous opioids,[96,97] or the idea that acupuncture works on more grossly networked pathways of neural innervations.[98] The exact mechanism remains elusive.

OTHER EASILY CONTROLLABLE, SUCCESSFUL AGING STRATEGIES
Exercise for Healthy Living

Exercise is essential. What is the best exercise? The one(s) that a person will do. The best time of day to exercise is the time that best fits into each individual's schedule. The ideal amount is 4 to 6 times per week for 1 hour, but that is something most people need to work up to if they are not already regular exercisers. Probably the best cardiopulmonary exercise is walking, especially for the out of shape. Speed walking, cross-country skiing, or low-impact aerobic workouts are excellent because they exercise the limbs as well as the heart and lungs. Running is a good exercise, too, but is not as beneficial in the long term if it is done on hard surfaces, because of the resulting stress on joints. It is estimated that it takes 18 to 254 days to establish automaticity with a given desired behavior, depending on its complexity.[99]

Sun Exposure Effects on Healthy Living

Avoiding damaging sun exposure reduces the incidence of skin cancer and the appearance of aging. Humans need sunlight to synthesize vitamin D and for a sense of well-being. How much an individual can tolerate without damage is related to previous sun exposure, melanin levels, and genetics. It has been shown that mtDNA mutations are induced in the human skin by repetitive ultraviolet light exposure.[100] Recent research indicates that moderate sun exposure is essential. Dr Edward Giovannucci,[101] a Harvard University professor of medicine and nutrition research, suggests that vitamin D might help prevent 30 deaths for each death caused by skin cancer. "I would challenge anyone to find an area or nutrient or any factor that has such consistent anticancer benefits as vitamin D," Dr Giovannucci[101] claims. Sunlight is beneficial but needs to be in amounts that do not cause damage.

Sensible Lifestyle Choices

Make generally sensible lifestyle choices: for example, do not drink and drive or ride with someone who does; drive safely according to conditions; whenever possible, choose a safe neighborhood in which to live.

MULTIMODAL APPROACHES AND OUTCOMES: EXAMINING THE ROLE AND POWER OF THE PHYSICIAN IN PATIENT EDUCATION

Can the physician be a teacher of successful longevity? Does the physician not suffer from the same shortcomings the general population (ie, knowing what to do but having difficulty/lacking the motivation to actually do it)? Must physicians be doing, rather than saying, the behavior they are trying to teach? Must the physician be a positive role model in order to motivate others? Does the physician have time to educate patients in the course of the day?

Individuals who are practicing the advice that they give are more believable and motivating to the recipient of that advice. Physicians who are struggling to better their own behaviors are more believable than those who willfully practice bad habits. Whatever the state of a physician's own behaviors, patients need encouragment to use strategies that will lead them toward successful longevity. In one study of 2710 current smokers, only 48.8% stated that their physicians had ever advised them to smoke less or stop smoking.[102] Advice from doctors helps people who smoke to quit. Even when doctors provide brief simple advice about quitting smoking, this increases the likelihood that someone who smokes will successfully quit and remain a nonsmoker 12 months later.[103]

"I was counseling one of my neurosomatic therapy patients to quit smoking," relates author Kyrras Conrad, RN. "The client seemed reluctant to quit smoking on my say-so but said he had always said he would quit smoking if his doctor advised it, so I told him to ask his doctor on his next appointment a few days away (a vascular surgeon whom he was seeing for peripheral arterial disease). When he came back to see me the following week I asked him if he had mentioned it to his doctor. He told me he had and that the doctor said 'I can hardly tell you to quit smoking since I smoke myself.'" What a missed opportunity by the physician! Even if you are not the perfect role model (and no one is), do not miss an opportunity to provide guidance to others.[104,105] If you are obese and think that you are not in a position to give nutrition advice, give it anyway, and then refer the patient to a holistic nutritionist.

SUMMARY

This article examines current research on aging, distills nutritional advice to manageable guidelines, introduces an effective soft tissue therapy that reduces sequelae of aging through postural correction, and discusses the physician as a powerful force to influence patients to live better lives.

In summary, maintain proper nutrition, strive to maintain an appropriate weight, avoid tobacco use, limit alcohol, avoid damaging sun exposure, maintain good posture, exercise, simplify your lifestyle and reduce stress, nurture a support system, wash your hands often and well, make other sensible lifestyle choices, and try to get at least 8 hours of sleep in a 24-hour period. Endeavor to teach your patients these precepts as much as possible, and practice what you can.

REFERENCES

1. Pommier JP, Lebeau J, Ducray C, et al. Chromosomal instability and alteration of telomere repeat sequences. Biochimie 1995;77(10):817–25.
2. Shay JW, Wright WE. Telomerase activity in human cancer. Curr Opin Oncol 1996;8(1):66–71.
3. Seidman MD. Effects of dietary restriction and anitoxidants on presbyacusis. Laryngoscope 2000;110:727–38.
4. Sohal RS, Allen RG. Relationship between metabolic rate, free radicals, differentiation and aging: a unified theory. Basic Life Sci 1985;35:75–104.
5. Southorn PA, Powis G. Free radicals in medicine. I: Chemical nature and biologic reactions. Mayo Clin Proc 1988;63:381–9.
6. Seidman MD, Khan MJ, Bai U, et al. Biologic activity of mitochondrial metabolites on aging and age-related hearing loss. Am J Otol 2000;21:161–7.
7. Nelson SK, Bose SK, Grunwald GK, et al. The induction of human superoxide dismutase and catalase in vivo: a fundamentally new approach to antioxidant therapy. Free Radic Biol Med 2006;40(2):341–7.
8. Donovan EL, McCord JM, Reuland DJ, et al. Phytochemical activation of Nrf2 protects human coronary artery endothelial cells against an oxidative challenge. Oxid Med Cell Longev 2012;2012:132931.

9. Hybertson BM, Gao B, Bose SK, et al. Oxidative stress in health and disease: the therapeutic potential of Nrf2 activation. Mol Aspects Med 2011;32(4–6):234–46.

10. Joddar B, Reen RK, Firstenberg MS, et al. Protandim attenuates intimal hyperplasia in human saphenous veins cultured ex vivo via a catalase-dependent pathway. Free Radic Biol Med 2011;50(6):700–9.

11. Robbins D, Zhao Y. The role of manganese superoxide dismutase in skin cancer. Enzyme Res 2011;2011:409295.

12. Qureshi MM, McClure WC, Arevalo NL, et al. The dietary supplement protandim decreases plasma osteopontin and improves markers of oxidative stress in muscular dystrophy Mdx mice. J Diet Suppl 2010;7(2):159–78.

13. Lim J, van der Pol S, Drexhage J, et al. Nrf2 activators: a novel strategy to promote oligodendrocyte survival in multiple sclerosis? 5th Joint triennial congress of the European and Americas Committees for Treatment and Research in Multiple Sclerosis. Amsterdam: 2011. Abstract Available at: http://registration.akm.ch/einsicht.php?XNABSTRACT_ID=137548&XNSPRACHE_ID=2&XNKONGRESS_ID=150&XNMASKEN_ID=900. Accessed January 23, 2013.

14. Gold R, Kappos L, Arnold DL, et al. Placebo-controlled phase 3 study of oral BG-12 for relapsing multiple sclerosis. N Engl J Med 2012;367(12):1098–107.

15. Seidman MD, Bai U, Khan MJ, et al. Association of mitochondrial DNA deletions and cochlear pathology: a molecular biologic tool. Laryngoscope 1996;106(6):777–83.

16. Ueda N, Oshima T, Ikeda K, et al. Mitochondrial DNA deletion is a predisposing cause for sensorineural hearing loss. Laryngoscope 1998;108:580–4.

17. Seidman MD, Bai U, Khan MJ, et al. Mitochondrial DNA deletions associated with aging and presbyacusis. Arch Otolaryngol Head Neck Surg 1997;123(10):1039–45.

18. Fischel-Ghodsian N. Mitochondrial mutations and hearing loss: paradigm for mitochondrial genetics. Am J Hum Genet 1998;62(1):15–9.

19. Prazma J, Carrasco VN, Butler B, et al. Cochlear microcirculation in young and old gerbils. Arch Otolaryngol Head Neck Surg 1990;116:932–6.

20. Gacek RR, Schuknecht HF. Pathology of presbyacusis. Int J Audiol 1969;8:199–209.

21. Harkins SW. Effects of age and interstimulus interval on the brainstem auditory evoked potential. Int J Neurosci 1981;15:107–18.

22. Rosenhall U, Pederson DM. Effects of presbyacusis and other types of hearing loss on auditory brainstem response. Scand Audiol 1986;15:179–85.

23. Hoeffding V, Feldman ML. Changes with age in the morphology of the cochlear nerve in rats: light microscopy. J Comp Neurol 1988;276:537–46.

24. Semsei I, Szeszak F, Nagy I. In vivo studies on the age-dependent decrease of the rates of total and mRNA synthesis in the brain cortex of rats. Arch Gerontol Geriatr 1982;1:29–42.

25. Semsei I, Rao G, Richardson A. Changes in the expression of superoxide dismutase and catalase as a function of age and dietary restriction. Biochem Biophys Res Commun 1989;165:620–5.

26. Richardson A, Butler JA, Rutherford MS, et al. Effects of age and dietary restriction on the expression of alpha-2u-globulin. J Biol Chem 1987;262:12821–5.

27. Fraser GE, Shavlik DJ. Ten years of life: is it a matter of choice? Arch Intern Med 2001;161:1645–52.

28. Campbell TM II, Campbell TC. The China Study: the most comprehensive study of nutrition ever conducted and the startling implications for diet, weight loss and long-term health. Dallas (TX): BenBella Books; 2004.

29. Selye H. The stress of life. New York: McGraw-Hill; 1978.
30. Simonton OC, Creighton J, Simonton SM. Getting well again: the bestselling classic about the Simontons' revolutionary lifesaving self- awareness techniques. New York: Bantam; 1992.
31. Vaillant GE, Mukamal K. Successful aging. Am J Psychiatry 2001;158(6): 839–47.
32. Forman JP, Stampfer MJ, Curhan GC. Diet and lifestyle risk factors associated with incident hypertension in women. JAMA 2009;302(4):401–11.
33. Djoussé L, Driver JA, Gaziano JM. Relation between modifiable lifestyle factors and lifetime risk of heart failure. JAMA 2009;302(4):394–400.
34. Dunn AL, Marcus BH, Kampert JB, et al. Comparison of lifestyle and structured interventions to increase physical activity and cardiorespiratory fitness: a randomized trial. JAMA 1999;281(4):327–34.
35. Heilbronin LK, de Jonge L, Frisard M, et al. Effect of six-month caloric restriction on biomarkers of longevity, metabolic adaptation and oxidative stress in over-weight individuals. JAMA 2006;295:1539–48.
36. Weindruch R, Walford RL. The retardation of aging in mice by dietary restriction: longevity, cancer, immunity and lifetime energy intake. J Nutr 1986;116:641–54.
37. Pearson KJ, Baur JA. Resveratrol delays age-related deterioration and mimics transcriptional aspects of dietary restriction without extending life span. Cell Metab 2008;8:157–68.
38. Baur JA, Pearson KJ. Resveratrol improves health and survival of mice on a high-calorie diet. Nature 2006;444(7117):337–42.
39. Kochanek KD, Xu J, Murphy S, et al. Centers for Disease Control and Prevention's National Vital Statistics Reports 2011;59(4):5.
40. Knekt P, JaYvinen R, SeppSnen R, et al. Dietary Flavonoids and the Risk of Lung Cancer and Other Malignant Neoplasms. Am J Epidemiol 1997;146(3): 223–30.
41. Anand P, Kunnumakkara AB, Sundaram C, et al. Cancer is a preventable disease that requires major lifestyle changes. Pharm Res 2008;25(9):2097–116.
42. Sasco AJ, Secretan MB, Straif K. Tobacco smoking and cancer: a brief review of recent epidemiological evidence. Lung Cancer 2004;45(2):S3–9.
43. World Cancer Research Fund/American Institute for Cancer Research. Food, nutrition, physical activity, and the prevention of cancer: a global perspective. Washington, DC: AICR; 2007.
44. The global alliance against chronic respiratory diseases of the world health organization. General meeting report. Toronto, June 1–2, 2010.
45. Norrving B, Kissela B. The global burden of stroke and need for a continuum of care. Neurology 2013;80(3 Suppl 2):S5.
46. Gu Y, Nieves JW, Stern Y, et al. Food combination and Alzheimer disease risk: a protective diet. Arch Neurol 2010;67(6):699–706.
47. Micik SH, Yuwiler J. Injuries–the neglected disease of modern society. West J Med 1990;152(3):288.
48. Committee on Trauma and Committee on Shock, Division of Medical Sciences, National Academy of Sciences, National Research Council. Accidental death and disability: the neglected disease of modern society. Washington, DC: Institute of Medicine, National Academy of Sciences; 1966. p. 10, 11.
49. de la Monte SM, Neusner A, Chu J, et al. Epidemiological trends strongly suggest exposures as etiologic agents in the pathogenesis of sporadic Alzheimer's disease, diabetes mellitus, and non-alcoholic steatohepatitis. J Alzheimers Dis 2009;17(3):519–29.

50. Dubnov-Raz G, Berry EM. The dietary treatment of obesity. Med Clin North Am 2011;95(5):939–52.
51. Anderson J, Young L, Long E. Diet and hypertension. Colorado State University Extension 11/98; revised 8/08. Fact Sheet No.9.318 Food and Nutrition Series, Health. Available at: http://www.ext.colostate.edu/pubs/foodnut/09318.html. Accessed January 23, 2013.
52. Johnson RJ, Sanchez-Lozada LG, Nakagawa T. The effect of fructose on renal biology and disease. J Am Soc Nephrol 2010;21:2036–9.
53. Lieber CS. Relationships between nutrition, alcohol use, and liver disease. Bethesda, MD: National Institute on Alcohol Abuse and Alcoholism/NIH; 2004.
54. McDougall JD. The Free McDougall Program. 2012. Available at: http://www.drmcdougall.com/free.html. Accessed January 23, 2013.
55. Lautermann J, Crann SA, McLaren J, et al. Glutathione-dependent antioxidant systems in the mammalian inner ear: effects of aging, ototoxic drugs and noise. Hear Res 1997;114(1–2):75–82.
56. Shi Q, Gibson GE. Oxidative stress and transcriptional regulation in Alzheimer's disease. Alzheimer Dis Assoc Disord 2007;21(4):276–91.
57. Constant J. Alcohol, ischemic heart disease, and the French paradox. Coron Artery Dis 1997;8(10):645–9.
58. Belguendouz L, Fremont L, Linard A. Resveratrol inhibits metal ion-dependent and independent peroxidation of porcine low-density lipoproteins. Biochem Pharmacol 1997;53(9):1347–55.
59. Fauconneau B, Waffo-Teguo P, Huguet F, et al. Comparative study of radical scavenger and antioxidant properties of phenolic compounds from Vitis vinifera cell cultures using in vitro tests. Life Sci 1997;61(21):2103–10.
60. Olas B, Wachowicz B, Saluk-Juszczak J, et al. Effect of resveratrol, a natural polyphenolic compound, on platelet activation induced by endotoxin or thrombin. Thromb Res 2002;107(3–4):141–5.
61. Bertelli AA, Ferrara F, Diana G, et al. Resveratrol, a natural stilbene in grapes and wine, enhances intraphagocytosis in human promonocytes: a co-factor in antiinflammatory and anticancer chemopreventive activity. Int J Tissue React 1999;21(4):93–104.
62. Tredici G, Miloso M, Nicolini G, et al. Resveratrol, map kinases and neuronal cells: might wine be a neuroprotectant? Drugs Exp Clin Res 1999;25(2–3):99–103.
63. Virgili M, Contestabile A. Partial neuroprotection of in vivo excitotoxic brain damage by chronic administration of the red wine antioxidant agent, trans-resveratrol in rats. Neurosci Lett 2000;281(2–3):123–6.
64. Draczynska-Lusiak B, Doung A, Sun AY. Oxidized lipoproteins may play a role in neuronal cell death in Alzheimer disease. Mol Chem Neuropathol 1998;33(2):139–48.
65. Zini R, Morin C, Bertelli A, et al. Effects of resveratrol on the rat brain respiratory chain. Drugs Exp Clin Res 1999;25(2–3):87–97.
66. Manna SK, Mukhopadhyay A, Aggarwal BB. Resveratrol suppresses TNF-induced activation of nuclear transcription factor NF-kappa B, activator protein-1, and apoptosis: potential role of reactive oxygen intermediates and lipid peroxidation. J Immunol 2000;164(12):6509–19.
67. Shimada T, Hiraishi H, Terano A. Hepatocyte growth factor protects gastric epithelial cells against ceramide-induced apoptosis through induction of cyclo-oxygenase-2. Life Sci 2000;68(5):539–46.
68. Nogawa S, Zhang F, Ross ME, et al. Cyclo-oxygenase-2 gene expression in neurons contributes to ischemic brain damage. J Neurosci 1997;17(8):2746–55.

69. Ho L, Pieroni C, Winger D, et al. Regional distribution of cyclooxygenase-2 in the hippocampal formation in Alzheimer's disease. J Neurosci Res 1999;57(3): 295–303.
70. Almer G, Guegan C, Teismann P, et al. Increased expression of the pro-inflammatory enzyme cyclooxygenase-2 in amyotrophic lateral sclerosis. Ann Neurol 2001;49(2):176–85.
71. Shirahama T, Sakakura C. Overexpression of cyclooxygenase-2 in squamous cell carcinoma of the urinary bladder. Clin Cancer Res 2001;7(3):558–61.
72. Hayek MG, Mura C, Wu D, et al. Enhanced expression of inducible cyclooxyge-nase with age in murine macrophages. J Immunol 1997;159(5):2445–51.
73. Govoni S, Masoero E, Favalli L, et al. The cycloxygenase-2 inhibitor SC58236 is neuroprotective in an in vivo model of focal ischemia in the rat. Neurosci Lett 2001;303(2):91–4.
74. Kim JW, Baek BS, Kim YK, et al. Gene expression of cyclooxygenase in the aging heart. J Gerontol A Biol Sci Med Sci 2001;56(8):B350–5.
75. Collis DK, Ponseti IV. Long-term follow-up of patients with idiopathic scoliosis not treated surgically. J Bone Joint Surg Am 1969;51:425–45.
76. Branthwaite MA. Cardiorespiratory consequences of unfused idiopathic scoliosis. Br J Dis Chest 1986;80:360–9.
77. Travell J, Simons D. 1st edition. Myofascial pain and dysfunction: a trigger point manual, vol. I. Baltimore (MD): Williams & Wilkins; 1983. p. 4, 15, 18–19, 103.
78. Mense S, Simons DG, Russell IJ. Muscle pain: understanding its nature, diag-nosis, and treatment. Baltimore (MD): Lippincott Williams & Wilkins; 2000. p. 151.
79. Levine RA, Mandel SS, Seidman MD, et al. Randomized controlled clinical trial testing complementary and alternative medicine therapies to alleviate chronic low back pain. North American Research Conference. Edmonton, May 24–26, 2006.
80. Levine RA, St John P, Eckert E, et al. St John neurosomatic therapy is effective in reducing symptoms of intractable headache: a complementary and integrative medicine pilot study. North American Research Conference. Edmonton, May 24–26, 2006.
81. Unschuld P. Medicine in China, a history of ideas. Berkeley (CA): University of California Press; 1985. p. 109–15.
82. Sima Qian, Dawson R. The first Emperor. Selections from the Historical Records. NY: Oxford University Press; 2007. p. 74–5, 119, 148–9.
83. Correa-Velez I, Clavarino A, Eastwood H. Surviving, relieving, repairing, and boosting up: reasons for using complementary/alternative medicine among patients with advanced cancer: a thematic analysis. J Palliat Med 2005;8(5): 953–61.
84. Gupta D, Lis CG, Birdsall TC, et al. The use of dietary supplements in a commu-nity hospital comprehensive cancer center: implications for conventional cancer care. Support Care Cancer 2005;13(11):912–9.
85. Evans M, Shaw A, Thompson EA, et al. Decisions to use complementary and alternative medicine (CAM) by male cancer patients: information-seeking roles and types of evidence used. BMC Complement Altern Med 2007;4(7):25.
86. Barnes PM, Bloom B, Nahin RL. Complementary and alternative medicine use among adults and children: United States, 2007. Natl Health Stat Report 2008;10(12):1–23.
87. Verhoef MJ, Balneaves LG, Boon HS, et al. Reasons for and characteristics associated with complementary and alternative medicine use among adult cancer patients: a systematic review. Integr Cancer Ther 2005;4(4):274–86.

88. Halliwell B. Dietary polyphenols: good, bad, or indifferent for your health? Cardiovasc Res 2007;73(2):341–7.
89. Shahidi F, Janitha PK, Wanasundara PD. Phenolic antioxidants. Crit Rev Food Sci Nutr 1992;32:67–103.
90. Halliwell B, Rafter J, Jenner A. Health promotion by flavonoids, tocopherols, tocotrienols, and other phenols: direct or indirect effects? Antioxidant or not? Am J Clin Nutr 2005;81(Suppl 1):268S–76S.
91. Li YJ, Gong M, Konishi T. Antioxidant synergism among component herbs of traditional Chinese medicine formula ShengMai San studied in vitro and in vivo. J Health Sci 2007;53:692–9. Available at: http://jhs.pharm.or.jp/data/53%286%29/53_692.pdf. Accessed January 24, 2013.
92. Konishi T. Brain oxidative stress as basic target of antioxidant traditional oriental medicines. Neurochem Res 2009;34:711–6.
93. Larkey L, Jahnke R, Etnier J, et al. Meditative movement as a category of exercise: implications for research. Not Found In Database 2009;6:230–8.
94. Jahnke R, Larkey L, Rogers C, et al. A comprehensive review of health benefits of qigong and tai chi. Am J Health Promot 2010;24(6):e1–25.
95. Langevin HM, Bouffard NA, Badger GJ, et al. Subcutaneous tissue fibroblast cytoskeletal remodeling induced by acupuncture: evidence for a mechanotransduction-based mechanism. J Cell Physiol 2006;207:767–74.
96. Pomeranz BJ. Acupuncture and the raison d'être for alternative medicine. Altern Ther Health Med 1996;2(6):85–91.
97. Han JS. Acupuncture: neuropeptide release produced by electrical stimulation of different frequencies. Trends Neurosci 2003;26(1):17–22.
98. Wang SM, Kain ZN, White P. Acupuncture analgesia: I. The scientific basis. Anesth Analg 2008;106(2):602–10.
99. Lally P, Van Jaarsveld C, Potts HWW, et al. How are habits formed: modelling habit formation in the real world. Eur J Soc Psychol 2010;40:998–1009.
100. Berneburg M, Plettenberg H, Medve-König K, et al. Induction of the photoaging-associated mitochondrial common deletion in vivo in normal human skin. J Invest Dermatol 2004;122:1277–83.
101. Giovannucci EL. The role of vitamin D in cancer prevention: what do we really know? Amer Ass Canc Research 101st Ann Mtg, Washington, DC. April 20, 2010.
102. Frank E, Winkleby MA, Altman DG, et al. Predictors of physicians' smoking cessation advice. JAMA 1991;266(22):3139–44.
103. Stead LF, Bergson G, Lancaster T [review]. Cochrane Collaboration. Physician advice for smoking cessation, vol. 4. Oxford (United Kingdom): John Wiley; 2008. p. 4. Available at: http://www.ncbi.nlm.nih.gov/pubmed/18425860. Accessed January 23, 2013.
104. Watts MS. Physicians as role models in society. West J Med 1990;152(3):292.
105. Schwenk T. Physicians as role models. Am Fam Physician 2007;75(7):1089–90. Available at: http://www.aafp.org/afp/2007/0401/p1089.html. Accessed January 23, 2013.

Complementary and Integrative Treatments
Allergy

Grant Garbo, MD[a],*, Belachew Tessema, MD[b],
Seth M. Brown, MD, MBA[b]

KEYWORDS

- Allergic rhinitis • Immunotherapy • Allergy treatment • Integrative medicine

KEY POINTS

- Allergic rhinitis is a treatable disease with multiple options at the physician's disposal.
- Current pharmacologic treatment regimens include nasal saline irrigation, antihistamines, cell membrane stabilizers, leukotriene inhibitors, and steroids.
- Immunotherapy is a common method of treatment, with ongoing studies evaluating the efficacy of sublingual versus subcutaneous regimens.
- Multiple complementary therapies are currently being investigated, with several proving to be efficacious, such as butterbur extract, bioflavonoid, Spirulina, and other herbs.
- Acupuncture has not been definitively shown to be effective in treating allergic rhinitis compared with placebo.

OVERVIEW

Allergy is the clinical manifestation of an unwanted immune response after repeated contact with normally innocuous substances, such as

- Pollen
- Mold spores
- Animal dander
- Dust mites
- Foods
- Stinging insects

One clinical manifestation, allergic rhinitis (AR), is an inflammation of the nasal mucous membranes caused by an IgE-mediated reaction to the allergen. AR affects between 20% and 25% of the population in the United States.[1] This is a disease commonly found in childhood with increasing prevalence. A US study of 4- to 7-year-old

[a] University of Connecticut School of Medicine, 263 Farmington Avenue, Farmington, CT 06030, USA; [b] Connecticut Sinus Institute, University of Connecticut School of Medicine, 21 South Road, Farmington, CT 06032, USA
* Corresponding author.
E-mail address: ggarbo@resident.uchc.edu

Otolaryngol Clin N Am 46 (2013) 295–307
http://dx.doi.org/10.1016/j.otc.2012.12.005
0030-6665/13/$ – see front matter © 2013 Elsevier Inc. All rights reserved.

children revealed a prevalence of AR between 30% and 40%, with rates increasing into college years.[2] Allergy is also characterized by sneezing, itching, and congestion and can be associated with asthma, otitis media with effusion, rhinosinusitis, and nasal polyps.

PHYSIOLOGY AND ANATOMY
The Immune System

The immune system is responsible for identifying and destroying elements foreign to the body while recognizing and protecting self, termed *self-tolerance*. It comprises the innate and adaptive immune systems.

The innate immune system is the first line of defense against potential invaders and is composed of barrier mechanisms, such as tight junctions along with cilia, defensins, lysozyme, and cells. Neutrophils, monocytes, mast cells, eosinophils, basophils, and dendritic cells work together through pattern recognition receptors to opsonize bacteria, activate coagulation and complement cascades, induce phagocytosis, and implement proinflammatory signaling pathways. This system is activated by foreign bodies and works quickly to help rid the body of infection.

The adaptive immune system is a more specific approach to protecting the body from infection. It is triggered when a pathogen evades the innate immune system. A new foreign antigen is presented to T cells and recognized as nonself, leading to the secretion of cytokines to recruit fresh macrophages, neutrophils, and other lymphocytes to the site of infection or spur the growth of additional T cells. T cells also secrete various molecules to induce B cells to produce specific antibodies via interleukin 4 (IL-4), or opsonizing antibodies via interferon γ (INF-γ).

Allergy Reactions

Allergy is caused by a type I hypersensitivity reaction, also termed an *atopic reaction*. This reaction is caused by excess production of IgE and begins with sensitization to the allergen, inducing IgE antibody production through T- and B-cell cascades. A family history of atopy, including asthma, eczema, hay fever, and urticaria, is a risk factor for the development of AR, asthma, and atopic dermatitis. Having one allergic parent leads to a 30% increased risk of having children with atopy, whereas having 2 allergic parents leads to an increased risk of 50%. Other risk factors include

- Genetic susceptibility
- Environmental factors
- Exposure to allergens
- Passive exposure to tobacco smoke
- Exposure to diesel exhaust[3]

Allergy reactions are split into 2 phases: early (humeral reaction) and late (cellular reaction). The early phase occurs within 10 to 15 minutes of exposure. Allergens deposited on mucosal surfaces are sampled by dendritic cells and migrated to lymph nodes for presentation to T cells for sensitization. Subsequent exposure results in antigen attachment to 2 IgE antibodies on mast cells, resulting in degranulation of histamine. High levels of mast cells in the mucosa of the respiratory and gastrointestinal tracts, the subconjunctiva of the eye, and the subcutaneous layer of the skin increases susceptibility at these sites. The inflammatory response leads to the release of histamine, leukotrienes, cytokines, prostaglandins, and platelet-activating factors. The histamine released is responsible for sneezing, rhinorrhea, itching, vascular permeability, vasodilation, and glandular secretions.

The late phase occurs 4 to 6 hours after exposure and is mostly a result of various cytokines and leukotrienes released from mast and T cells. These factors cause an influx of eosinophils through chemotaxis and can prolong symptoms and enhance the allergic cascade for up to 48 hours.[3]

Hygiene Hypothesis

Several theories describe the pathophysiology of allergies, with the most prominent currently being the "hygiene hypothesis." The hygiene hypothesis describes children raised in modern metropolitan lifestyles being relatively devoid of the natural microbial burdens seen by previous generations. These burdens may have prompted early immune maturation and prevented allergic disease and asthma from developing. Lack of immune maturation may be causing understimulated immune systems in infancy, allowing the "allergic march."[4]

The allergic march is a subset of allergic disorders, such as atopic dermatitis or eczema, food allergies, AR, and allergy-associated asthma. It is thought that nature may immunize against the allergic march through various microbial exposures of the respiratory and gastrointestinal tracts. As immune systems mature, the production of T lymphocytes increases. These increased numbers of T lymphocytes result in the increased formation of IFN-γ, which may inhibit mucous gland and smooth muscle hyperplasia, the fibrotic repair process, and mast cell activation.[4]

Various studies have shown that increased exposure to various allergens may actually help decrease the incidence of allergic responses. A study performed by Svanes and colleagues[5] showed that cat ownership helped decrease the number of atopic individuals developing asthma and dog ownership protected against the development of allergic asthma.

Classification and Symptoms

AR is separated into seasonal and perennial types. Seasonal AR is associated with various seasons depending on the allergen; the spring air is full of tree pollen, grasses dominate the air as summer begins, and weeds and molds fill the air in autumn. Symptoms vary throughout the year and are somewhat based on the pollen count; they consist predominantly of sneezing, congestion, watery rhinorrhea, and itchy eyes and nose.

Perennial AR is a more constant disease process. It is usually the result of allergies to dust mites, animal dander, mold spores, or cockroaches. The symptoms differ slightly from those of seasonal AR, with less sneezing, rhinorrhea, and eye involvement. This classification can be further divided into intermittent, with symptoms lasting for less than 4 days per week or less than 4 weeks, or persistent, with symptoms lasting for greater than 4 days per week or greater than 4 weeks.

MEDICAL TREATMENT APPROACHES AND OUTCOMES

Approaches to treatments of allergy consist of avoidance, various pharmacotherapy, immunotherapy, and integrated and alternative remedies, including herbal treatment. These therapies are aimed at decreasing inflammation and histamine release. When selecting a treatment option, it is important to consider the main symptoms, symptom severity, quality of life, cost of therapy, side effects of the treatment, and the allergens involved.

Antihistamines

First-line medical therapy for allergy is usually antihistamines, which come in oral and nasal spray form. These drugs work as an H1 receptor antagonist, preventing histamine-induced reactions, such as vascular permeability, smooth muscle contraction, mucous production, and pruritus. Antihistamines have a good effect on early-phase reactions, but little effect on congestion. The first-generation oral antihistamines are notorious for causing sedation and impairing performance secondary to their lipophilicity, allowing easy crossing of the blood–brain barrier. These medications also cause significant anticholinergic side effects, including dry mouth, blurred vision, and thickened mucous. Second-generation antihistamines are generally less sedative, have a rapid onset within 1 hour, and produce fewer anticholinergic side effects. These medications do not cross the blood–brain barrier as easily, causing less sedation than their predecessors. However, these medications can still be sedative with increased dosage. Second-generation antihistamines are thought to change the conformation of the histamine receptor, deactivating it and providing longer symptomatic relief.

Intranasal antihistamine sprays, such as azelastine or olopatadine, have been approved for the treatment of allergies and vasomotor rhinitis. These drugs show rapid onset and good potency, with limited side effects, such as mild sedation and bitter taste. In a double-blind placebo-controlled study, Yamamoto and colleagues[6] were able to show equal efficacy between oral and nasal antihistamines in regard to sneezing, rhinorrhea, and nasal congestion. However, olopatadine was more effective in controlling eye itching and watering. Hoyte and Katial[7] evaluated various studies in their review and were able verify that these sprays were as efficacious or superior to oral second-generation antihistamines. Several recent studies comparing antihistamine nasal spray and nasal steroid sprays have shown increased efficacy of the antihistamine spray. Yañez and Rodrigo[8] were able to show improved benefit in regard to ocular symptoms and nasal congestion when comparing intranasal antihistamines and intranasal steroids. No difference was seen between olopatadine and fluticasone when analyzing the total nasal symptom score (TNSS), including congestion, runny nose, sneezing, itchy nose, and ocular symptoms. However, olopatadine did display a faster onset of action, recorded by Patel and colleagues as less than 30 minutes compared with mometasone's onset of action of 8 hours.[9,10] These studies have shown nasal antihistamines to be superior to nasal steroids in the management of some symptoms; however, the combination of the 2 medications was shown to be superior to monotherapy with either medication in the reduction of TNSS.[11]

Corticosteroids

Corticosteroids have long been considered to be the most effective pharmacotherapy for the treatment of AR. Intranasal versions have been shown to relieve sneezing, itching, rhinorrhea, and nasal congestion. Relief from these symptoms is usually achieved after 1 to 2 weeks of therapy, although effectiveness depends on regular use and adequate nasal airway for application. Nasal corticosteroids have no significant systemic absorption and some have been approved for use in patients aged 2 years and older. Side effects include dryness and epistaxis, which can be reduced through careful patient education. Occasional case reports have linked glaucoma with intranasal steroid use; however, a case-controlled study performed by Garbe and colleagues[12] found no association. Systemic corticosteroids are often used for severe intractable symptoms in a tapering dose.

Decongestants

Decongestants are α-adrenergic receptor agonists that cause vasoconstriction, reducing turbinate congestion and improving patency of the airway. However, these medications have no effect on rhinorrhea, pruritus, or sneezing. Topical decongestant therapy is recommended for no more than 5 days because prolonged use can lead to rhinitis medicamentosa. Oral decongestants have less potential to elicit rebound rhinitis but have a broad range of side effects, including insomnia, anxiety, nervousness, irritability, tremulousness, restlessness, and headache. These medications should be avoided in patients with hypertension, arrhythmias, angina, urinary retention, or glaucoma.

Others

Intranasal saline irrigation has long been used as single-modality or adjuvant therapy for the treatment of AR. It has been found to be particularly useful in the presence of crusted nasal secretions secondary to chronic, thick drainage. A randomized study by Wang and colleagues[13] examined the impact of nasal irrigation in children with acute sinusitis and found significant improvement in rhinorrhea, nasal congestion, throat itching, sleep quality symptoms, and nasal airflow. Another study of children found nasal irrigation to be additive to the use of intranasal glucocorticoids.[14]

Intranasal anticholinergics, such as ipratropium bromide, help to control rhinorrhea but have little to no effect on other allergy symptoms. These medications act through blocking parasympathetic input to the nasal mucosa and relieving symptoms of rhinorrhea.

Mast cell stabilizers, such as cromolyn sodium (oral) and cromolyn sodium nasal solution, act through stabilizing the membranes of mast cells, thereby limiting the amount of histamine released during the early phase of an allergic response. The caveat to this medication regimen is that it must be used before the onset of symptoms and be continued throughout the entire exposure, usually every 6 hours.

Leukotriene inhibitors, such as montelukast, a specific antagonist of leukotriene receptors, are generally less effective than antihistamines and intranasal steroids but more effective than placebo.

Recombinant human monoclonal antibody to IgE, or anti-IgE therapy, with omalizumab, acts through binding circulating IgE molecules. The thought is that fewer molecules of IgE will be available to bind to mast cell receptors to precipitate an allergic reaction. This therapy is costly and the US Food and Drug Administration (FDA) currently approves its use only for moderate to severe persistent asthma in adults and children older than 12 years who have not experienced an adequate response to inhaled glucocorticoids.

One randomized trial evaluated patient response to omalizumab. Patients were randomly assigned to either subcutaneous placebo or various dosages of omalizumab every 4 weeks before ragweed season. Rhinitis symptoms were significantly improved in the highest-dosage experimental group. A dose-dependent decrease in free IgE levels was also seen with omalizumab use.[15] Another trial randomized children to placebo or omalizumab after subcutaneous immunotherapy treatment and showed significantly lowered leukotriene release in the omalizumab plus immunotherapy group.[16] These studies suggest the efficacy of using anti-IgE therapy to treat allergies.

Subcutaneous and Sublingual Immunotherapy

Immunotherapy has been used as a method to increase the threshold level of the appearance of symptoms after aeroallergen exposure though gradually increasing dosages of antigen. This method of treatment is indicated in patients who have inadequate control of symptoms with pharmacotherapy and/or allergen sensitivities. If no clinical improvement is seen in 1 year, reasons for lack of efficacy should be evaluated, such as ongoing significant allergenic exposures, continued exposure to nonallergen triggers, missing of clinically relevant allergens, and/or failure to treat with adequate dosages of allergens. If no reason can be found, the therapy should be discontinued.

Cox and Wallace[17] recently published a review of immunotherapy articles. Subcutaneous immunotherapy (SCIT) has been used for a longer period, and therefore more information has been published on its use compared with sublingual immunotherapy (SLIT). Multiple trials have shown the efficacy of SCIT, and it is an accepted form of allergic therapy. However, larger concerns have been expressed regarding its safety. SCIT adverse reactions range from local to systemic. The local reactions of erythema, pruritus, and swelling are fairly common, occurring in 26% to 82% of patients and associated with 0.7% to 4.0% of injections.[18–20] Systemic reactions can range from mild rhinitis to life-threatening anaphylaxis and occur in 2% to 7% of patients and with 0.2% of injections.[21]

SLIT has become much more common in Europe than the United States. The benefits of SLIT are improved safety and the ability to home-administer compared with SCIT. American otolaryngologists were surveyed twice regarding reasons for not using SLIT, and responded with the lack of FDA approval as the number one cited reason, at 61.7% to 86.3%, and unknown effective dose as a distant second, at 27.5% to 43.9%. Although the effective dose has not yet been established, it is usually in the range of 300 times greater than SCIT dosing.[21] Few studies have been performed comparing SLIT dosing frequency regimens, and none have compared the same dose administered at different frequencies.

In a meta-analysis analyzing 979 patients undergoing SLIT in 22 trials, Wilson and colleagues[22] reported a significant reduction in symptoms and medication use. Furthermore, Penagos and colleagues[23] was able to establish a significant reduction in symptoms and medication use in the pediatric population undergoing grass pollen SLIT therapy. SLIT has been shown to be safer than SCIT therapy, with a lower rate of systemic reactions overall and severe systemic reactions being very uncommon. However, local reactions are more common, with increased rates of oropharyngeal pruritus and/or mouth edema (46% and 18%, respectively).[24] SLIT has also been associated with complaints of occasional abdominal pain, vomiting, uvular edema, and urticaria. In all of the trials and treatments, no deaths and only rare cases of anaphylaxis have been associated with SLIT.

In the treatment of grass pollen allergens, SCIT and SLIT are equally efficacious. In a comparison of 3 large clinical trials of grass tablets versus 1 large SCIT trial, when evaluating clinical parameters of SCIT and SLIT compared with placebo, reductions in symptoms of the immunotherapy arms were seen at 32% and 21% to 37%, respectively. Reductions in the use of pharmacotherapy of 41% and 29% to 46%, respectively, were also seen.[25–28]

The mechanisms behind the effect of immunotherapy are unclear but are thought to be related to the production of blocking antibodies or a regulation of immune cascade. A review of various SCIT articles showed that most patients treated with immunotherapy show an increase in specific IgE with therapy.[17] Various immunologic effects have been shown, including an increase in specific IgG, IgE-blocking antibodies, and specific IgE, with blunting of further seasonal increases in IgE, all or none of which may be responsible for the decreased response to allergen. Early events after immunotherapy include generation of T-regulatory cells, which may produce cytokines such as IL-10, IL-12, or transforming growth factor β.[21]

Regardless of mechanism, studies have been able to link AR as a risk factor for the development of asthma, with up to 40% of patients with AR developing asthma later in life. Polosa and colleagues[29] was able to show a significantly lowered incidence of asthma in patients treated with SCIT compared with pharmacotherapy alone 7 years after discontinuation of treatment. Another study evaluated 113 children with either

SLIT or pharmacotherapy for 3 years and was able to show a 3.8-times greater risk of developing asthma in the pharmacotherapy group.[30]

PATIENT SELF-TREATMENTS

The idea of patient self-treatment revolves around the idea of avoidance and environmental controls. To be successful in avoiding allergens, patients should undergo an allergy test. Patients with pollen allergies are advised to avoid outdoor activities during relevant pollen seasons. These individuals should concentrate on staying indoors and using the air conditioner if available. Reducing the household humidity to less than 50% helps stave off mold and mildew. Patients with allergies to dust and/or pets should thoroughly wash bed linens in hot water; remove carpets and pets; encase pillows, mattresses, and box springs with hypoallergenic covering; clean ducts; and eliminate cockroaches. Through these methods, some patients are able to achieve good control of their allergies without introducing pharmacotherapy.

INTEGRATIVE TREATMENT APPROACHES AND OUTCOMES

Complementary and integrative medicine (CIM) therapies are frequently used to treat various chronic diseases such as AR. Nearly 50% of American adults experiencing asthma or rhinosinusitis have tried CIM treatments.[31] The scientific community has evaluated the claims of various CIM therapies for the treatment of allergy. Many more therapies are being studied in addition to those mentioned herein. This article includes the more commonly used therapies and those that have shown a high likelihood of success (**Table 1**).

Honey

Local honey has long been held as a natural remedy for the treatment of seasonal allergies caused by pollen. A study performed by Rajan and colleagues[32] randomly assigned participants to either corn syrup with honey flavoring or locally or nationally collected honey. After tracking allergy symptoms using a diary, neither honey group experienced a decrease in allergy symptoms compared with the corn syrup group after 10 days.

Butterbur

Petasites hybridus, or butterbur extract, has also been getting much attention for its antileukotriene biosynthetic and antihistamine activity. These effects are thought to be from petasin, a component of the extract. Butterbur is an herbaceous plant native to Europe, northern Africa, and southwestern Asia and has been used for years to treat bronchial asthma, smooth muscle spasms, and headaches. Multiple studies of butterbur have been performed, with most showing favorable results in the treatment of AR compared with placebo or even established antihistamine pharmacotherapy.

Schapowal[33] published multiple studies proclaiming the effects of butterbur on AR. A prospective randomized double-blind study (RDBS) assessing changes in symptoms, physician's global assessment, and responder rate found butterbur and fexofenadine to be significantly better at controlling AR compared with placebo. However, no significant difference was seen between the antihistamine and the butterbur. In another RDBS, Schapowal[34] evaluated butterbur versus cetirizine and found no significant differences between the treatments, and showed that trends favored butterbur for the treatment of AR. Other published papers with different authors have found similar trends.[35–38] However, Gray and colleagues[36] compared the effects on AR of butterbur versus placebo and were unable to observe a significant difference. Overall,

Table 1
Overview of alternative herbal therapies for AR[a]

Therapy	Ingredient	Mechanism of Action	Evidence
Local Honey	Local pollen	Allows the body to build up tolerance to offending allergens (pollen)	No supporting evidence
Butterbur extract	Petasin	Antileukotriene biosynthesis and antihistamine properties	Studies displayed butterbur's equal efficacy with several antihistamine drugs
Spirulina	Dried biomass of *Arthrospira platensis*	Inhibition of mast cell release of histamine and possible increased IFN-γ levels	Randomized double-blind study showed significant reduction in IL-4 levels
Bioflavonoid	Quercetin	Inhibits basophil and mast cell degranulation	Twice as effective as sodium cromolyn in reducing LT production
Flavonolignan	Silymarin	Stabilizes cell membrane	Addition of silymarin to cetirizine improved clinical symptoms
Saccharomyces cerevisiae	Oral yeast	Unknown	Showed reduction in nasal congestion
Baikal skullcap root	*Scutellaria baicalensis*	Unknown	Decreased serum IgE and IL-5 levels
Soy sauce	Shoyu polysaccharides	Unknown	Reduced runny nose, sore throat, and itchy eyes
Xin-yi-san	Unknown Chinese herb	Unknown	Improvements in nasal symptoms and congestion, suppressed serum IgE levels, and increased IL-10 and IL-8 levels

Abbreviations: IFN, interferon; IL, interleukin; LT, leukotriene.
[a] Various herbs have been studied and have shown positive results. All herbs listed are compared with placebo in the description of evidence.

there seems to be a trend toward acceptance of butterbur as a treatment option for AR, but further studies must be performed.

When considering the use of butterbur for AR, one must remember the possible side-effect profile. Many preparations contain unsaturated pyrrolizidine alkaloids (UPA), which is considered to be hepatotoxic, nephrotoxic, mutagenic, carcinogenic, and associated with venoocclusive disease. Therefore, it is important for patients to use preparations that are certified to be free of UPA.[39]

Spirulina

Spirulina is the dried biomass of *Arthrospira platensis*, a photosynthetic bacterium found in fresh and salt water. This supplement has been touted as an effective treatment of AR. Mao and colleagues[40] evaluated its effects and cited inhibition of histamine release from mast cells and increased INF-γ levels as possible mechanisms.

This RDBS compared its effects versus placebo and showed significantly reduced IL-4 levels in the experimental group, but it did not evaluate symptoms.

Bioflavonoids

Bioflavonoids and flavonolignans are naturally occurring chemical compounds. Quercetin is a bioflavonoid found in many vegetables and fruits that is believed to inhibit basophil and mast cell degranulation. Several studies have reliably validated this claim. Huang and colleagues[41] examined the effects of quercetin on dendritic cell activation and function and found that it inhibited dendritic cell activity through reduced production of proinflammatory cytokines and chemokines. Quercetin was also seen to block endocytosis by dendritic cells and limited its immunostimulatory ability. Otsuka and colleagues[42] showed that quercetin was almost twice as effective as sodium cromolyn in reducing neutrophil lysosomal enzyme secretion and leukotriene production. Silymarin extracted from milk thistle is made up of 3 flavonolignans, silibinin, silydianin, and silychristin, and is also thought to stabilize the cell membrane. A recent study evaluated the effects of silymarin versus placebo using the sinonasal outcome test 20 (SNOT-20) as an evaluation tool. Both groups received cetirizine in addition to the placebo or silymarin, and both groups showed significant improvement in clinical symptom severity. However, the study group showed a significantly larger improvement in SNOT-20 when comparing pretreatment and posttreatment numbers.[43]

Saccharomyces cerevisiae is an oral yeast-derived compound currently being evaluated for its effects on AR. In an RDBS comparing the compound with placebo, Moyad and colleagues[44] noted a significant reduction in nasal congestion and rhinorrhea, a reduced number of days with nasal congestion, and an improved quality of life based on questionnaire responses.

Baikal Skullcap Root

Baikal skullcap root, or Scutellaria baicalensis, has long been used in Asian countries as a treatment for various illnesses, including AR. Kim and colleagues[45] evaluated the effects of Scutellaria baicalensis on IgE and cytokine levels in mice and found sizable decreases in plasma IgE and IL-5 levels, although neither was statistically significant.

Shoyu Polysaccharides

The Japanese have introduced Shoyu polysaccharides as a possible treatment option for AR. Kobayashi and colleagues[46] has been leading the research in identifying quality of life improvement with soy sauce ingredients, Shoyu polysaccharides. He performed an RDBS comparing oral supplementation of Shoyu polysaccharides versus placebo and was able to show a significant reduction in symptom scores for runny nose, sore throat, and itchy eyes in treated individuals.

Traditional Chinese Medicine

Chinese herbal medicine

The Chinese populations have a long history of using herbal medicine to treat ailments of all types, including AR. Xue and colleagues[47] evaluated a Chinese herbal medicine containing 18 herbs and compared it with placebo treatment. The study was able to establish significant reduction in symptoms in the treated group. In an RDBS examining Xin-yi-san, Yang and colleagues[48] showed improvement in nasal symptoms and congestion, suppressed serum IgE levels, and increased IL-10 and IL-8 levels in patients receiving the herb.

Acupuncture

Some studies have been able to show positive results in the treatment of AR with acupuncture, whereas others have refuted the claims of allergy symptom relief. A large nonblinded study of more than 5000 patients evaluated the Rhinitis Quality of Life Questionnaire over 3 months of weekly acupuncture sessions and showed a significant improvement in the quality of life of the experimental group compared with the control group.[49]

An RDBS performed by Ng and colleagues[50] was also able to show a decrease in daily rhinitis scores and increased symptom-free days in subjects undergoing acupuncture compared with sham acupuncture. Furthermore, in systematic review of acupuncture, Lee and colleagues[51] determined that it failed to show effects in subjects experiencing seasonal AR but did significantly lower rhinitis and nasal symptoms in subjects with perennial AR.

Ear acupressure

Another method of controlling AR symptoms is ear acupressure. In a recent systematic review evaluating 7 papers, which were "poor quality" for not including details of randomization or using blinding, Zhang and colleagues[52] determined that ear acupressure is as effective in treating AR as body acupuncture or antihistamines. However, the researchers were unable to recommend these treatments because of the poor quality of the studies being reviewed.

SUMMARY

AR is a common disease that affects millions of people worldwide. Various cultures and civilizations have been using numerous methods to combat these symptoms in an effort to find relief. Within the medical community, several proven treatments are available, ranging from innocuous nasal saline irrigation to immunotherapy to tamper with the immune system. Beyond pharmacotherapy are other options for treating AR, some questionable and others on their way to being validated. A great need still exists for further study in integrative therapies to determine how best to incorporate them into the current regimen.

REFERENCES

1. Jarvis D, Burney P. ABC of allergies: the epidemiology of allergic disease. BMJ 1998;316:607.
2. Zeiger RS, Heller S, Mellon MH, et al. Effect of combined maternal and infant food-allergen avoidance on development of atopy in early infancy: a randomized study. J Allergy Clin Immunol 1989;84:72–89.
3. Bailey B. Head and neck surgery – otolaryngology. 4th edition. New York: Lippincott Williams & Wilkins; 2006.
4. Liu A. Hygiene theory and allergy and asthma prevention. Paediatr Perinat Epidemiol 2007;21(Suppl 3):2–7.
5. Svanes C, Heinrich J, Jarvis D, et al. Pet-keeping in childhood and adult asthma and hay fever: European community respiratory health survey. J Allergy Clin Immunol 2003;112:289–300.
6. Yamamoto H, Yamada T, Kubo S, et al. Efficacy of oral olopatadine hydrochloride for the treatment of seasonal allergic rhinitis: a randomized, double-blind, placebo-controlled study. Allergy Asthma Proc 2010;31(4):296–303.
7. Hoyte FC, Katial RK. Antihistamine therapy in allergic rhinitis. Immunol Allergy Clin North Am 2011;31:509–43.

8. Yañez A, Rodrigo G. Intranasal corticosteroids versus topical H1 receptor antagonists for the treatment of allergic rhinitis: a systematic review with meta-analysis. Ann Allergy Asthma Immunol 2002;89:479–84.

9. Kaliner MA, Storms W, Tilles S, et al. Comparison of olopatadine 0.6% nasal spray versus fluticasone propionate 50 microg in the treatment of seasonal allergic rhinitis. Allergy Asthma Proc 2009;30:255–62.

10. Patel D, D'Andrea C, Sacks HJ. Onset of action of azelastine nasal spray compared with mometasone nasal spray and placebo in subjects with seasonal allergic rhinitis evaluated in an environmental exposure chamber. Am J Rhinol 2007;21:499–503.

11. Ratner P, Hampel F, VanBavel J, et al. Combination therapy with azelastine hydrochloride nasal spray and fluticasone propionate nasal spray in the treatment of patients with seasonal allergic rhinitis. Ann Allergy Asthma Immunol 2008;100:74–81.

12. Garbe E, LeLorier J, Boivin JF, et al. Inhaled and nasal glucocorticoids and the risks of ocular hypertension or open-angle glaucoma. JAMA 1997;277:722–7.

13. Wang YH, Yang CP, Ku MS, et al. Efficacy of nasal irrigation in the treatment of acute sinusitis in children. Int J Pediatr Otorhinolaryngol 2009;73:1696.

14. Li H, Sha Q, Zuo K, et al. Nasal saline irrigation facilitates control of allergic rhinitis by topical steroid in children. ORL J Otorhinolaryngol Relat Spec 2009;71:50.

15. Casale TB, Condemi J, LaForce C, et al. Effect of omalizumab on symptoms of seasonal allergic rhinitis: a randomized controlled trial. JAMA 2001;286:2956.

16. Kopp MV, Brauburger J, Riedinger F, et al. The effect of anti-IgE treatment on in vitro leukotriene release in children with seasonal allergic rhinitis. J Allergy Clin Immunol 2002;110:728.

17. Cox L, Wallace D. Specific allergy immunotherapy for allergic rhinitis: subcutaneous and sublingual. Immunol Allergy Clin North Am 2011;31(3):561–99.

18. Nelson BL, Dupont LA, Reid MJ. Prospective survey of local and systemic reactions to immunotherapy with pollen extracts. Ann Allergy 1986;56(4):d331–4.

19. Prigal SJ. A ten-year study of repository injections of allergens: local reactions and their management. Ann Allergy 1972;30(9):529–35.

20. Tankersley MS, Butler KK, Butler WK, et al. Local reactions during allergen immunotherapy do not require dose adjustment. J Allergy Clin Immunol 2000;106(5): 840–3.

21. Cox L, Larenas-Linnemann D, Lockey RF, et al. Speaking the same language: the World Allergy Organization subcutaneous immunotherapy systemic reaction grading system. J Allergy Clin Immunol 2010;125(3):569–74, 574.e1–e7.

22. Wilson DR, Lima MT, Durham SR. Sublingual immunotherapy for allergic rhinitis: systematic review and meta-analysis. Allergy 2005;60(1):4–12.

23. Penagos M, Compalati E, Tarantini F, et al. Efficacy of sublingual immunotherapy in the treatment of allergic rhinitis in pediatric patients 3 to 18 years of age: a meta-analysis of randomized, placebo-controlled, double-blind trials. Ann Allergy Asthma Immunol 2006;97(2):141–8.

24. Dahl R, Kapp A, Colombo G, et al. Efficacy and safety of sublingual immunotherapy with grass allergen tablets for seasonal allergic rhinoconjunctivitis. J Allergy Clin Immunol 2006;118(2):434–40.

25. Frew AJ, Powell RJ, Corrigan CJ, et al. Efficacy and safety of specific immunotherapy with SQ allergen extract in treatment-resistant seasonal allergic rhinoconjunctivitis. J Allergy Clin Immunol 2006;117(2):319–25.

26. Durham SR, Yang WH, Pedersen MR, et al. Sublingual immunotherapy with once-daily grass allergen tablets: a randomized controlled trial in seasonal allergic rhinoconjunctivitis. J Allergy Clin Immunol 2006;117(4):802–9.

27. Didier A, Malling HJ, Worm M, et al. Optimal dose, efficacy, and safety of once-daily sublingual immunotherapy with a 5-grass pollen tablet for seasonal allergic rhinitis. J Allergy Clin Immunol 2007;120:1338–45.

28. Dahl R, Kapp A, Colombo G, et al. Sublingual grass allergen tablet immuno-therapy provides sustained clinical benefit with progressive immunologic changes over 2 years. J Allergy Clin Immunol 2008;121(2):512–518.e2.

29. Polosa R, Al-Delaimy WK, Russo C, et al. Greater risk of incident asthma cases in adults with allergic rhinitis and effect of allergen immunotherapy: a retrospective cohort study. Respir Res 2005;6:153.

30. Novembre E, Galli E, Landi F, et al. Coseasonal sublingual immunotherapy reduces the development of asthma in children with allergic rhinoconjunctivitis. J Allergy Clin Immunol 2004;114(4):851–7.

31. Resnick E, Bielory B, Bielory L. Complementary therapy in allergic rhinitis. Curr Allergy Asthma Rep 2008;8:118–25.

32. Rajan TV, Tennen H, Lindquist RL, et al. Effect of ingestion of honey on symptoms of rhinoconjunctivitis. Ann Allergy Asthma Immunol 2002;88(2):198–203.

33. Schapowal A. Treating intermittent allergic rhinitis: a prospective, randomized, placebo and antihistamine-controlled study of Butterbur extract Ze 339. Phyt-other Res 2005;19(6):530–7.

34. Schapowal A. Randomised controlled trial of butterbur and cetirizine for treating seasonal allergic rhinitis. BMJ 2002;324(7330):144–6.

35. Schapoal A. Butterbur Ze339 for the treatment of intermittent allergic rhinitis: dose-dependent efficacy in a prospective, randomized, double-blind, placebo-controlled study. Arch Otolaryngol Head Neck Surg 2004;130:1381–6.

36. Gray RD, Haggart K, Lee DK, et al. Effects of butterbur treatment in intermittent allergic rhinitis: a placebo-controlled evaluation. Ann Allergy Asthma Immunol 2004;93(1):56–60.

37. Lee DK, Haggart K, Robb FM, et al. Butterbur, a herbal remedy, attenuates aden-osine monophosphate induced nasal responsiveness in seasonal allergic rhinitis. Clin Exp Allergy 2003;33:885–6.

38. Lee DK, Gray RD, Robb FM, et al. A placebo-controlled evaluation of butterbur and fexofenadine on objective and subjective outcomes in perennial allergic rhinitis. Clin Exp Allergy 2004;34:646–9.

39. Seidman MD. Complementary and alternative medications and techniques. In: Benninger MS, Murry T, editors. The Singer's voice. Plural Publishing; 2008. p. 103–16.

40. Mao TK, Van de Water J, Gershwin ME. Effects of a Spirulina-based dietary supplement on cytokine production from allergic rhinitis patients. J Med Food 2005;8:27–30.

41. Huang RY, Yu YL, Cheng WC, et al. Immunosuppressive effect of quercetin on dendritic cell activation and function. J Immunol 2010;184:6815–21.

42. Otsuka H, Inaba M, Fujikura T, et al. Histochemical and functional characteris-tics of metachromatic cells in the nasal epithelium in allergic rhinitis: studies of nasal scrapings and their dispersed cells. J Allergy Clin Immunol 1995;96: 528–36.

43. Bakhshaee M, Jabbari F, Hoseini S, et al. Effect of silymarin in the treatment of allergic rhinitis. Otolaryngol Head Neck Surg 2011;145(6):904–9.

44. Moyad MA, Robinson LE, Zawada ET, et al. Immunogenic yeast-based fermenta-tion product reduces allergic rhinitis-induced nasal congestion: a randomized, double-blind, placebo-controlled trial. Adv Ther 2009;26(8):795–804.

45. Kim J, Lee I, Park S, et al. Effects of Scutellariae radix and Aloe vera gel extracts on immunoglobulin E and cytokine levels in atopic dermatitis NC/Nga mice. J Ethnopharmacol 2010;132:529–32.
46. Kobayashi M, Matsushita H, Shioya I, et al. Quality of life improvement with soy sauce ingredients, Shoyu polysaccharides, in perennial allergic rhinitis: a double-blind placebo-controlled clinical study. Int J Mol Med 2004;14(5):885–9.
47. Xue CC, Thien FC, Zhang JJ, et al. Treatment for seasonal allergic rhinitis by Chinese herbal medicine: a randomized placebo controlled trial. Altern Ther Health Med 2003;9(5):80–7.
48. Yang SH, Yu CL, Chen YL, et al. Traditional Chinese medicine, Xin-yi-san, reduces nasal symptoms of patients with perennial allergic rhinitis by its diverse immunomodulatory effects. Int Immunopharmacol 2010;10(8):951–8.
49. Brinkhaus B, Witt CM, Jena S, et al. Acupuncture in patients with allergic rhinitis: a pragmatic randomized trial. Ann Allergy Asthma Immunol 2008;101(5):535–43.
50. Ng DK, Chow PY, Ming SP, et al. A double-blind, randomized, placebo-controlled trial of acupuncture for the treatment of childhood persistent allergic rhinitis. Ann Allergy Asthma Immunol 2008;101(5):535–43.
51. Lee MS, Pittler MH, Shin BC, et al. Acupuncture for allergic rhinitis: a systematic review. Ann Allergy Asthma Immunol 2009;102(4):269–79 [quiz: 279–81, 307].
52. Zhang CS, Yang AW, Zhang AL, et al. Ear-acupressure for allergic rhinitis: a systematic review. Clin Otolaryngol 2010;35(1):6–12.

Complementary and Integrative Treatments
Otitis Media

Jessica R. Levi, MD, Robert O'Reilly, MD*

KEYWORDS

- Acute otitis media • Homeopathic remedies
- Complementary and alternative medicine • Antibiotics

KEY POINTS

- Acute otitis media is quite common and is the main reason for antibiotic prescriptions in children.
- Symptomatic relief in acute otitis media may be obtained with use of herbal ear drops or homeopathic remedies.
- In children with acute otitis media, emphasis should be placed on prevention of future episodes with good nutrition and elimination of secondhand smoke exposure and bottle feeding. Probiotics and xylitol may be useful in preventing otitis media.
- For patients with chronic otitis media, politzerization may prove effective.

OVERVIEW

According to the American Academy of Pediatrics (AAP) and the American Academy of Otolaryngology and Head and Neck Surgery, acute otitis media (AOM) is defined as[1] a history of acute onset of signs and symptoms,[2] the presence of middle ear effusion, and[3] signs and symptoms of middle ear inflammation. As part of the treatment algorithm for AOM, it is important to consider it as part of a spectrum of disease processes. It should be differentiated from both recurrent acute otitis media (ROM, defined as acute otitis media at least 3 times within 6 months) and persistent otitis media with effusion (COM, defined as presence of middle ear fluid in the absence of symptoms for more than 8 weeks). AOM can also progress to intracranial (such as brain abscess) and extracranial (such as temporal bone abscess) complications as well.

AOM is diagnosed frequently in early childhood and peaks in incidence between 6 and 15 months of age. It typically results from a *Streptococcus pneumoniae*, *Haemophilus influenzae*, or *Moraxella catarrhalis* infection and is the most common reason for

Disclosures: None.
Division of Otolaryngology, Department of Surgery, Alfred I. duPont Hospital for Children, Nemours Children's Clinic, 1600 Rockland Road, Wilmington, DE 19803, USA
* Corresponding author.
E-mail address: roreilly@nemours.org

Otolaryngol Clin N Am 46 (2013) 309–327
http://dx.doi.org/10.1016/j.otc.2013.01.001
0030-6665/13/$ – see front matter © 2013 Elsevier Inc. All rights reserved.

oto.theclinics.com

physician visits and antibiotic prescriptions in children. Eighty percent of AOM cases resolve without treatment within 3 days, and the most sensitive and specific way to diagnose it is with pneumatic otoscopy. The cost of treating middle ear infections in the United States is approximately $2.0 billion to $3.5 billion per year.[1] Antibiotic therapy for AOM can result in significant expense in excess of $100 per episode.[1]

Today almost half of all antibiotic prescriptions are for children with otitis media. In a study in 2010, Arguedas and colleagues[2] interviewed 1800 physicians from France, Germany, Spain, Poland, Argentina, Mexico, South Korea, Thailand, and Saudi Arabia and found that although there was widespread concern over antibiotic resistance, 81% of physicians used antibiotics as first-line treatment for AOM.

The principle of observation or alternative treatments was popularized in the 1980s in areas of Western Europe. Van Buchem and colleagues[3] in the Netherlands found infants could initially be treated with an analgesic agent and nose or ear drops with antibiotics administered only if the signs and symptoms persisted for more than 3 days. It was not until 2004 that the AAP and the American Academy of Family Physicians (AAFP) advocated in their guidelines for initial observation rather than immediate antibiotics in the treatment of AOM in selected children (**Box 1**).[4] As a result of the push for early observation, many patients and families have turned to complementary methods for symptomatic relief or even for resolution of the disease process.

PHYSIOLOGY AND ANATOMY

Otitis media results from inflammation involving the middle ear space. The middle ear is a small air-filled cavity that is part of a larger functional system that includes the nasopharynx, Eustachian tube, and the mastoid air cells. The Eustachian tube is derived from the first pharyngeal pouch and is lined by respiratory mucosa (ciliated, pseudostratified, columnar epithelium). It is divided into an osseus intratemporal portion and a cartilaginous nasopharyngeal portion. It functions to protect the middle ear from reflux of nasopharyngeal secretions into the middle ear and provides aeration and pressure equalization to the middle ear. It is commonly believed that otitis media results in part from poor ventilation and clearance of secretions by the Eustachian tube (eg, Eustachian tube dysfunction). Infants and children have important anatomic differences in their Eustachian tubes compared with adults: the tube is shorter, and the cranial base is flatter in children than adults, describing a more horizontal course providing less protection. Through maturation, the angle of the cranial base increases and concomitantly the angle of the Eustachian tube increases, reaching adult size by age 7.[5,6]

The only active dilator of the Eustachian tube is thought to be the tensor veli palatini. It has been suggested that many of the age-related changes in Eustachian tube function (and, therefore, decreased rates of otitis media with age) are related to more efficient muscular activity resulting in improved middle ear aeration such that the

---

Box 1
Watchful waiting guidelines

In 2004, as part of their guidelines, the American Academy of Pediatrics and the American Academy of Family Physicians recommended initial observation of AOM in selected patients:

- 6 months to 2 years: nonsevere illness at presentation *and* uncertain diagnosis
- 2+ years: nonsevere illness at presentation *or* uncertain diagnosis
- If symptoms do not resolve in 24–48 hours, they should then be treated with antibiotics.

Eustachian tube is no longer a passive route for nasal secretions.[7] It is also believed that maturation of the immune system assists in preventing infection.

There are other known risk factors for AOM, such as large daycare centers, bottle feeding, and smoke exposure. Finally, Beery and colleagues[8] have shown there is a seasonal variation in otitis media and Eustachian tube dysfunction, with improvement in the spring and summer.

SYMPTOMS

The symptoms of otitis media can be quite variable in children depending on the acuity of disease and age of the child. AOM may result in tugging at the ears or increased "fussiness" (eg, crying more than usual, decreased oral intake, decreased sleep). This may be associated with fever, nausea, or diarrhea. Older children may complain of ear pain, and occasionally the tympanic membrane can rupture, resulting in bloody otorrhea. In some cases, children can have imbalance. Rarely, facial nerve paralysis or paresis can ensue because of the position of the facial nerve in the middle ear, particularly if it is dehiscent of its bony covering. In COM, the symptoms may be more subtle, such as hearing loss or painless otorrhea.

MEDICAL TREATMENT APPROACHES AND OUTCOMES

The mainstay of medical treatment for otitis media has traditionally been antibiotics. More recently, there has been an increasing interest in complementary or alternative medical treatments, which are discussed in later sections of this article. In the 1980s, AOM was almost exclusively treated with antibiotics. But with increased concern over side effects of antibiotics and resistance patterns of bacteria, there has been a shift in treatment patterns. In 2004, the AAP and the AAFP suggested initial observation in most patients and treatment only if it failed after 2 or 3 days (continued pain and fevers). Because of this change, there have been studies comparing treatment of AOM with either antibiotics or placebo. As AOM has a high rate of spontaneous resolution, a trial to prove any treatment effect must demonstrate rapid resolution of symptoms.

In a randomized controlled trial by Tähtinen and colleagues[9] in 2011, 319 children aged 6 to 35 months with a new diagnosis of AOM were randomized to receive either amoxicillin-clavulanate or placebo and evaluated for treatment failure defined by the condition of the patient and clinical otoscopic signs. Of the children receiving amoxicillin-clavulanate, 18.6% failed by day 7, whereas 44.9% of those receiving placebo failed. Overall, amoxicillin-clavulanate reduced the progression to treatment failure by 62% and the need for rescue treatment by 81%. However, 47.8% of the children in the amoxicillin-clavulanate group had diarrhea, compared with 26.6% in the placebo group; there was also a greater rate of eczema (8.7% vs 3.2%) in the antibiotic group. There was no significant difference in analgesic rates. In a similar study in 2011, Hoberman and colleagues[10] performed a randomized controlled trial of 291 children aged 6 to 23 months with AOM with 2 treatment groups: amoxicillin-clavulanate or placebo for 10 days. Treatment with antibiotics tended to reduce the time to resolution of symptoms, as well as overall symptom burden; it also reduced signs of acute infection on examination.

Amoxicillin is most commonly used as first-line antibiotic therapy (see **Box 2** for dosing). In allergic patients, trimethoprim and sulfamethoxazole (Bactrim), erythromycin, and clindamycin plus a sulfonamide may be used. Cephalosporins present another option (ceftriaxone, cefdinir, and cefpodoxime). A small percentage of patients do not improve on these regimens and after 3 days are deemed "resistant." In these

---

Box 2
Antibiotic dosing for otitis media

1. Amoxicillin:
   a. <3 months: 20–30 mg/kg/d divided every 12 hours
   b. >3 months: 40–50 mg/kg/d divided every 8–12 hours
2. For resistant cases, amoxicillin/clavulanate
   a. <3 months: 30 mg/kg/d divided every 12 hours
   b. >3 months: 25–45 mg/kg/d divided every 12 hours

---

cases, amoxicillin/clavulanic acid, cefuroxime, or ceftriaxone are typically effective. In cases of "resistant" AOM, targeted therapy via culture is often helpful because both *H influenzae* and *M catarrhalis* are often beta lactamase positive, and more than one-quarter of *S pneumoniae* are resistant.

In COM, medical treatments have been aimed at improving Eustachian tube function, with various results shown in the literature. Some approaches include the use of decongestants, nasal steroids, or treatment of underlying allergies. Sometimes topical or oral antibiotics are also used. The efficacy of these treatments continues to be studied.

SURGICAL TREATMENT APPROACHES AND OUTCOMES

Surgery for AOM is necessary only if it is accompanied by intracranial or extracranial complications, such as subperiosteal abscess or subdural abscess, or if a resistant organism is suspected. In recurrent AOM, myringotomy with pressure-equalizing tube placement may be indicated. In 2004, the AAFP, American Academy of Otolaryngology-Head and Neck Surgery, and AAP subcommittee on otitis media recommended surgery when 3 or more episodes of AOM occurred during the previous 6 months, or 4 or more episodes occurred during the previous year.

In COM, myringotomy tube placement is considered in children with 3 months or more of documented effusion, particularly if there is documented hearing loss or speech and language delays. In patients requiring a second myringotomy and tube placement, an adenoidectomy may also be considered.[11,12]

PATIENT SELF-TREATMENTS AND PREVENTION

Symptomatic relief of AOM is of paramount importance to patients and families. Many find relief with warm compresses and steam. Gargling salt water may help as well (it is theorized that the salt water can help reduce inflammation of swollen mucosa and thereby help drain the Eustachian tubes). Judicious use of over-the-counter nasal sprays also helps some people. Herbal ear drops are also used for symptomatic relief. The composition is quite variable, but they usually contain some combination of the following: *Calendula flores* (marigold), garlic (*Allium sativum*), mullein (*Verbascum thapsus*), St. John's wort (*Hypericum perforatum*), lavender, and vitamin E. In 2001, Sarrell and colleagues[13] compared Otikon Otic Solution (Healthy-On Ltd, Petach-Tikva, Israel), a naturopathic herbal extract containing *A sativum*, *V thapsus*, *C flores*, and *H perforatum* in olive oil, with anesthetic (ear drops containing ametocaine and phenazone in glycerin) and found comparable rates of analgesia in patients with AOM. A Cochrane systematic review in 2004[14] concluded that naturopathic ear drops were "modestly therapeutic" for ear pain associated with otitis media with no safety concerns. But a subsequent Cochrane review in 2006[15] evaluated 4 trials and found there was insufficient evidence to know whether naturopathic ear drops were effective.

The identification of risk factors for otitis media has spurred research involving prevention ranging from lifestyle modification to immunization to diet. There are many well-documented studies that show increased rates of otitis media with bottle feeding compared with breast feeding. In a study by Sabirov and colleagues[16] in 2009, among children with AOM, the prevalence of nontypeable *H influenzae* (a known otitis media pathogen) was higher in bottle-fed infants compared with breast-fed infants. Furthermore, they showed that specific immunoglobulin G antibodies to nontypeable *H influenzae* were lower in formula-fed infants, intermediate in breast-fed and bottle-fed infants, and highest in exclusively breast-fed infants. It has also been hypothesized that the position of the infant while feeding may make a difference in terms of nasopharyngeal reflux. Additionally, smoking inside the home or outside the home but wearing the same clothes around children can also play a role in AOM. Large day care settings and pacifier use have also been implicated (**Table 1**).

Recently there has been interest in the role of nutrition and food allergies in the pathogenesis of otitis media. There have been reports that nutritional supplements can help prevent otitis media, and reports that nutritional deficiencies are associated with increased incidence of otitis media. In a recent study by Lasisi in 2008,[17] patients with acute suppurative otitis media and COM were found to have retinol/vitamin A levels that were lower than in age-matched controls. The levels were also significantly lower in patients with recurrent AOM compared with those with a single episode of AOM. In a meta-analysis in 2009, Elemraid and colleagues[18] reviewed rates of AOM or COM and vitamin supplementation. They found some evidence that deficiencies of zinc or vitamin A, or both, may lead to increased rates of otitis media. Abba and colleagues[19] in 2010 reviewed 12 randomized controlled trials in which zinc was given at least once a week for at least once a month versus placebo. They examined rates of otitis media and found conflicting reports regarding the efficacy of treatment but did not find any serious adverse events with zinc supplementation.

Food allergies may also have a role in otitis media, and, thus, decreased consumption of allergenic foods may reduce the number of episodes of otitis media, although the precise pathogenesis remains speculative. Interestingly, nutrition as it relates to obesity may also affect the rate of otitis media. In a report by Nelson and colleagues[20]

Table 1			
Risk factors for recurrent acute otitis media (AOM)			
Risk Factor	Risk for	RR	P Value
Family history of AOM	AOM	2.6	<.001
Day care outside home	AOM	2.5	.003
Not breastfeeding at all	Recurrent AOM	2.1	<.001
At least one sibling	Recurrent AOM	1.9	.001
Child care outside home	Recurrent AOM	1.8	.004
Parental smoking	AOM	1.7	<.001
Family day care	AOM	1.6	.002
Pacifier use	AOM	1.2	.008
Breast feeding <3 mo	AOM	1.2	.003

Abbreviations: AOM, acute otitis media; RR, risk ratio.
From Uhari M, Mäntysaari, K, Niemelä, M. Meta-analytic review of the risk factors for acute otitis media. Clin Infect Dis 1996;22(6):66; with permission.

in 2011, elevated body mass index in children was associated with an increase in otitis media requiring tympanostomy tubes.

In 2001, the Centers for Disease Control and Prevention recommended that the PCV7 (initial Prevnar vaccine) be administered to all infants and young children; this produced significant shortages that were not fully resolved until 2004. Research since then has shown an overall decrease in rates of otitis media caused by pneumococcus. Cost analyses have suggested that immunization of all healthy infants with this vaccine could prevent more than 1 million episodes of AOM and 12,000 cases of invasive pneumococcal disease. The Finnish Otitis Media Study Group demonstrated that not only was there a decreased incidence of pneumococcal AOM but also a decreased rate of tympanostomy tube placement for recurrent disease.[21] Stamboulidis and colleagues[22] showed an increased rate of penicillin-resistant pneumococcal strains causing otitis media (4% vs 13%) but a decrease in the proportion resistant to macrolides (44% vs 35%). They also found a decrease of 38% in rates of otorrhea visits per 10,000 emergency room visits. A second-generation 13-valent pneumococcal conjugate vaccine (PCV13) was licensed and recommended for universal immunization of children through age 5 years in 2010. Its introduction is intended to address the residual burden of pneumococcal diseases that persists a decade after the introduction of PCV7.

Otitis media often follows upper respiratory infections or other viral illnesses, such as influenza. In a study by Block and colleagues[23] in 2011, influenza vaccination was thought to be protective for otitis media. They compared live attenuated influenza vaccine (approved for children older than 2 years) with placebo and found overall efficacy against influenza-associated AOM was 85%.

INTEGRATIVE TREATMENT APPROACHES AND OUTCOMES

Although there has been much research into the effectiveness and safety of many complementary and integrative medical (CIM) treatments of otitis media, most of the studies have significant methodological flaws, making definitive conclusions difficult. Furthermore, studies of the cost-effectiveness of such treatments need to be performed. Through a family questionnaire, Marchisio and colleagues[24] found that 46% of children aged 1 to 7 years with 3 or more episodes of AOM in 6 months used some component of CIM. Interestingly, they found many fewer were PCV7 or influenza vaccinated (34% and 15%, respectively). Patients spent between Euro 25 and Euro 50 per month in 27.6% of cases and Euro 50 per month or more in 16%.

Homeopathy

Homeopathy is based on the principle that "like cures like" (eg, any substance that produces symptoms in a healthy patient can relieve those same symptoms in an ill patient). Homeopathic remedies used for otitis media are dilute and generally are regarded as "safe" (see **Table 2** for a list of the most common homeopathic remedies and their uses). There have been reports of an initial aggravation of symptoms in approximately 10% to 20% of patients.[25] In one study, however, there were 3 cases of severe adverse events in one practice of homeopathic care over 7 years (1 perforation of a tympanic membrane, 1 cholesteatoma, and 1 case of mastoiditis), although it is unclear if these are necessarily directly attributable.[26]

Findings from 3 randomized controlled trials and 2 observational studies suggest homeopathy may result in a more rapid reduction of symptoms, shorter duration of pain, a reduction in recurrence, and a reduction in antibiotic use. In a small, non-blinded, randomized controlled trial by Harrison and colleagues[27] in 1999, 33 children

Table 2
List of common homeopathic remedies used to treat otitis media and conditions for which they are used

Homeopathic Remedy	Condition
Aconitum/Aconite/Aconitum napellus[a]	For throbbing ear pain that comes on suddenly after exposure to cold or wind and in children with high fever and whose ears are bright red or tender to the touch. Better in the initial stages of an ear infection.
Belladonna[a]	For throbbing and sharp pain accompanied by fever, intense heat, and flushing in the outer ear and along the side of the face. Some suggest it is better for the right ear. It comes from an extract from a poisonous plant of the nightshade family and should be used with caution.
Capsicum	Treats heat and inflammation, along with significant pain.
Chamomilla[a]	For children with otitis media who are very irritable, in great pain, and can't be consoled.
Ferrum phosphoricum	In early otitis media, this a common remedy used; gradual onset of symptoms; patient has flushed face, doesn't like noise, wants to lie still.
Hepar sulphuricum	Pain in ears especially with swallowing; yellowish-green discharge, wind or draft aggravates pain.
Kali muraticum	Popping and crackling sound heard in ear when swallowing and with nose blowing, hearing may be decreased, feeling of fullness and congestion in the ear. Also used to clear Eustachian tubes when fluid persists after acute otitis media.
Lycopodium	For right-side ear pain that is worse in the late afternoon and early evening; fullness of the ears, ringing or buzzing of the ears.
Magnesia phosphorica	Earache, especially after exposure to cold wind and drafts. May not be an infection at all, but rather nerve irritation, more right ear than left; pain relieved by heat, feels better with rubbing.
Mercurius	Good for chronic ear infections; for pain that is worse at night and may extend down into the throat; relief comes from nose blowing; earache may occur when damp or fog or weather changes occur, may salivate or sweat.
Pulsatilla[a]	For infection following exposure to cold or damp weather; the ear is often red and may have a yellowish/greenish discharge from ear or nose; ear pain may worsen after sleep and with warmth, may be alleviated by cool compresses.
Silica	For chronic or late-stage infection when the child feels chilly, weak, and tired; sweating may also be present.
Verbascum	Especially left-sided otitis media, may have a cough or laryngitis as well.

[a] Most commonly used.

(aged 18 months to 8 years) with otitis media with effusion, abnormal tympanograms, and hearing loss of more than 20 dB were randomized to receive either homeopathic therapy or watchful waiting. More patients in the group receiving homeopathic remedies had normal tympanograms after treatment (75% vs 31%, $P = .015$). There was a trend toward improvement in hearing, lower antibiotic use, and lower referral rates to specialists in the homeopathic group.

In a nonrandomized study by Friese and colleagues[28] in 1997, 131 children with AOM (aged 6 months to 11 years) received either homoeopathic single remedies (*Aconitum napellus*, *Apis mellifica*, *Belladonna*, *Capsicum*, Chamomilla, *Kalium bichromicum*, *Lachesis*, *Lycopodium*, *Mercurius solubilis*, Okoubaka, *Pulsatilla*, Silicea) or nasal drops, antibiotics, secretolytics, or antipyretics, or a combination of the 4. Median duration of therapy was significantly less in the homeopathically treated group (4 days vs 10 days), with an associated shorter duration of pain (2 days vs 3 days) and less recurrence of otitis media (70.7% free of recurrence vs 56.5% free of recurrence).

In another randomized controlled trial by Jacobs and colleagues[29] in 2001, 75 children diagnosed with AOM (as defined by middle ear effusion plus ear pain or fever, or both, for less than 36 hours) were randomized to either homeopathic therapy or placebo administered 3 times daily for 5 days. The homeopathic group had a decrease in symptoms at 24 and 64 hours after treatment ($P<.05$). There was a trend toward fewer treatment failures at 5 days, 2 weeks, and 6 weeks. Frei and Thurneysen in 2001[26] also looked at symptomatic improvement in a group of 230 children with AOM who received an initial dose of homeopathic medicine and found 39% had pain control after 6 hours. After a subsequent dose, an additional 33% had pain control at 12 hours. They also found homeopathic remedies to be 14% less expensive than traditional remedies. More recently, in 2005, Wustrow[30] looked at symptomatic improvement and antibiotic use in 390 children (aged 1–10 years) with AOM self-selected to receive either "conventional treatment" (decongestant nose drops, mucolytics, analgesics, and antibiotics) or homeopathic remedies (Otovowen [Weber & Weber, Germany]). Patients taking "conventional therapy" overall took more antibiotics (80.5% vs 14.4%; χ^2 test, $P<.001$) and more analgesics (66.8% vs 53.2%; χ^2 test, $P = .007$) than patients taking homeopathic remedies. Time to recovery was similar in the 2 groups. Furthermore, although these treatments are found over the counter, it is recommended that any treatment decisions be discussed with someone educated in homeopathy and its interactions with other medications. Clearly, larger randomized controlled and blinded studies are required to accurately assess the efficacy and safety of these treatments.

Other Natural Health Products

There is conflicting research on the efficacy of natural health products such as Echinacea, cod liver oil, and xylitol. Linday and colleagues[31] in 2002 suggested a rationale for the effectiveness of some of these products: they found children with ROM had lower blood cell concentrations of an omega 3 fatty acid (called EPA), vitamin A, and selenium, which are believed to have important properties in immune function. Subsequently, they enrolled 8 children to take 1 teaspoon of lemon-flavored cod liver oil (containing EPA and vitamin A) plus half a tablet of multivitamin supplement (containing selenium) for 7 months. During this period, 12% fewer days of antibiotics were prescribed than before study enrollment ($P<.05$). It has been suggested that these products can prevent otitis media.

Although there are many natural health products available (see **Table 3** for a more complete list), one of the most common herbs taken in the United States is Echinacea, which is generally taken for or to prevent the common cold; its effectiveness for otitis media has not been well studied. In a double-blind randomized controlled trial by Cohen and colleagues[32] in 2004, 430 children aged 1 to 5 years ingested either 5.0 mg/mL or 7.5 mg/mL of a mixture containing Echinacea, propolis, and vitamin C or placebo twice daily for 12 weeks. The mixture reduced the number of AOM

Table 3
List of common natural health products used to treat otitis media

Natural Health Product	Use
Chamomile (*Matricaria chamomilla*)	It is thought to have antiviral properties and has been used for infant colic, digestive upset, and diarrhea. The oil fraction is believed to have the anti-infective properties, whereas the flavonoids are thought to be anti-inflammatory. There is little evidence for its use in otitis media. It comes as a tincture (1–3 mL, 3 times a day; infants: 1–3 drops per pound of body weight 3 times a day) and a tea (1 cup of boiling water over 1 heaping tablespoon of flowers). Occasionally patients are allergic to it.
Cleavers	Used to assist lymphatic clearance of debris during AOM or with serous otitis media. Tincture 0.5–2 mL 3 times daily. Tea is also used: 1 cup 2 or 3 times per day.
Cod liver oil	A source of omega-3 fatty acids and vitamins A and D. It has been shown that patients with ROM have low blood levels of some omega-3 fatty acids, vitamin A, and selenium. Safety of long-term consumption of cod liver oil is not known; studies have shown adverse health effects from polychlorinated biphenyls and dioxin residues found in fish oil.
Echinacea (*Echinacea purpurea*)	Its activity is believed to be nonspecific activation of the immune system (including activating natural killer cells and macrophages and increasing circulating levels of alpha interferon), but there is some evidence that the caffeic esters are antibacterial and antiviral and the polyacetylenes may be bacteriostatic. It is most commonly used for treatment of upper respiratory infections, but it is not well studied for otitis media specifically. Dose of Echinacea: tinctures, either in alcohol or glycerites, are available. Children: 1–5 mL 3–5 times daily, infants: 1 or 2 drops per pound of body weight 3 times a day. Tablets, capsules, and whole herb taken as tea or infusion are also used orally.
Elder flower/berry (*Sambucus nigra*), European alder (*Sambucus canadensis*), or American elder (Caprifoliaceae)	Used to dry excessive nasal secretions, also has antiviral activity, best during AOM, especially if an upper respiratory tract infection is present. Tincture 0.5–3.0 mL 3 times daily. Tea is also used: 1 cup 2 or 3 times per day.
Elecampane root *(Inula helenium)*	It has bacteriostatic and antiviral activity and may strengthen resistance of mucosal lining. Can be used in AOM or chronic serous otitis media. Tincture 0.5–2.0 mL 3 times daily.
Eucalyptus	Is administered usually as steam inhalation and is used mostly late in the course of AOM.
Goldenseal (*Hydrastis canadensis*)	Used only during AOM when there is evidence of purulence. Tincture 0.5–2.0 mL 3 times daily.
Marshmallow (*Althea officinalis*)	Used for soothing inflamed mucous membranes and helps loosen and moisten thick mucus. In otitis media, it is used particularly to help open the Eustachian tube. Tincture: 1 drop per 2 pounds of body weight (up to 2 mL) 3–6 times daily. Decoction: 1 tablespoon root simmered in 1 cup of water for 10 minutes; 1 to 3 tablespoons of the strained liquid is taken 2–6 times daily. If taking with prescription medications, take the medications at least 1 hour before or 2 hours after taking marshmallow root, because the herb may decrease the absorption of drugs.

(*continued on next page*)

Table 3 *(continued)*	
Natural Health Product	**Use**
Mullein (*Verbascum thapsus*)	Decreases phlegm and strengthens the respiratory mucosa and acts topically as a local anti-inflammatory. It can be used as topical ear oil for otitis externa. For otitis media, it is chosen to unblock the Eustachian tube and to decrease inflammation. Tincture: 1 drop per 2 pounds of body weight every 4 hours. Tea: 1 to 2 teaspoons herb/cup of boiling water, steeped covered 10–15 minutes, and strained; 1 to 4 cups per day.
Usnea (*Usnea barbata*)	Has antiviral and antibacterial properties, used during acute episodes of otitis media. Tincture 0.5–5.0 mL 3 times daily.
Xylitol	Used as an artificial sweetener in chewing gum and has been shown to inhibit the growth of *Streptococcus pneumoniae* by changing the ultrastructure of the bacterial capsule. Many studies show effectiveness of xylitol (gum > syrup) in preventing otitis media when given 5 times daily. It can cause abdominal pain and loose stools, which leads to large dropout rates from many studies and difficulty drawing meaningful conclusions. It also prevents dental caries.

Abbreviations: AOM, acute otitis media; ROM, recurrent otitis media.

episodes per child by 68% (*P*<.001). Side effects involving mild gastrointestinal and palatability symptoms were reported in 9 children, including 7 from the mixture group and 2 from the placebo group (*P* = .54).

Xylitol is a natural sugar found in strawberries, raspberries, rowanberries, and plums, often used as a sweetener in chewing gum, and has been studied for its effectiveness in preventing otitis media. In an article by Uhari and colleagues[33] in 2000, xylitol was shown to inhibit the growth of *S pneumoniae* as well as inhibit the attachment of both *S pneumoniae* and *H influenzae* to the nasopharyngeal cells. Kurola and colleagues[34] in 2009 offered a possible explanation for this: exposure to xylitol lowered cpsB (pneumococcal capsular locus) gene expression levels significantly compared with those in the control (*P* = .035) and glucose (*P* = .011) media, thus changing the ultrastructure of the pneumococcal capsule. Perhaps more clinically relevant, Uhari and colleagues[35] in 1996 found in a randomized controlled trial that xylitol (8.4 g/d in divided doses 5 times daily) reduced the occurrence of AOM by 41% (95% confidence interval [CI]: 4.6%–55.4%). In addition, fewer of the children receiving xylitol required antibiotics during that study period (18.5% vs 28.9%, *P* = .032). In 1998,[36] the same group demonstrated a 40% reduction of otitis media in patients receiving xylitol gum, 30% reduction in those receiving syrup, and 20% reduction in those receiving xylitol lozenge, compared with controls, and, in 2000,[33] they further corroborated these findings in a study looking at chewing gum versus syrup versus controls and found the 2-month to 3-month efficacy was 40% with chewing gum and 30% with syrup. Interestingly, it was ineffective in children with indwelling tympanostomy tubes. Although most studies show some efficacy of xylitol in preventing AOM, Tapiainen and colleagues[37] compared control mixture, xylitol mixture, control chewing gum, xylitol chewing gum, or xylitol lozenges used during an active upper respiratory infection and found no preventive effect of xylitol.

Most studies report a 5-times-a-day dosing schedule, which likely limits full compliance and, thus, reasonable conclusions. To address some of these concerns, Hautalahti and colleagues[38] looked at whether xylitol administered 3 times daily over 3 months was effective (9.6 g/d divided into 3 doses) and found no preventive effect of xylitol over control solutions/gum in preventing otitis media. Furthermore, xylitol has common side effects, including abdominal pain and diarrhea, which often lead to high dropout rates. In general, many of these natural health products have side effects and can interact with other herbs or medications; thus, it is important to consult a physician when taking these medications.

Probiotics

Probiotics are microorganisms (most commonly lactobacilli or bifidobacteria, or both) that are often added to foods and are thought to confer health benefits by restoring microbial balance. In general, they are thought to be safe in immunocompetent individuals but, like other drugs and herbs, have the potential to interact with other medications and, thus, should be used with the supervision of a physician. In immunocompromised patients, there are reports of adverse health effects, such as pneumonia, meningitis, and sepsis. Probiotics are thought to reduce upper respiratory tract colonization with pathogenic bacteria by stimulating antibody production and enhancing the phagocytic activity of blood leukocytes.[39]

There is conflicting evidence on the effectiveness of probiotics in preventing AOM. In a randomized controlled study by Hatakka and colleagues[40] in 2001, 571 children were randomized to receive milk supplemented with *Lactobacillus rhamnosus* or without supplement 3 times daily, 5 days a week, for 7 months. There was a significant decrease in the number of days absent from day care in the probiotic group but only a slight trend toward fewer episodes of AOM. In a later study by Hatakka and colleagues[41] in 2007, children were randomized to receive a probiotic capsule (*L rhamnosus* GG [LGG] and *L rhamnosus* strain C705, *Bifidobacterium breve* 99, and *Propionibacterium freudenreichii* JS) or placebo daily for 24 weeks. Although there was a large dropout rate, they found that probiotics did not reduce the occurrence or recurrence of otitis media. They also obtained nasopharyngeal samples at 3 points in time and showed no reduction in the presence of *S pneumoniae* or *H influenzae* but did show increased prevalence of *M catarrhalis*.

Roos and colleagues[39] in 2001 reported on the use of a probiotic nasal spray (*Streptococcus sanguis, Streptococcus mitis,* and *Streptococcus oralis*) in children and found preventive effects on AOM and COM (42% without recurrence in the probiotic group vs 22% in the placebo group, $P = .02$). More recently, in 2009, Stecksén-Blicks and colleagues[42] showed milk supplemented with probiotics and fluoride (*Lactobacillus rhamnosus* LB21 [10(7) colony-forming units/mL)] and 2.5 mg fluoride per liter) consumed once daily, 5 days a week, for 21 months, had preventive effects on otitis media (0.4 days of otitis media vs 1.3 days of otitis media, $P<.05$). Rautava and colleagues[43] in 2009 looked at probiotics in infants by supplementing the formula of infants younger than 2 months with either probiotics (LGG and *Bifidobacterium lactis* Bb-12) or placebo daily until the age of 12 months. There was a significant reduction in the number of episodes of otitis media in the first 7 months of life (22% vs 50%, risk ratio [RR] 0.44 [95% CI 0.21–0.90]; $P = .014$) and a decrease in the amount of antibiotics prescribed (31% vs 60%, RR 0.52 [95% CI 0.29–0.92]; $P = .015$). These conflicting reports highlight the need for further research in this area.

Osteopathy

Osteopathy is a system of therapy founded in the nineteenth century based on the concept that the body can heal itself when it is in a normal structural relationship, has a normal environment, and has good nutrition. Osteopathy often includes chiropractics but is not limited to it. Craniosacral therapy, a practice in which the bones and tissues of the head and neck are manipulated, also is a component of osteopathy. According to some osteopathic practitioners, there are common patterns of cervical and cranial "osteopathic restrictions" that are found in children with otitis media, particularly with regard to the movement of the temporal bones. Other cranial and cervical restrictions of movement are also seen. Treatment in children is often more gentle than adults and may simply appear as though the practitioner is placing his or her hands on the child's head or neck with minimal or no motion.

A randomized controlled trial by Mills and colleagues[44] in 2003 evaluated osteo-pathic techniques (OMT), including "gentle techniques on areas of restriction consist-ing of articulation, myofascial release, balanced membranous tension, balanced ligamentous tension, facilitated positional release, and/or counter strain treatments" in the treatment of otitis media. Children aged 6 months to 4 years with recurrent AOM were randomized to either standard care, such as antibiotics, or to standard care and OMT over 6 months. Patients in the OMT group had fewer episodes of AOM per month ($P = .04$) and less need for tympanostomy tubes ($P = .03$). There was no difference in antibiotic use, parental satisfaction, or hearing results. Unfortu-nately, there was a large dropout rate (25%), making conclusions difficult. Meaningful conclusions were also difficult in a 2006 cohort study by Degenhardt and Kuchera,[45] in which children with recurrent AOM were given weekly OMT and antibiotics for 3 weeks and then evaluated 1 year later. Five (62.5%) of 8 subjects had no documented episode of AOM at the 1-year follow-up. Without a control group, it is difficult to inter-pret these results.

Osteopathic techniques can include the "Galbreath maneuver" or the "Muncie tech-nique" for treatment of otitis media. In 1929, Galbreath, a doctor of osteopathy, devel-oped a technique in which the ipsilateral mandible is forced downward and medially in a repetitive gentle fashion to help drain the middle ear. In this way, a pumping action is created on the Eustachian tube, which can help drain the middle ear. It is also possible that this maneuver alternately compresses and releases the pterygoid plexus of veins and lymphatics, allowing drainage of the middle ear.[46] More recently, in 1962 by Ruddy[47] and then again in 1995 by Heatherington,[48] the "Muncie technique" for treat-ing otitis media was described. In this maneuver, the physician places a fingertip cephalad and lateral to the Rosenmuller fossa and applies light repetitive pressure in this area, effectively pumping the Eustachian tube and allowing fluid to drain. This is often not tolerated well in children, and, therefore, Channell[49] offers the "modified Muncie technique," in which a finger is placed at the posterior tonsillar pillar and lateral, circular, repetitive motions are made in the soft tissue; motion is transmitted superiorly to the opening of the Eustachian tube. Effectiveness of these techniques is mainly anecdotal but may warrant future research.

Chiropractics

"Chiropractics" comes from the Greek word meaning hand and is based on the prin-ciple that the body can heal itself when the skeletal system is aligned. With regard to otitis media, practitioners state that chiropractic manipulation improves innervation and function of the tensor veli palatini.

Froehle[50] examined the effectiveness of chiropractic care in 46 children with AOM (who had a total of 95 AOM episodes) aged 5 years and younger. Patients were given 3 treatments per week for 1 week and then 2 treatments per week for 1 week and then 1 treatment per week with termination when parents, physicians, or chiropractic practi-tioner deemed the child improved. They found that overall 93% of AOM improved, with 75% occurring within 10 days and 43% with only 1 or 2 treatments. In 2004, Zhang and Synder[51] looked at rates of otitis media resolution in 21 children (aged 9 months to

9 years) diagnosed with AOM (defined as erythematous, bulging tympanic membranes and fever). These children were treated with "toftness" (low force) chiropractic adjustments over 14 days, and, overall, 95% had return of normal-appearing tympanic membranes and a decrease in their fevers. Fallon[52] examined 332 children (aged 27 days to 5 years) with a prior diagnosis of otitis media (acute and chronic) for effectiveness of chiropractic manipulation. Children who had AOM (n = 127) received an average of 4.00 ± 1.03 adjustments, attained normal otoscopic and tympanographic examination findings after 6.67 (±1.90) and 8.35 (±2.88) days, and had an overall recurrence rate of AOM of 11.02% in 6 months. Patients with chronic otitis media required 5.00 ± 1.53 adjustments, attained normal otoscopic examination results in 8.57 ± 1.96 days, and had normal tympanogram results in 10.18 ± 3.39 days. There is some concern over the safety of chiropractics in a pediatric population because of anatomic immaturity; pediatric patients may be at increased risk for injury following rapid rotational movements or forces. Rarely, serious adverse events have been reported, such as paraplegia and death.[53] The effectiveness of chiropractic medicine in treatment of otitis media is not known because there are few studies with methodological shortcomings.

Traditional Chinese and Japanese Medicine

Traditional Chinese medical (TCM) practices encompass many healing modalities including acupuncture, moxibustion (heat therapy), Anma (or Tuina, an ancient massage technique and the basis of Shiatsu therapy), diet, and herbal medicine and are predicated on the idea of disease prevention through moderation and harmony/balance within the body. Traditional Japanese medicine is referred to as Kampo and likely has its roots in TCM stemming from the fifth and sixth centuries, and, thus, it uses similar techniques to TCM. Diagnosis often relies both on patient history and examination of the tongue and pulses, and the provider determines the unique pattern of disharmony present in the patient at that point in time. For otitis media, often a combination of herbal therapy and acupuncture is used, although exact treatments are quite patient-specific and often practitioner-specific as well. Interestingly, both acupuncture and Chinese herbal medicine are approved by the World Health Organization as therapies to treat AOM or COM. In children who do not tolerate acupuncture with needles, acupressure, adhesive magnets on acupuncture points, or laser acupuncture is used instead.

Acupuncture is based on the notion that the body's energy force, "chi," travels known channels ("meridians") that can become blocked; small needles are inserted to correct the flow of the energy. In a study by Sanchez-Araujo and Puchi in 2011,[54] acupuncture was evaluated in dogs for the treatment of otitis media. Thirty-one dogs with ROM were randomized to receive conventional medicine and either sham acupuncture or actual acupuncture in 4 sessions. Over the subsequent year, 14 (93%) dogs in the acupuncture group were free of otitis, compared with 7 (50%) in the sham group (P<.01). There is little understanding why acupuncture may be effective in treating otitis media, but it is suggested that it has immunomodulatory properties that may play a role in clearance of middle ear fluid.

Many herbs and combinations of herbs exist in TCM and include skullcap (*Scutellaria baicalensis*), alisma (*Alisma plantago-aquatica*), plantain (*Plantago major*), bupleurum (*Bupleurum chinense*), and licorice (*Glycyrrhiza uralensis*). The research on both Chinese and Japanese traditional medicine is limited; there are few studies in English, and many are limited by sample size, randomization, and outcome measures. However, there is much research examining the use of some of these herbs in animals (few in English), showing that in the guinea pig "sairei-to" enhances mucociliary clearance[55] and prevents endotoxin-induced otitis.[56] According to Zhang and colleagues,[57] eryanling (EYL) liquid reduces the degree of inflammatory exudation and mucosal swelling in the guinea pig and may have a nonspecific enhancing effect on the immune system in mice. Sun and colleagues[58] in 2005 examined the use of Qingqiao capsule (QQC) in treating patients with otitis media. Patients were randomized to receive either QQC, 5 capsules, 3 times daily for 10 to 14 days or cefaclor capsules (20 mg/kg/d) for 10 to 14 days. Those receiving QQC had improved hearing ($P<.01$), but no difference was found with respect to ear pain. In a study by Jeong and colleagues[59] in 2002, Allergina, which is a combination of many traditional herbs, was compared with antibiotics in 17 children with otitis media and was found to decrease the signs of otitis media compared with antibiotics. Unfortunately, the study was limited by its small sample size and nonspecific outcome measure, as well as unclear randomization. Other reports suggest efficacy of other herbal compounds (such as that by Liu in 1990,[60] concluding efficacy of borneol-walnut oil over neomycin in the treatment of otitis media, and that of Liao and colleagues[61] in 1998, stating efficacy of Tongqiao in COM), but again are limited by sample size, randomization, and outcome measures.

Although Japanese traditional medicine (Kampo) bears many resemblances to TCM, needles are not inserted as deeply in Kampo acupuncture as in TCM, which may make it easier for children to tolerate. With respect to herbal medicinal therapies, an herb used in many TCM practices for treatment of otitis media, sairei-to, was studied in Japan in 1997 by Ikeda and colleagues[62] and was found to have promise in resolution of serous otitis media in 35 children who received it daily for 4 weeks. Again, with no control arm and unclear outcome measures, conclusions become difficult. In a more recent study by Maruyama and colleagues[63] in 2009, Juzen-taiho-to (JTT, TJ-48), given at 0.10 to 0.14 g/kg/d twice a day for 3 months, was evaluated in 24 otitis-prone infants. Infants receiving JTT had fewer hospital visits, antibiotics, and fevers than before JTT administration. Of the patients, 95.2% had no otitis media while taking JTT, but 66.7% experienced purulent otitis media following discontinuation. Interestingly, the frequency of otitis media increased significantly after stopping JTT ($P = .004$) and decreased again with JTT resumption ($P = .005$). It has been suggested that Kampo's effectiveness overall may be in part because of selective increase in ion transport across the ear epithelium.[62]

Other Therapies

Aromatherapy has also been used to treat otitis media. Lavender (Lavandula officinalis) essence may sometimes help to reduce the inflammation and pain of ear infections. Other oils used include chamomile (Matricaria recutita), cajuput, evening primrose oil (Oenothera biennis), fatty acid, flax oil, and borage. This has not been studied to date.

Ayurvedic medicine was developed in ancient India, is based on the principle of balance, and literally means knowledge for long life. In otitis media, Ayurvedic physicians massage the lymph nodes outside the ears to open the Eustachian tubes. Often a drink made with the herb amala is given also; amala contains vitamin C as well as antiviral and antibacterial properties.

Politzerization was first described by Professor Politzer in 1861 and involves inflating the middle ear by blowing air up the nose during swallowing. There has been research in this technique mainly for COM; there is no evidence that it is curative in the acute setting. Stangerup in 1998[64] reported in a meta-analysis that most studies show clearance of effusions in 52% to 62% of ears up to 9 months after the treatment. Furthermore, they recommend that politzerization be considered a first-line treatment of COM, before consideration of both antibiotics and surgery. More recently, in 2000, a study by Arick and Silman[65] showed politzerization twice a week for up to 6 weeks resolved air bone gaps in 70% of children treated compared with only 20% of controls.

MULTIMODAL APPROACHES AND RECOMMENDATIONS

According to the AAFP and AAP, management of AOM begins with watchful waiting. These recommendations are not always followed, and symptomatic treatment and early resolution are sought, often with antibiotic use (see **Fig. 1** for treatment algorithm). Herbal ear drops may be helpful in symptomatic relief. Homeopathic treatments may help decrease pain and other symptoms and may lead to a faster resolution of disease. More severe cases of otitis media, such as those with intracranial or extracranial complications, and those that fail to improve with observation or complementary/alternative medicine (after 48–72 hours) should be treated with antibiotics and, in some cases, surgical intervention. It is best to consult a physician when making these decisions for full guidance on risks and benefits of any treatment option.

Often, children do not simply have one episode of otitis media but go on to develop COM with effusion or recurrent AOM. In these cases, tympanostomy tubes are often used, but emphasis should also be placed on disease prevention. Irritants, such as bottle feeding or exposure to secondhand smoke, should be limited as much as possible. Children with poor nutrition are likely at greater risk, and parents should be counseled on the importance of nutrition and possible vitamin supplements (such as zinc, cod liver oil, and vitamins A, C, and D).

Politzerization may have a role in COM but has not been proven to be effective in preventing AOM. Osteopathic manipulation and chiropractic treatments have only had very limited study and require further investigations to prove efficacy. Probiotics and xylitol may be beneficial in preventing otitis media and decreasing antibiotic use. Of all of the complementary and alternative medical therapies, only xylitol has been

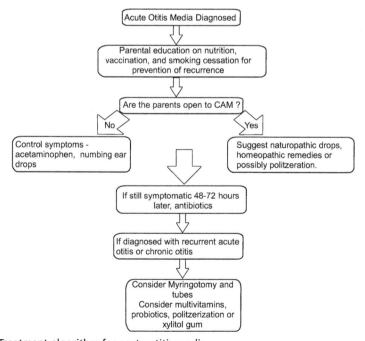

Fig. 1. Treatment algorithm for acute otitis media.

studied in well-designed, randomized, blinded trials; it has been shown to be effective but only in 5-times-daily dosing, which limits its applicability. Many methodologies have shown some positive trends in small groups, but few if any have yet shown benefit in double-blind randomized controlled studies and, thus, remain speculative.

REFERENCES

1. Stool SE, Field MJ. The impact of otitis media. Pediatr Infect Dis J 1989;8:S11–4.
2. Arguedas A, Kvaerner K, Liese J, et al. Otitis media across nine countries: disease burden and management. Int J Pediatr Otorhinolaryngol 2010;74: 1419–24.
3. Van Buchem FL, Peeters MF, van't Hof MA. Acute otitis media: a new treatment strategy. Br Med J (Clin Res Ed) 1985;290(6474):1033–7.
4. American Academy of Family Physicians, American Academy of Otolaryngology-Head and Neck Surgery, American Academy of Pediatrics Subcommittee on Otitis Media With Effusion. Otitis media with effusion. Pediatrics 2004;113: 1412–29.
5. Bluestone CD, Doyle WJ. Anatomy and physiology of Eustachian tube and middle ear related to otitis media. J Allergy Clin Immunol 1988;81(5 Pt 2):997–1003.
6. Sadler-Kimes D, Siegel MI, Todhunter JS. Age-related morphologic differences in the components of the Eustachian tube/middle ear system. Ann Otol Rhinol Laryngol 1989;98:854–8.
7. Bylander A. Function and dysfunction of the Eustachian tube in children. Acta Otorhinolaryngol Belg 1984;38:238–45.
8. Beery QC, Doyle WJ, Cantekin EI, et al. Longitudinal assessment of Eustachian tube function in children. Laryngoscope 1979;89(9 Pt 1):1446–56.
9. Tähtinen PA, Laine MK, Huovinen P, et al. A placebo-controlled trial of antimicrobial treatment for AOM. N Engl J Med 2011;364:116–26.
10. Hoberman A, Paradise JL, Rockette HE, et al. Treatment of AOM in children under 2 years of age. N Engl J Med 2011;364:105–15.
11. Gates GA, Avery CA, Prihoda TJ, et al. Effectiveness of adenoidectomy and tympanostomy tubes in the treatment of chronic otitis media with effusion. N Engl J Med 1987;317:1444–51.
12. Paradise JL, Bluestone CD, Rogers KD, et al. Efficacy of adenoidectomy for recurrent otitis media in children previously treated with tympanostomy-tube placement. Results of parallel randomized and nonrandomized trials. JAMA 1990;263:2066–73.
13. Sarrell EM, Mandelberg A, Cohen HA. Efficacy of naturopathic extracts in the management of ear pain associated with AOM. Arch Pediatr Adolesc Med 2001;155:796–9.
14. Glasziou PP, Del Mar CB, Sanders SL, et al. Antibiotics for acute otitis media in children. Cochrane Database Syst Rev 2004;(1):CD000219.
15. Foxlee R, Johansson A, Wejfalk J, et al. Topical analgesia for acute otitis media. Cochrane Database Syst Rev 2006;(3):CD005657.
16. Sabirov A, Casey JR, Murphy TF, et al. Breast-feeding is associated with a reduced frequency of AOM and high serum antibody levels against NTHi and outer membrane protein vaccine antigen candidate P6. Pediatr Res 2009;66:565–70.
17. Lasisi AO. The role of retinol in the etiology and outcome of suppurative otitis media. Eur Arch Otorhinolaryngol 2009;266(5):647–52.
18. Elemraid MA, Mackenzie IJ, Fraser WD, et al. Nutritional factors in the pathogenesis of ear disease in children: a systematic review. Ann Trop Paediatr 2009;29:85–99.

19. Abba K, Gulani A, Sachdev HS. Zinc supplements for preventing otitis media [review]. Cochrane Database Syst Rev 2010;(2):CD006639.
20. Nelson HM, Daly KA, Davey CS, et al. Otitis media and associations with overweight status in toddlers. Physiol Behav 2011;102:511–7.
21. Eskola J, Kilpi T, Palmu A, et al. Efficacy of a pneumococcal conjugate vaccine against acute otitis media. N Engl J Med 2001;344:403–9.
22. Stamboulidis K, Chatzaki D, Poulakou G, et al. The impact of the heptavalent pneumococcal conjugate vaccine on the epidemiology of AOM complicated by otorrhea. Pediatr Infect Dis J 2011;30:551–5.
23. Block SL, Heikkinen T, Toback SL, et al. The efficacy of live attenuated influenza vaccine against influenza-associated acute otitis media in children. Pediatr Infect Dis J 2011;30:203–7.
24. Marchisio P, Bianchini S, Galeone C, et al. Use of complementary and alternative medicine in children with recurrent AOM in Italy. Int J Immunopathol Pharmacol 2011;24:441–9.
25. Dantes F, Rampes H. Do homeopathic medicines provoke adverse effects? Br Homeopath J 2000;89:S35–8.
26. Frei H, Thurneysen A. Homeopathy in AOM in children: treatment effect or spontaneous resolution? Br Homeopath J 2001;90:178–9.
27. Harrison H, Fixsen A, Vickers A. A randomized comparison of homoeopathic and standard care for the treatment of glue ear in children. Complement Ther Med 1999;7:132–5.
28. Friese KH, Kruse S, Lüdtke R, et al. The homeopathic treatment of otitis media in children—comparisons with conventional therapy. Int J Clin Pharmacol Ther 1997;35:296–301.
29. Jacobs J, Springer DA, Crothers D. Homeopathic treatment of AOM in children: a preliminary randomized placebo-controlled trial. Pediatr Infect Dis J 2001;20: 177–83.
30. Wustrow TP. Naturopathic therapy for acute otitis media. An alternative to the primary use of antibiotics. HNO 2005;53:728–34 [in German].
31. Linday LA, Dolitsky JN, Shindledecker RD, et al. Lemon-flavored cod liver oil and a multivitamin-mineral supplement for the secondary prevention of otitis media in young children: pilot research. Ann Otol Rhinol Laryngol 2002;111: 642–52.
32. Cohen HA, Varsano I, Kahan E, et al. Effectiveness of an herbal preparation containing Echinacea, propolis, and vitamin C in preventing respiratory tract infections in children: a randomized, double-blind, placebo-controlled, multicenter study. Arch Pediatr Adolesc Med 2004;158:217–21.
33. Uhari M, Tapiainen T, Kontiokari T. Xylitol in preventing AOM. Vaccine 2000; 19(Suppl 1):S144–7.
34. Kurola P, Tapiainen T, Kaijalainen T, et al. Xylitol and capsular gene expression in Streptococcus pneumoniae. J Med Microbiol 2009;58(Pt 11):1470–3.
35. Uhari M, Kontiokari T, Koskela M, et al. Xylitol chewing gum in prevention of AOM: double-blind randomised trials. Br Med J 1996;313:1180–4.
36. Uhari M, Kontiokari T, Niemela M. A novel use of xylitol sugar in preventing AOM. Pediatrics 1998;102:879–84.
37. Tapiainen T, Luotonen L, Kontiokari T, et al. Xylitol administered only during respiratory infections failed to prevent acute otitis media. Pediatrics 2002; 109(2):E19.
38. Hautalahti O, Renko M, Tapiainen T, et al. Failure of xylitol given three times a day for preventing AOM. Pediatr Infect Dis J 2007;26:423–7.

39. Roos K, Hakansson EG, Holm S. Effect of recolonisation with "interfering" alpha streptococci on recurrences of acute and secretory otitis media in children: randomised placebo controlled trial. BMJ 2001;322:210–2.
40. Hatakka K, Savilahti E, Ponka A, et al. Effect of long-term consumption of probiotic milk on infections in children attending day care centres: double blind, randomised trial. Br Med J 2001;322:1327–9.
41. Hatakka K, Blomgren K, Pohjavuori S, et al. Treatment of AOM with probiotics in otitis-prone children-a double-blind, placebo-controlled randomised study. Clin Nutr 2007;26:314–21.
42. Stecksén-Blicks C, Sjöström I, Twetman S. Effect of long-term consumption of milk supplemented with probiotic lactobacilli and fluoride on dental caries and general health in preschool children: a cluster-randomized study. Caries Res 2009;43:374–81.
43. Rautava S, Salminen S, Isolauri E. Specific probiotics in reducing the risk of acute infections in infancy—a randomised, double-blind, placebo-controlled study. Br J Nutr 2009;101:1722–6.
44. Mills MV, Henley CE, Barnes LL, et al. The use of osteopathic manipulative treatment as adjuvant therapy in children with recurrent AOM. Arch Pediatr Adolesc Med 2003;157:861–6.
45. Degenhardt BF, Kuchera ML. Osteopathic evaluation and manipulative treatment in reducing the morbidity of otitis media: a pilot study. J Am Osteopath Assoc 2006;106:327–34.
46. Pratt-Harrington D. Galbreath technique: a manipulative treatment for otitis media revisited [review]. J Am Osteopath Assoc 2000;100:635–9.
47. Ruddy TJ. Osteopathic manipulation in eye, ear, nose, and throat disease. AAO Yearbook 1962;133–40.
48. Heatherington JS. Manipulation of the Eustachian tube. AAO Journal 1995;5:27–8.
49. Channell MK. Modified Muncie technique: osteopathic manipulation for Eustachian tube dysfunction and illustrative report of case. J Am Osteopath Assoc 2008;108:260–3.
50. Froehle RM. Ear infection: a retrospective study examining improvement from chiropractic care and analyzing for influencing factors. J Manipulative Physiol Ther 1996;19:169–77.
51. Zhang JQ, Synder BJ. Effect of toftness chiropractic adjustments for children with acute otitis media. J Vertebral Subluxation Res 2004;29:1–4.
52. Fallon JM. The role of the chiropractic adjustment in the care and treatment of 332 children with otitis media. J Clin Chiropract Pediatr 1997;2:167–83.
53. Lee KP, Carlini WG, McCormick GF, et al. Neurologic complications following chiropractic manipulation: a survey of California neurologists. Neurology 1995;45:1213–5.
54. Sánchez-Araujo M, Puchi A. Acupuncture prevents relapses of recurrent otitis in dogs: a 1-year follow-up of a randomised controlled trial. Acupunct Med 2011;29:21–6.
55. Sugiura Y, Ohashi Y, Nakai Y. The herbal medicine, sairei-to, enhances the mucociliary activity of the tubotympanum in the healthy guinea pig. Acta Otolaryngol Suppl 1997;531:17–20.
56. Sugiura Y, Ohashi Y, Nakai Y. The herbal medicine, sairei-to, prevents endotoxin-induced otitis media with effusion in the guinea pig. Acta Otolaryngol Suppl 1997;531:21–33.
57. Zhang H, Li S, Liu R. Clinical and experimental study on treatment of acute catarrhal otitis media with eryanling oral liquid. Zhongguo Zhong Xi Yi Jie He Za Zhi 2000;20:743–6 [in Chinese].

58. Sun YD, Chen LH, Hu WJ, et al. Evaluation of the clinical efficacy of Qingqiao capsule in treating patients with secretory otitis media. Chin J Integr Med 2005;11:243–8.
59. Jeong HJ, Hong SH, Kim SC, et al. Effects of Allergina on the treatment of otitis media with effusions. Inflammation 2002;26:89–95.
60. Liu SL. Therapeutic effects of borneol-walnut oil in the treatment of purulent otitis media. Zhong Xi Yi Jie He Za Zhi 1990;10:93–5, 69. [in Chinese].
61. Liao Y, Huang Y, Ou Y. Clinical and experimental study of Tongqiao tablet in treating catarrhal otitis media. Zhongguo Zhong Xi Yi Jie He Za Zhi 1998;18:668–70 [in Chinese].
62. Ikeda K, Furukawa M, Tanno N, et al. Increase of Cl- secretion induced by Kampo medicine (Japanese herbal medicine), Sai-rei-to, in Mongolian gerbil middle ear epithelium. Jpn J Pharmacol 1997;73:29–32.
63. Maruyama Y, Hoshida S, Furukawa M, et al. Effects of Japanese herbal medicine, Juzen-taiho-to, in otitis-prone children—a preliminary study. Acta Otolaryngol 2009;129:14–8.
64. Stangerup SE. Autoinflation: historical highlights and clinical implications. Ear Nose Throat J 1998;77(737):740–2.
65. Arick DS, Silman S. Treatment of otitis media with effusion based on politzerization with an automated device. Ear Nose Throat J 2000;79:290–2, 294, 296 passim.

Complementary and Integrative Treatments Adenotonsillar Disease

Kathleen R. Billings, MD[a,b],*, John Maddalozzo, MD[a,b]

KEYWORDS

- Adenotonsillar disease • Integrative medicine
- Complementary and alternative medicine • Streptococcal tonsillitis

KEY POINTS

- Treatment of patients with sore throat and tonsillitis is essentially geared toward pain management and often antibiotic therapy.
- Herbs and dietary supplements are some of the most common complementary and alternative medicine therapies employed for respiratory ailments.
- Homeopathic and herbal remedies have been shown to have minimal adverse effects, but their potential benefits are not clear due to lack of consistent use of similar remedies by treating clinicians and lack of standardization of dosing.
- The use of acupuncture as a viable pain management tool cannot be denied, although its use for managing sore throat pain in those with acute tonsillitis is not proven.

Throat infections are among the most common reasons to see a primary care physician, along with other complaints of the ear, nose, and throat such as respiratory infections and otitis media. These result in substantial cost for outpatient visits and for the treatments prescribed, such as antibiotics. Indirect costs associated with throat infections (eg, missing school or work for the patient or caregiver) can be high as well.[1] Although sore throats are a common reason for patients to seek medical care, it is estimated that 4 to 6 times as many people suffering sore throat do not seek medical care.[2] Sore throat often improves spontaneously, but the associated discomfort may be a reason for some to seek complementary and integrative medicine (CIM) approaches for treatment. Musculoskeletal complaints are the most common reason for patients to seek CIM therapies; however, head and chest colds, of which sore throat may be a primary symptom, were a common reason in a study by Barnes and colleagues,[3] although the incidence of seeking these therapies decreased

Funding Sources and Conflict of Interest: None.
[a] Division of Pediatric Otolaryngology, Department of Surgery, Ann and Robert H. Lurie Children's Hospital of Chicago, Northwestern University, Chicago, IL, USA; [b] Division of Otolaryngology-Head and Neck Surgery, Ann and Robert H. Lurie Children's Hospital of Chicago, Box #25, Chicago, IL 60611-2605, USA
* Corresponding author.
E-mail address: kbillings@luriechildrens.org

Otolaryngol Clin N Am 46 (2013) 329–334
http://dx.doi.org/10.1016/j.otc.2012.12.006
0030-6665/13/$ – see front matter © 2013 Elsevier Inc. All rights reserved.

between 2002 and 2007. This article discusses conventional treatment of adenoton-sillar disease and focuses on research looking at CIM options for treatment of this disease process and primary symptom.

PHYSIOLOGY AND ANATOMY

Throat infection is defined as sore throat caused by viral or bacterial infection of the pharynx, palatine tonsils, or both, which may or may not be culture positive for group A *Streptococcus*.[1] Watchful waiting for recurrent throat infections if there have been fewer than 7 episodes in the past year, fewer than 5 episodes per year in the past 2 years, or fewer than 3 episodes per year in the past 3 years is the current recommen-dation to clinicians.[1,4]

Good documentation during each episode of the symptoms, physical findings, culture results, days of school absence, and quality of life issues are helpful to the otolaryngologist when making treatment recommendations. In addition, a 12-month period of observation is recommended before consideration for tonsillectomy as an intervention, given a tendency for these infections to improve over time.[4] In the mean-time, treatment of patients with sore throat and tonsillitis is essentially geared toward pain management and often antibiotic therapy.

MEDICAL TREATMENT APPROACHES AND OUTCOMES IN SORE THROAT

The role of antibiotic therapy in treating a sore throat is not clear, as patients generally recover within 3 to 4 days (although some develop complications). In a Cochrane review of the use of antibiotics for sore throat, antibiotics were found to shorten the illness by an average of about 1 day and to reduce the chance of rheumatic fever in communities where this complication is common.[2] Analysis showed that sore throat and fever were reduced with the use of antibiotics by about half, and the greatest difference was seen by 3 days of illness. In a comparison of *Streptococcus*-positive and -negative throat swabs, antibiotics were more effective against symptoms at day 3 for patients with *Streptococcus*-positive swabs. The authors concluded that antibiotics confer benefits in the treatment of sore throat, but the absolute benefit was modest. Many will require treatment with antibiotics to protect against nonsuppurative and suppurative compli-cations of sore throat for one to see a benefit.[2] It is up to the clinician to educate patients about the option to avoid antibiotic usage when treating sore throats.

SURGICAL TREATMENT APPROACHES AND OUTCOMES FOR SORE THROAT AND TONSILLITIS

The mainstay of surgical treatment of tonsillitis is tonsillectomy if the frequency criteria described by Paradise[4] are met (7 tonsillitis infections in 1 year, 5 infections each year for 2 years, or 3 infections each year for 3 years), and there is documentation in the medical record for each sore throat of

- Temperature >38.3°C
- Cervical adenopathy
- Tonsillar exudate
- Positive test for group A beta-hemolytic streptococci

Supportive clinical documentation may include

- Absence from school or work
- Spread of infection within the family
- Family history of rheumatic heart disease or glomerulonephritis

Other variables may favor surgical intervention, including

- Antibiotic allergy or intolerance
- Periodic fever, aphthous stomatitis, pharyngitis, and adenitis
- History of a peritonsillar abscess[1]

Studies have shown that patients suffered fewer infections following surgery, resulting in fewer antibiotics and physician visits, and an overall improved quality of life. Nonetheless, the risks of tonsillectomy, including postoperative hemorrhage, dehydration, postoperative pulmonary edema, and velopharyngeal insufficiency, need to be considered when making recommendations.

INTEGRATIVE TREATMENT APPROACHES AND OUTCOMES FOR SORE THROAT AND TONSILLITIS

Clearly not all patients with sore throat or tonsillitis are candidates for medical or surgical intervention. Therefore, the remainder of this discussion will focus on CIM options for treating sore throat and tonsillitis.

The 5 subgroups of CIM therapies are (1) integrative medical systems, (2) mind–body intervention, (3) biologically based therapies, (4) manipulative and body-based methods, and (5) energy therapies.[3]

Specific studies looking at all categories as they pertain to the treatment of adenotonsillar disease are not available in the literature. Those CIM therapies that have been assessed are reviewed.

Homeopathy for Respiratory Ailments

In a multicenter comparison of homeopathic and conventional treatment for acute respiratory and ear complaints, Haidvogl and colleagues[5] did not find homeopathic approaches to be inferior to conventional treatment. Homeopathy is a system of medical practices based on the theory that any substance that can produce symptoms of disease or illness in a healthy person can cure those symptoms in a sick person (like cures like).[3] In this study, sore throat was the most common complaint (43.4%) of the adults enrolled and second most common complaint (24.6%), after cough, for the children participating. The patients were not randomized to their treatment arm, as many of the patients in the homeopathic group had a strong treatment preference. The primary outcome measure of the study was complete recovery, or major improvement after 14 days. The authors found the response rates at 7, 14, and 28 days between the 2 groups to be similar for both adults and children. Sixty-two different homeopathic remedies were prescribed by the treating physicians across this study, based on their personal preference. The most common were belladonna, pulsatilla, hepar sulphuris, and byronia alba.

These are all plant derivatives, but they are not the same as herbal remedies for illness. Conventional treatments were most often antibacterial agents, nasal preparations, and analgesics.

Despite the large number of treatments used, the percentage of adverse reactions was not significantly different in 2 treatment arms (2% for homeopathy and 2.4% for conventional).

Using an homeopathic approach to treating disease processes clearly requires special training to gain an understanding of the best uses and adverse effects of the prescribed treatments. All the physicians participating in the previously mentioned study had special training and years of experience.[5] Not all studies have shown a favorable advantage to a homeopathic approach in treating respiratory tract infections. A reduction in the use of antibiotics occurred both in those treated with homeopathic remedies and the placebo controls in De Lange's study.[6] The authors felt this could be related to the natural development of the children in the study, potential lifestyle and dietary changes, and reduction of stress and anxiety created by open medical expectations.[6] Regardless, any use of homeopathic treatment for sore throat and tonsillitis should be by a qualified specialist who is familiar with the benefits and limitations of such remedies.

Herbs and Dietary Supplements for Respiratory Ailments

Herbs and dietary supplements, other than vitamins and minerals, are some of the most common CIM therapies employed for respiratory ailments, and they have been widely used by healers and health care practitioners around the world.[7,8] Some of the common herbal remedies include echinacea, ginkgo biloba, and ginseng. There are clearly large differences in herbs available in different regions across the world, making it difficult to standardize their use as health care remedies. A German study looked at the efficacy of an herbal compound of *Phytolacca*, *Guajacum*, and *Capsicum* for the treatment of patients diagnosed with acute tonsillitis. This was an observational study, which showed an improvement in moderate or severe difficulty swallowing by 5 days of treatment.[9] No controls were used in this study to demonstrate whether, with no treatment or placebo, the symptoms may have resolved spontaneously.

Another group looked at the efficacy of using an extract of *Pelargonium sidoides* (umckaloabo), a member of the geranium family, for treatment of acute nongroup A beta-hemolytic *Streptococcus* tonsillitis in children.[10] The study showed that those patients receiving the herbal remedy had reduced severity of their symptoms and shortened duration of illness by about 2 days compared with the placebo group. The exact mechanism of action of umckaloabo is not clear, but it may exert antibacterial effects against a wide range of gram-negative and gram-positive bacteria. Few adverse effects caused by umckaloabo have been reported, and they are usually skin related. It also may have an anticoagulant effect, however. Therefore, care must be taken in suggesting this mode of therapy to those with disorders of coagulation or in those who are already taking anticoagulants. Other studies have shown evidence of improved symptoms in those with bronchitis or the common cold who are taking this remedy.[11] A concern with this and other herbal remedies is lack of standard preparation and dosing guidelines, which may impact the clinical effects. Close monitoring of symptom response to treatment and adverse effects is suggested.

Outcomes for Use of Herbs for Sore Throat Treatment

Looking for herbal CIM treatments for sore throat may lead many to an Internet search. The Natural Medicine Comprehensive Online Database lists and describes natural medicines for the management of colds and influenza.[12] Specifically, there are natural products promoted to boost or support the immune system, like astralagas, echinacea, garlic, and ginseng. Astralagas is a Chinese herb promoted to prevent colds and influenza by stimulating lymphocyte production, although it is not recommended for prophylactic use. Echinacea, on the other hand, may reduce the risk of the common cold when taken continuously for 2 months, and it is thought to have immunostimulant properties. Similarly, ginseng preparations may reduce respiratory symptom severity and duration of symptoms when taken regularly in the influenza season. Garlic may have immunostimulant and antiviral activity, and limited evidence may show a reduction in the number of colds in winter months compared with those taking placebo. Other herbal remedies that may act as immunomodulators include andrographis, elderberry, goldenseal, and boneset, to name a few. The use of such remedies for the prevention or treatment of sore throat and tonsillitis is not clear, although generally the risk and adverse affects is small. Again, the physician should use caution in recommending these therapies given the lack of strong evidence to support their benefits, particularly in pregnant patients and those taking other medications that may cross-react to these remedies.

A Cochrane review was updated in 2010 assessing the role of Chinese medicinal herbs in treating sore throats.[8] The use of medicinal herbs in China and among Chinese people worldwide is common, and the authors sought to evaluate the efficacy and safety of these remedies. Seven trials involving over 1200 participants were included in their analysis. The studies were found to be of methodologically poor quality, and the herbal preparations were not specifically characterized and only used in 1 trial (the herbs were not standardized across multiple trials). In 3 of the studies reviewed, the herbal remedy was found to be superior to the control in improving recovery from sore throat, whereas in the other 4 studies, the response to the herbal therapy was similar to the control group. None of the studies reported any adverse events. Ultimately, based on the existing evidence, the authors could not recommend Chinese medicinal herbs as an effective remedy for sore throat. Concerns were again raised regarding the lack of standardization and variability in preparation of the herbal remedies, which might provide a consistent effect. Clearly, studies using a standard preparation of a specific herbal therapy, along with appropriate controls, are needed.

Acupuncture for Sore Throat Treatment

The studies described thus far have focused on homeopathic and herbal treatments of adenotonsillar disease and sore throat. Another potential integrative treatment for sore throat pain is the use of acupuncture. Acupuncture has been used for centuries as a means of treating a wide number of illnesses, and it can be an effective resource for pain management practitioners. Fleckenstein and colleagues[13] studied a single-point acupuncture treatment for the management of sore throat in patients with acute tonsillitis and pharyngitis. The study involved patients who received either acupuncture or sham laser acupuncture at a single point in the large intestine meridian on the forearm. A change in pain intensity on swallowing a sip of water, measured by a visual analog scale 15 minutes after treatment, was evaluated. A significant difference between the 2 groups was not seen, and patient satisfaction was high in both groups. The authors commented that a response to palpation of the forearm area in the sham group may have elicited the positive effect. In addition, the perceived expectations of treatment success by the patients might have improved their reaction. The use of acupuncture as a viable pain management tool cannot be denied, although its use for managing sore throat pain in those with acute tonsillitis is not proven.

SUMMARY

In conclusion, although antibiotics may shorten duration of illness for those with tonsillitis and sore throat, many patients will improve spontaneously. The adverse effects of antibiotic treatment and potential lack of efficacy may be a reason to seek CIM therapies. Homeopathic and herbal remedies have been shown to have minimal adverse effects, but their potential benefits are not clear due to lack of consistent use of similar remedies by treating clinicians and lack of standardization of dosing.

The widespread use of these treatments by many cultures around the world, and the interest by patients in this country in seeking CIM approaches to therapy, suggest that continued research is needed. Health care providers who are not familiar with the benefits and potential risks of these therapies should be cautious in their recommendations. Given that most patients with sore throat do not seek medical attention, the use of CIM treatments in this country is likely vastly underestimated.

REFERENCES

1. Baugh RB, Archer SM, Mitchell RB, et al. Clinical practice guideline: tonsillectomy in children. Otolaryngol Head Neck Surg 2011;144(Suppl 1):S1–30.
2. Del Mar CB, Glasziou SA, Spinks AB. Antibiotics for sore throat. Cochrane Database Syst Rev 2006;4:CD000023.
3. Barnes PM, Bloom B, Nahin RL. Complementary and alternative medicine use among adults and children: United States, 2007. Natl Health Stat Report 2008;(12):1–24.
4. Paradise JL, Bluestone CD, Bachman RZ, et al. Efficacy of tonsillectomy for recurrent throat infection in severely affected children: results of parallel randomized and nonrandomized clinical trials. N Engl J Med 1984;310:674–83.
5. Haidvogl M, Riley DS, Heger M, et al. Homeopathic and conventional treatment for acute respiratory and ear complaints: a comparative study on outcome in the primary care setting. BMC Complement Altern Med 2007;7:7.
6. de Lange de Klerk ES, Blommers J, Kuik DJ, et al. Effect of homeopathic medicines on daily burden of symptoms in children with recurrent upper respiratory infections. BMJ 1994;309:1329–32.
7. Njoroge GN, Bussman RW. Traditional management of ear, nose, and throat (ENT) diseases in central Kenya. J Ethnobiol Ethnomed 2006;2:54.
8. Shi Y, Gu R, Liu C, et al. Chinese medicinal herbs for sore throat. Cochrane Database Syst Rev 2007;3:CD004877.
9. Rau E. Treatment of acute tonsillitis with a fixed-combination herbal preparation. Adv Ther 2000;17(4):197–203.
10. Bereznoy VV, Riley DS, Wassmer G, et al. Efficacy of extract of *Pelargonium sidoides* in children with acute non-group A beta-hemolytic *Streptococcus* tonsillopharyngitis: a randomized, double-blind, placebo-controlled trial. Altern Ther Health Med 2003;9(5):68–70.
11. Natural Standards Research Committee. Umckaloabo (*Pelargonium sidoides*). Natural Standard Monograph 2011;1–13.
12. Natural medicines in the clinical management of colds and flu. Natural Medicines Comprehensive Database. NIH Publication No. 10–6248, revised June 2010.
13. Fleckenstein J, Lill C, Ludtke R, et al. A single point acupuncture treatment at large intestine meridian: a randomized controlled trial in acute tonsillitis and pharyngitis. Clin J Pain 2009;25(7):624–31.

Complementary and Integrative Treatments
Upper Respiratory Infection

Jessica R. Weiss, MD[a],*, Belachew Tessema, MD[b],
Seth M. Brown, MD, MBA[b]

KEYWORDS

- Upper respiratory tract infection • Common cold • Alternative therapy
- Complementary therapy

KEY POINTS

- The current theory regarding upper respiratory tract infections (URIs) holds the inflammatory response to viral infection, rather than the virus itself, responsible for the symptoms.
- Treatment of URI remains focused on symptom management and the tincture of time.
- Antibiotics and surgery have no role in the treatment of an uncomplicated URI.
- Nasal decongestants offer modest but significant relief of nasal congestion, with a low incidence of adverse effects.
- Insufficient evidence supports the use of vitamin and herbal remedies in the prevention and/or treatment of URIs, although some studies have shown significant benefits in symptom reduction.
- Evidence supporting the use of acupuncture for URIs is too limited to offer a recommendation regarding this treatment.

OVERVIEW

The combination of nasal congestion, rhinorrhea, sore throat, cough, and malaise is the symptomatic profile that constitutes an uncomplicated upper respiratory tract infection (URI), also known as the common cold. It is a pervasive illness; approximately 25 million people in the United States visit their doctor every year seeking treatment for a URI.[1] Nationally, the economic burden of URI is estimated to be approximately $40 billion per year, including $22 billion from nearly 200 million lost work days every year.[2] Because no known cure exists for the common URI, numerous products are available for treatment, each marketed with the promise of alleviating the associated symptoms and/or shortening the duration of illness. The evidence supporting these

[a] Deparment of Surgery, Division of Otolaryngology-Head and Neck Surgery, University of Connecticut School of Medicine, 263 Farmington Avenue, Farmington, CT 06030, USA; [b] Deparment of Surgery, Division of Otolaryngology-Head and Neck Surgery, Connecticut Sinus Institute, University of Connecticut School of Medicine, 21 South Road, Suite 112, Farmington, CT 06032, USA
* Corresponding author.
E-mail address: jweiss@resident.uchc.edu

Otolaryngol Clin N Am 46 (2013) 335–344
http://dx.doi.org/10.1016/j.otc.2012.12.007
0030-6665/13/$ – see front matter © 2013 Elsevier Inc. All rights reserved.

oto.theclinics.com

claims is variable and is the focus of this article, with an emphasis on complementary and integrative therapies because these are being used with increasing frequency in the United States.[3]

PATHOPHYSIOLOGY AND ANATOMY

URIs are caused by a plethora of viruses, with rhinovirus being the most common causative agent.[4,5] Other responsible viruses include coronavirus, parainfluenza, respiratory syncytial virus, adenovirus, and enterovirus.[4,5] It is even likely that a portion of URIs are caused by viruses that have not yet been identified.[4]

The pathophysiology of a URI begins with transmission of the offending agent, which may occur via 3 routes: touching one's nose or eyes after contacting either an infected person or a contaminated object, inhalation of small particle aerosols that were produced by the cough of an infected person, or the sneeze of an infected person resulting in large particle aerosols landing on the nasal mucosa or conjunctiva.[4,5] The viral agent travels from the eye to the nasal mucosa via the nasolacrimal duct. Once the virus infects the nasal mucosa, it is propelled to the nasopharynx through mucociliary action of the respiratory epithelium lining the nasal cavities. The virus then binds to epithelial cell receptors, which allow it to gain entrance into these cells. Within the epithelial cells rapid viral replication occurs.

The current theory regarding URIs holds the inflammatory response to viral infection, rather than the virus itself, responsible for the symptoms. In response to viral infection of the nasal epithelial cells, an upregulation of inflammatory mediators occurs, including cytokines such as interleukins 6 and 8,[4,5] which drive the host's inflammatory response. As a result, there is an influx of neutrophils, vasodilation, and an increase in vascular permeability that results in the leakage of plasma proteins into the nasal cavity. Additionally, parasympathetic stimulation occurs, which causes production of excess mucous.[4] This process translates into nasal congestion, rhinorrhea, and sneezing.[4,5]

One reason people are susceptible to recurrent URIs year after year is challenges to immunity. Some virus types, including respiratory syncytial virus, parainfluenza, and coronavirus, do not produce lasting immunity. Other viruses, including rhinovirus, adenovirus, and enterovirus, do produce lasting immunity but so many serotypes exist that one is still susceptible to recurrent infection. These challenges are also the reason that no antiviral medications are available that are effective in treating URIs. Thus, treatment of URIs remains focused on symptom management and the tincture of time.

SYMPTOMS

The symptoms of the common URI include nasal congestion, sneezing, rhinorrhea, sore throat, headache, myalgia, and malaise. Fever may be present but is more common in children than adults.[4] Symptom duration is usually 7 to 10 days but can be as long as 3 weeks.[4] Drainage from rhinorrhea often begins clear but then may become thicker and discolored. Yellow or green nasal discharge is not an indication of a bacterial infection but rather of neutrophil infiltration, which is the hallmark of the immune system response.[5]

MEDICAL TREATMENT APPROACHES AND OUTCOMES
Antibiotics

Antibiotics have no role in the treatment of an uncomplicated URI with or without purulent rhinorrhea.[6] Specifically, antibiotics do not decrease severity or duration of symptoms and commonly are associated with adverse effects, most commonly gastrointestinal issues, such as diarrhea.[6] In the United States, unnecessary prescription of antibiotics results in an economic burden of nearly $800 million per year and puts the patient and society at risk for developing antibiotic-resistant strains of bacteria.[1]

Oral and Intranasal Decongestants

Nasal congestion is one of the most common and bothersome symptoms of a URI, and therefore many over-the-counter cold remedies are geared toward relieving this symptom. Common oral decongestants include pseudoephedrine and phenylephrine. Phenylpropanolamine was previously used in over-the-counter preparations but has been removed from the market because of an associated risk of intracranial hemorrhage.[5] Pseudoephedrine, a popular over-the-counter remedy for nasal congestion, has come under scrutiny recently because of its use in the illicit manufacturing of methamphetamines. Although still available over-the-counter, it is now only accessible behind pharmacy counters and its purchase is monitored.[5]

A review of the current literature was completed in 2009 by Taverner and Latte[7] to assess the efficacy of topical and oral decongestants in relieving nasal congestion. Only randomized, placebo-controlled trials were included in their review. Their analysis indicated that nasal decongestants offer modest but significant relief of nasal congestion with a low incidence of adverse effects. Symptomatic relief was supported by a physiologic response of a significant reduction in nasal airway resistance. The evidence supports recommending a single dose trial of decongestants for patients with a URI. Those who experience improvement in symptoms of nasal congestion should be encouraged to continue treatment for 3 to 5 days. It is important to inform patients to discontinue use of topical decongestants after this period because of the risk of a rebound increase in congestion, as is seen with rhinitis medicamentosa. Patients with hypertension and/or benign prostatic hypertrophy should be closely monitored if using oral decongestants because the α-adrenergic properties may exacerbate these conditions.

Intranasal Steroids

Topical steroid sprays used intranasally have been shown to have significant benefit in treatment of nasal inflammation that is characterized by a dominantly eosinophilic infiltration, such as allergic rhinitis and nasal polyposis. They have not, however, proven beneficial in the treatment of infectious nasal inflammation, such as the common cold/URI.[8,9]

Intranasal Ipratropium Bromide

Ipratropium bromide is an anticholinergic agent that when used intranasally can decrease rhinorrhea associated with the common cold.[10] It has not been shown to have an effect on nasal congestion.[10] It is generally well tolerated, with nasal dryness, blood tinged mucous, and epistaxis being the most commonly reported adverse effects.[10] For patients with a URI whose chief complaint is rhinorrhea, use of intranasal ipratropium bromide could be of benefit.

Antihistamines

Although antihistamines have a proven role in the treatment of allergy-associated nasal symptoms, they do not offer benefit in relief of sneezing, rhinorrhea, or nasal congestion associated with a URI.[11] The main adverse affect is sedation, which is seen more commonly with first-generation antihistamines. The use of antihistamines is not recommended for the treatment of nasal symptoms associated with URI.[11]

Nonsteroidal Anti-Inflammatory Agents

Nonsteroidal anti-inflammatory agents are known for their analgesic, antipyretic, and anti-inflammatory properties and have widespread use for a variety of ailments. For the common cold they have proven effective for reducing pain-related symptoms, including myalgias, headache, and otalgia.[12] Despite their anti-inflammatory properties, a literature review completed by Kim and colleagues[12] did not support the theory that they might be helpful in reducing respiratory symptoms associated with URI, such as cough, sneezing, or rhinorrhea.

Guaifenesin

Limited evidence is available on the utility of the expectorant guaifenesin in treating URI symptoms. In a review of 2 studies, Smith and colleagues[13] identified conflicting data. In one study, patients reported no difference in cough but did report a decrease in the thickness of mucous; in the second study patients did experience a decrease in cough frequency. Because side effects are minimal, it is reasonable for patients to trial guaifenesin to determine if they experience benefit. Further study is needed to determine the overall effectiveness of guaifenesin in the treatment of URIs.

SURGICAL TREATMENT APPROACHES AND OUTCOMES

Surgical intervention has no role in the management of an uncomplicated URI.

PATIENT SELF-TREATMENTS
Nasal Saline Irrigation

Nasal saline irrigation is often used as an adjunctive treatment for URIs. It can be used in the form of an atomized spray or lavage irrigation. The utility of nasal saline lies in its ability to clear excess mucous from the nasal cavities, improve mucociliary clearance, and reduce cough associated with postnasal drip.[14] In general, studies on the use of nasal saline are limited because of the difficulty using an adequate control and thus inability to perform a blinded study. Additionally, numerous formulations and delivery methods are available for nasal saline, making comparisons between studies more difficult. Finally, outcomes are often based on patients subjectively reporting symptoms, allowing the introduction of bias.

In 2010, Kassel and colleagues[14] performed an exhaustive literature review to assess the efficacy of nasal saline irrigation in the treatment of symptoms associated with URIs, the duration and severity of these symptoms, and the incidence of adverse effects associated with nasal saline use. Although evidence was limited, they found no statistically significant improvement in symptom severity or duration associated with the use of nasal saline. However, a reduction in time off of work and a trend toward decreased antibiotic use were seen. Adverse effects were minor, with approximately one-third of subjects reporting a dry or irritated nose. In the adult population, none of these effects was significant enough to cease treatment with nasal saline. Overall, the authors concluded that nasal saline may offer some benefit to adults with a URI. However, the current evidence is not sufficiently convincing to make it a routine intervention.

Heated Humidified Air

Inhalation of heated, humidified air has long been used as home remedy for the common cold. It is thought to provide symptomatic relief of nasal congestion through improving mucous drainage, and the rise in temperature may impede viral replication.[15] The current literature shows conflicting data evaluating its efficacy, with some studies finding improvement of nasal symptoms after inhalation of warm humidified air, and other studies not.[15] A review by Singh and Singh[15] in 2011 pooled the results of randomized controlled trials on the topic and did not find that steam inhalation offered any consistent benefit to sufferers of the common cold. A large-scale, double-blinded study producing evidence of benefit is needed before heated, humidified air can be recommended as standard intervention.

INTEGRATIVE TREATMENT APPROACHES AND OUTCOMES
Zinc

Zinc supplementation has long been regarded as a potentially beneficial adjunct in the treatment and prevention of URIs. In the ionized form, zinc has demonstrated direct antiviral activity.[16] Available forms include syrup, tablet, or lozenge. It was previously marketed as an intranasal spray, but this product is no longer available because it was linked to irreversible anosmia.[17] If zinc supplementation is initiated within 24 hours of symptom onset, it has been shown to be beneficial in reducing the duration and severity of cold symptoms.[18] If it is taken in a prophylactic manner for a 5-month period, it has been shown to reduce the incidence of the common cold.[18] Adverse effects are more likely associated with the lozenge and include nausea and bad taste. Further research is needed to determine to optimal dosing regimen.[18]

Vitamin C

The use of vitamin C, also known as ascorbic acid, has been widely popular for the treatment and prevention of URIs since the 1970s when it was endorsed by Nobel laureate Linus Pauling.[19] A literature review and meta-analysis performed by Hemila and colleagues[19] in 2010 evaluated the strength of the evidence supporting the benefit of vitamin C. Their research concluded that when taken prophylactically, it was not effective in reducing the incidence of common cold in the general population. It did, however, have a beneficial effect on the severity and duration of symptoms. In a population consisting of people who performed strenuous physical activity and/or were subjected to significant cold stress, it can reduce the incidence of URIs when taken prophylactically.[19] When vitamin C was taken after the onset of cold symptoms, it did not exhibit a benefit on the severity or duration of symptoms, but this is an area that requires further study.[19]

Vitamin D

Vitamin D is known to play a role in immune system regulation. Studies have shown that vitamin D deficiency may result in more missed work days because of URIs.[20] Therefore, questions regarding its potential role in preventing or treating infection have been raised. A randomized controlled trial comparing vitamin D_3 supplementation versus placebo completed over 12 weeks during winter revealed no benefit in reducing the incidence of URIs or the severity of symptoms with vitamin supplementation.[21] However, the authors postulated that they could have failed to detect a benefit because of small sample size and late initiation of vitamin D supplementation during winter. They suggest that initiating supplementation during the fall could be more effective because it coincides with the time year when sunlight exposure deceases and would allow more time for vitamin D levels to stabilize.[21] Therefore, further study seems warranted.

Probiotics

Probiotics are live microorganisms that may be found and consumed in dietary supplements and fermented foods, such as yogurt. Although the mechanism is unclear, probiotics are theorized to provide potential health benefits through modulation of the immune system. One area of potential health benefit is in prevention and treatment of URIs. In 2011, Hao and colleagues[22] performed a literature review and meta-analysis to assess the effectiveness and safety of probiotics in preventing URIs. Their findings suggested that probiotics may decrease the rate of URIs, the number of subjects who experience URIs, and the use of antibiotics for URIs when compared with placebo. Hatakka and colleagues[23] showed similar results in a double-blind, randomized, controlled trial evaluating the use of probiotics in nearly 600 children who attended day care regularly in Finland. Adverse effects of probiotics are usually minor and consist of gastrointestinal discomfort.[22] Although more study is needed, the current, albeit limited, evidence supports the use of probiotics for preventing URIs, but the specific regimen has yet to be determined.

Garlic

Garlic (*Allium sativum*) has been theorized to have antimicrobial, antiviral, and antifungal properties. Therefore, it has been alleged that garlic supplementation may have use in preventing and treating the common cold, but the literature lacks solid evidence supporting this claim.[24] One randomized controlled trial conducted by Josling[25] in 2001 indicated a decreased incidence of the common cold in the study group taking garlic supplement over a 3-month period. However, further studies with larger sample sizes and clear outcome measures are needed before one can confidently conclude that garlic supplementation is effective in preventing and/or treating the common cold.[24,25]

Pelargonium sidoides

Pelargonium sidoides is a root from which an herbal supplement is prepared. This root has been shown to have immune system modulatory capabilities in vitro.[26] In one randomized controlled trial, this supplement proved to have benefit in treating the common cold, with decreased symptom severity, shorter symptom duration, fewer lost work days, and minimal associated adverse effects.[26] Because evidence is limited, this supplement cannot yet be recommended as a standard intervention but does show promise as an effective treatment.

Ginseng

Panax quinquefolius (North American ginseng) is a popular-selling root extract, partly because of claims of its efficacy in improving fatigue, depression, stress, sexual energy, and digestion; the promotion of general well-being; and the treatment and prevention of URIs.[16] Data validating these claims regarding URIs are limited. A systematic review performed by Seida and colleagues[27] in 2008 revealed that *P quinquefolius* does seem to be effective in decreasing the duration of cold symptoms when taken prophylactically for 2 to 4 months, but insufficient evidence showed a decrease in the incidence of URIs or severity of symptoms. However, no significant published studies have evaluated the short-term use of ginseng extract for treating URIs. Furthermore, the potential adverse effects of long-term ginseng therapy have not been investigated thoroughly. Therefore, long-term prophylactic use or short-term therapeutic use of North American ginseng for URIs cannot be recommended until further studies are completed.

Kan Jang

Kan Jang is a standardized extract that contains both *Andrographis paniculata* and *Acanthopanax senticosus*, which are theorized to provide benefit in the treatment of URIs because of their anti-inflammatory and immune-stimulatory properties.[28] Although, evidence supporting this is limited, it has been shown to improve symptoms of cough, throat irritation, and muscle soreness when taken 3 times daily for 3 days within 36 hours of symptom onset.[28] Thus, Kan Jang extract shows promise in providing symptomatic relief for URIs, but additional studies with larger sample size and assessment of associated adverse effects are needed before it may be recommended as standard treatment.

Echinacea

A plethora of Echinacea preparations made from a variety of species and methods is available. This heterogeneity makes comparative evaluation of the effects of Echinacea difficult. A recent review of the literature by Linde and colleagues[29] revealed that Echinacea has not proven effective in preventing URIs. However, the pressed juice of the aerial parts of the species *Echinacea purpurea* may be effective in decreasing the severity and duration of cold symptoms if initiated early in the disease course.[29] This is an area that warrants further study.

Quercetin

Quercetin (3,3′,4′,5,7-pentahydroxyflavone) is an antioxidant whose in vitro antiviral properties have made it a subject of study for possible efficacy in treating and preventing viral URIs.[30] It may be consumed as a supplement or within foods, such as broccoli, apples, berries, onions, and tea.[31] In mice it has been shown to counteract the increased URI susceptibility that is associated with exercise stress[32] and to decrease viral replication, expression of cytokines, and airway hyperresponiveness.[31] Its efficacy in humans was evaluated in a prospective, randomized, double-blind, placebo-controlled trial in which a supplement containing quercetin, vitamin C, and niacin was taken prophylactically for a 12-week period.[30] Within a subgroup of subjects aged 40 years and older with above-average fitness, a reduction in total sick days and symptom severity was seen.[30] However, the study did not include a control group consuming quercetin alone, without niacin or vitamin C, making it difficult to tie possible efficacy to quercetin alone. Additionally, when considering all subjects, an affect on URI rates, symptom severity, or symptom duration was not appreciated.[30]

Multimodal Approaches

Acupuncture

Sinus and nasal symptoms are ailments frequently treated by licensed acupuncturists who report good efficacy.[33] However, evidence supporting the use of acupuncture for URIs is limited, and therefore, a well-designed randomized control trial is needed.

Summary box: treatment recommendations	
Treatment	**Recommendation**
Antibiotics	Not recommended for treatment of upper respiratory tract infection (URI)
Decongestants	Both oral and topical preparations may provide modest improvement in nasal congestion
Intranasal steroids	Not recommended for treatment of URI
Intranasal ipratropium bromide	Beneficial in treatment of rhinorrhea associated with URI
Antihistamines	Not recommended for treatment of URI
Nonsteroidal anti-inflammatory drugs	Beneficial in treatment of pain symptoms associated with URI
Guaifenesin	No clear benefit, but individual patients may trial to see if they experience benefit
Nasal saline irrigation	No clear benefit, but individual patients may trial to see if they experience benefit
Heated humidified air	No clear benefit, but individual patients may trial to see if they experience benefit
Zinc	When taken therapeutically, may reduce duration and severity of symptoms. When taken prophylactically, may reduce incidence of URI
Vitamin C	When taken therapeutically, has not been shown to reduce duration or severity of symptoms. When taken prophylactically, may reduce incidence of URI in those exposed to significant physical and/or cold stress
Vitamin D	No clear benefit, further study is needed
Probiotics	When taken prophylactically, may reduce incidence of URI
Garlic	No clear benefit, further study is needed
Pelargonium sidoides	When taken therapeutically, may reduce duration and severity of symptoms, but evidence is limited and further study is needed
Ginseng	When taken prophylactically, has not been shown to reduce incidence of URI but may decrease duration of symptoms; evidence is limited and further study is needed
Quercetin	Limited evidence showing benefit when taken in conjunction with Vit C and Niacin in a subset of subjects but further study is needed
Kan Jang	When taken therapeutically, may reduce severity of symptoms but evidence is limited and further study is needed
Acupuncture	Very limited evidence, further study is needed

REFERENCES

1. Gonzales R, Malone DC, Maselli JH, et al. Excessive antibiotic use for acute respiratory infections in the United States. Clin Infect Dis 2001;33:757–62.
2. Fendrick AM, Monto AS, Nightengale B, et al. The economic burden of non-influenza-related viral respiratory tract infection in the United States. Arch Intern Med 2003;163:487–94.
3. Roehm C, Tessema B, Brown S. The role of alternative medicine in rhinology. Facial Plast Surg Clin North Am 2011;20(1):73–81.
4. Heikkinen T, Järvinen A. The common cold. Lancet 2003;361:51–9.
5. Pappas DE, Hendley JO. The common cold and decongestant therapy. Pediatr Rev 2011;32:47–55.

6. Arroll B, Kenealy T. Antibiotics for the common cold and acute purulent rhinitis. Cochrane Database Syst Rev 2005;(3):CD000247.
7. Taverner D, Latte J. Nasal decongestants for the common cold. Cochrane Database Syst Rev 2007;(1):CD001953.
8. Mygind N, Andersson M. Topical glucocorticosteroids in rhinitis: clinical aspects. Acta Otolaryngol 2006;126:1022–9.
9. Qvarnberg Y, Valtonen H, Laurikainen K. Intranasal beclomethasone dipropionate in the treatment of common cold. Rhinology 2001;39:9–12.
10. Albalawi ZH, Othman SS, Alfaleh K. Intranasal ipratropium bromide for the common cold. Cochrane Database Syst Rev 2011;(7):CD008231.
11. Sutter AI, Lemiengre M, Campbell H, et al. Antihistamines for the common cold. Cochrane Database Syst Rev 2003;(3):CD001267.
12. Kim SY, Chang YJ, Cho HM, et al. Non-steroidal anti-inflammatory drugs for the common cold. Cochrane Database Syst Rev 2009;(3):CD006362.
13. Smith SM, Schroeder K, Fahey T. Over-the-counter medications for acute cough in children and adults in ambulatory settings. Cochrane Database Syst Rev 2008;(1):CD001831.
14. Kassel JC, King D, Spurling GK. Saline nasal irrigation for acute upper respiratory tract infections. Cochrane Database Syst Rev 2010;(3):CD006821.
15. Singh M, Singh M. Heated, humidified air for the common cold. Cochrane Database Syst Rev 2011;(5):CD001728.
16. Seidman MD. Complementary and alternative medications and techniques. In: Benninger M, Murry T, editors. The performer's voice. San Diego: Plural Publishing; 2006. p. 163–76.
17. Davidson TM, Smith WM. The Bradford Hill criteria and zinc-induced anosmia: a causality analysis. Arch Otolaryngol Head Neck Surg 2010;136:673–6.
18. Singh M, Das RR. Zinc for the common cold. Cochrane Database Syst Rev 2011;(2):CD001364.
19. Douglas B, Hemilä H, Chalker E, et al. Vitamin C for preventing and treating the common cold. Cochrane Database Syst Rev 2007;(3):CD000980.
20. Laski I, Ruohola JP, Tuohimaa P, et al. An association of serum vitamin D concentrations <40 nmol/L with acute respiratory tract infection in young Finnish men. Am J Clin Nutr 2007;86:714–7.
21. Li-Ng M, Aloia JF, Pollack S, et al. A randomized controlled trial of vitamin D3 supplementation for the prevention of symptomatic upper respiratory tract infections. Epidemiol Infect 2009;137:1396–404.
22. Hao Q, Lu Z, Dong BR, et al. Probiotics for preventing acute upper respiratory tract infections. Cochrane Database Syst Rev 2011;(9):CD006895.
23. Hatakka K, Savilahti E, Ponka A, et al. Effect of long term consumption of probiotic milk on infections in children attending day care centres: double blind, randomized trial. BMJ 2001;322(1298):1327–9.
24. Lissiman E, Bhassale AL, Cohen M. Garlic for the common cold. Cochrane Database Syst Rev 2009;(3):CD006206.
25. Josling P. Preventing the common cold with a garlic supplement: a double blind, placebo-controlled survey. Adv Ther 2001;18(4):189–93.
26. Lizogub VG, Riley DS, Heger M. Efficacy of a pelargonium sidoides preparation in patients with the common cold: a randomized, double blind, placebo-controlled clinical trial. Explore (NY) 2007;3:573–84.
27. Seida JK, Durec T, Kuhle S. North American (Panax quinquefolius) and Asian ginseng (Panax ginseng) preparations for prevention of the common cold in healthy adults: a systematic review. Evid Based Complement Alternat Med 2009;2011:1–7.

28. Melchior J, Spasov AA, Ostrovskij OV, et al. Double-blind, placebo-controlled pilot and phase III study of activity of standardized *Andrographis paniculata* Herba Nees extract fixed combination (Kan jang) in the treatment of uncomplicated upper-respiratory tract infection. Phytomedicine 2000;7(5):341–50.
29. Linde K, Barrett B, Bauer R, et al. Echinacea for preventing and treating the common cold. Cochrane Database Syst Rev 2006;(1):CD000530.
30. Heinz S, Henson DA, Austin MD, et al. Quercetin supplementation and upper respiratory tract infection: a randomized controlled trial. Pharmacol Res 2010; 62:237–42.
31. Ganesan S, Faris AN, Comstock AT, et al. Quercetin inhibits rhinovirus replication *in vitro* and *in vivo*. Antiviral Res 2012;94:258–71.
32. Davis JM, Murphy EA, McClellan JL, et al. Quercetin reduced susceptibility to influenza infection following stressful exercise. Am J Physiol Regul Integr Comp Physiol 2008;295:505–9.
33. Pletcher SD, Goldber AN, Lee J, et al. Use of acupuncture in the treatment of sinus and nasal symptoms: results of a practitioner survey. Am J Rhinol 2006; 20(2):235–7.

Complementary and Integrative Treatments
Rhinosinusitis

Malcolm B. Taw, MD[a],*, Chau T. Nguyen, MD[b],
Marilene B. Wang, MD[b]

KEYWORDS

- Rhinosinusitis • Sinusitis • Integrative medicine • Traditional Chinese medicine
- Complementary and alternative medicine • Herbal medicine • Acupuncture

KEY POINTS

- Rhinosinusitis is characterized by inflammation of the mucosa involving the paranasal sinuses. It is one of the most common and significant health care problems in the United States.
- Evidence demonstrates that antibiotics provide very little clinical benefit and that although most patients will experience improvement following endoscopic sinus surgery, a significant proportion will not.
- The goals of treatment are to improve drainage, remove obstruction, promote mucociliary function, eradicate infection, reduce inflammation, and prevent complications.
- There is evidence for beneficial integrative treatment using herbal supplements, especially for *Pelargonium sidoides*, Sinupret, and Sinfrontal.
- There is evidence for beneficial integrative treatment using traditional Chinese medicine, including acupuncture and Chinese herbal medicine (*Xanthii fructus* and *Flos magnoliae*).

OVERVIEW

Rhinosinusitis (RS) is characterized by inflammation of the mucosa involving the paranasal sinuses and the nasal cavity and is the preferred term for sinusitis because this is almost always accompanied by concurrent nasal airway inflammation.[1,2] It is one of the most common and significant health care problems in the United States, with approximately 31 million Americans affected annually, prompting nearly 13 million physician office visits and more than 600 000 ambulatory surgical procedures per

Disclosure: The authors have no relevant financial interests pertaining to this article.
[a] UCLA Center for East-West Medicine, Department of Medicine, 2336 Santa Monica Boulevard, Suite 301, Santa Monica, CA 90404, USA; [b] UCLA Department of Head and Neck Surgery, 200 UCLA Medical Plaza, Suite 550, Los Angeles, CA 90095, USA
* Corresponding author.
E-mail address: mtaw@mednet.ucla.edu

Otolaryngol Clin N Am 46 (2013) 345–366
http://dx.doi.org/10.1016/j.otc.2013.02.002
0030-6665/13/$ – see front matter Published by Elsevier Inc.

oto.theclinics.com

year.[3–6] Quality of life can be adversely impacted, and emotional and daily functioning can be significantly impaired.[7,8] It is estimated that direct health care costs of more than $8.6 billion and indirect costs of approximately 73 million days of restricted activity are incurred annually.[9,10]

RS is the fifth leading diagnosis treated with antibiotics, with 21% of adults receiving prescriptions for this condition.[11] Despite this, an increasing amount of evidence demonstrates that antibiotics provide very little clinical benefit, with an average adverse event rate of 15% to 40% among different classes of antibiotics and severe adverse events in 3.5% of patients.[12–15] The enormous use of antibiotics can also contribute to the emergence of antibiotic-resistant bacteria.[16,17] Surgical interventions are used when patients have failed to respond appropriately to medical therapy. However, although most patients will experience improvement in symptoms and quality-of-life measures following endoscopic sinus surgery, a significant proportion (nearly 30%) will not, particularly those undergoing revision surgery.[18]

The causes of RS include infectious and allergic components but also involve environmental, general host, and local anatomic factors. Psychiatric conditions, such as depression, have also been found to be significant factors in the outcomes of patients treated with chronic RS.[19,20] Current standard treatment modalities commonly use multiple therapeutic methods to break the cycle of chronic disease. However, to date, there is no consensus as to the optimal treatment algorithm for patients with chronic RS.[21] Success in the treatment of chronic RS, unlike in acute RS, is variable and prone to relapse. Therefore, it is important to find other safe and effective treatments of RS.

There has been an explosion in the use of complementary and integrative medicine (CIM) in general over the last few decades; more than a third of Americans use some form of CIM, with annual out-of-pocket expenditures estimated to exceed $27 billion.[22–24] Surveys have also demonstrated that there is an increasing amount of interest in the use of CIM modalities specifically for the treatment of RS both in the United States[25–28] and internationally.[29–31] This finding seems to be true along the continuum of care for RS, whether before seeing an otolaryngologist or after aggressive medical and surgical therapy. There is also a wide range of therapies sought, including herbal medicine, acupuncture, homeopathy, and massage.

This article focuses on an integrative approach to RS.

PHYSIOLOGY AND ANATOMY
Diagnosis

RS can be categorized by duration of symptoms: acute (up to 4 weeks), subacute (4–12 weeks), and chronic (more than 12 weeks). Acute RS can be further categorized into viral RS or acute bacterial RS, with 4 or more episodes per year described as recurrent acute bacterial RS.[2,32–35]

Anatomy

The boundaries of the nasal cavity are the cribriform plate superiorly and the palatine processes of the maxilla inferiorly. Located on the lateral wall of the nose are the inferior, middle, superior turbinates, and, in some individuals, the supreme turbinates. The ostia for the anterior ethmoid sinuses and maxillary sinuses are beneath the middle turbinate, whereas the nasolacrimal duct opens beneath the inferior turbinates. The sphenoid ostium is located between the posteromedial border of the superior turbinate and the nasal septum. The nasal septum divides the nasal cavity and is comprised of both cartilage and bone and lined by respiratory mucosa.

The paranasal sinuses are comprised of 4 paired sinuses: maxillary, ethmoid, sphenoid, and frontal. The roof of the ethmoid sinus is the fovea ethmoidalis, which forms the floor of the anterior cranial cavity and slopes upward at an angle from the midline to extend 2 to 3 mm above the cribriform plate. The lateral wall of the ethmoid is the lamina papyracea, which is also the medial wall of the orbit. The ethmoid sinuses are comprised of numerous small air cells, which develop from evaginations of the lateral nasal wall in the embryo. There are an average of 9 ethmoid air cells present, although the number varies widely.

The ethmoid sinus can be divided into anterior and posterior groups of air cells. The anterior group of ethmoid cells includes the frontal recess, bullar, and infundibular cells. The infundibulum is the site of drainage for the frontal sinus and anterior ethmoid cells and is located lateral to the middle turbinate and anterior to the bulla. The bullar cells drain into the middle meatus via the hiatus semilunaris, a large cleft in the lateral nasal wall. The uncinate process, which forms the anterior border of the hiatus semilunaris, is a ridge of bone extending from the ascending process of the maxilla. The remaining anterior ethmoid cells drain into the middle meatus, whereas the posterior cells drain into the sphenoethmoidal recess. The vascular supply for the ethmoid sinuses is from the anterior and posterior ethmoidal arteries, and innervation of the sinuses comes from the orbital division of the fifth cranial nerve.

The maxillary sinuses are roughly triangular in shape, with boundaries of the orbital floor superiorly, the lateral nasal wall medially, and the bony lateral wall. The sinus drains into the natural ostium on the superior medial wall, which flows into the hiatus semilunaris. There may also be accessory maxillary sinus ostia in the medial sinus wall.

The frontal sinus originates from the frontal recess cells of the anterior ethmoid and at birth is often indistinguishable from these cells. The frontal sinus is usually well formed by 12 years of age but does not reach adult size until 18 to 20 years of age. The anterior table is twice as thick as the posterior table when measured in the midsagittal plane inferiorly. An intersinus septum separates the two sinuses. The sinuses drain through a nasofrontal recess into the hiatus semilunaris beneath the middle turbinate. In most adults, this recess is a mucous membrane–lined bony canal measuring 3 mm or greater.

The ostiomeatal complex includes the middle turbinate, uncinate process, middle meatus, hiatus semilunaris, and infundibulum. The drainage pathways for the frontal, anterior ethmoid, and maxillary sinuses all flow through the ostiomeatal complex. Obstruction of this relatively narrow path from polyps or other mass lesions, inflammatory edema, or purulence will result in postobstructive sinusitis involving one or more of the aforementioned sinuses.

The sphenoid sinuses originate as evaginations from the sphenoethmoidal recess. They are present at birth but do not begin to pneumatize until about 3 years of age. The development of the sinuses may continue through adulthood, and the size may vary greatly because of differences in the degree of development. The midline is often an irregularly shaped intersinus septum. Drainage is into the sphenoethmoidal recess medial to the superior turbinate. The superior boundary is the sella and pituitary fossa, whereas the lateral walls contain the optic nerve, carotid artery, and cavernous sinus. There may be bony dehiscence of the lateral wall over these structures.

Histology

The paranasal sinuses are lined by respiratory epithelium, which consists of pseudostratified ciliated columnar epithelium with goblet cells. Numerous mucous and serosanguinous glands are present. In addition to mucus, the sinus glands also secrete immunoglobulins, interferons, and lysozyme. The anterior portion of the nares and nasal septum are covered by skin with adnexa. The roof of the nasal cavity contains specialized olfactory epithelium with bipolar olfactory neurons.

Physiology

The sinus epithelium forms a mucociliary system, which supplies the nose with a mucous covering to warm and humidify inspired air. Both parasympathetic and sympathetic nerves supply this mucous blanket, which is renewed every 10 to 15 minutes.[36,37] The cilia beat 10 to 15 times per second and move the mucous blanket toward the natural ostia of the sinuses. Environmental factors influence ciliary function; humidity increases the activity, whereas dehydration and cold temperatures decrease flow.[38] Bacterial and viral proliferation may increase when there is dysfunction of the cilia and relative stasis of the mucous blanket. In addition to mucociliary dysfunction, any condition that obstructs the drainage of the sinuses (eg, polyps, inflammation, or edema of the nasal mucosa) will lead to sinusitis. Benign and malignant tumors of the nasal cavity, paranasal sinuses, and skull base can also lead to a postobstructive sinusitis of one or more of the paranasal sinuses.

Pathophysiology

A variety of host and environmental factors play a role in the development of RS. Host factors can be divided into general (genetic factors and immune deficiency), local (anatomic abnormalities, mucosal and bone inflammation), and environmental factors (air pollution, smoke, allergens, viruses, bacteria, and fungi).[39] The pathophysiology leading to RS of the maxillary and frontal sinuses usually involves a constellation of changes that lead to the obstruction of the ostiomeatal complex, including mucosal swelling and inflammation, mucous stasis, impaired mucociliary function, and microbial infection.

Lately, several different theories have emerged to describe the pathophysiology involved in chronic RS, especially of a recalcitrant nature, including inflammation, fungal-mediated hypersensitivity, bacterial biofilms, osteitis, and superantigens, with novel therapies targeted toward each of these specific areas.[40–46]

Other conditions to consider that can mimic chronic RS include gastroesophageal reflux disease, adenoiditis, Thornwaldt cyst, dental infection, granulomatous disorders, and neoplasia.[47]

SYMPTOMS

The signs and symptoms of RS can differ depending upon contributing factors and the overall duration. Acute RS often presents with purulent nasal discharge with nasal obstruction and facial pain or pressure. Additional symptoms can include hyposmia/anosmia, headache, fever, cough, aural fullness, halitosis, fatigue, and dental pain.[32] Because purulent nasal discharge cannot be used as a sole factor to distinguish between viral and bacterial infection, the illness pattern and duration should be used instead, with viral RS usually lasting less than 10 days, but acute bacterial RS being more persistent.[2,48] Chronic RS exists if these symptoms continue for greater than 12 weeks.

MEDICAL TREATMENT APPROACHES

The goals of treatment are to improve drainage, remove obstruction, promote mucociliary function, eradicate infection, reduce inflammation, and prevent complications.

Medical therapies for RS can include any of the following: intranasal or systemic steroids, topical or oral antibiotics, nasal saline irrigation, topical or systemic decongestants, antihistamines, leukotriene antagonists, mucolytics, expectorants, immunotherapy, and analgesics. If these conventional therapies are not effective and symptoms become refractory, other medical options that have been used include antifungals, proton-pump inhibitors, bacterial lysates, immunomodulators, and immunostimulants.[47,49–52] Long-term, low-dose macrolide therapy may also have a role in the treatment of chronic RS, given its demonstrated antiinflammatory effects.[53–55]

SURGICAL TREATMENT APPROACHES

Endoscopic sinus surgery is indicated for 2 reasons: (1) failed medical treatment or (2) potential or actual complications, such as the development of a mucocele, mucopyocele, orbital abscess, invasive fungal sinusitis, anatomic obstruction caused by polyps or mass lesion, or suspicion of malignancy. Substantial evidence exists that supports surgical intervention in reducing symptoms and improving quality of life in patients with RS.[56]

INTEGRATIVE TREATMENT APPROACHES AND OUTCOMES
Herbal Supplements (Single)

Pelargonium sidoides EPs 7630
In South Africa, *Pelargonium sidoides (P sidoides)* has historically been used to treat a variety of ailments, including upper respiratory tract infections like bronchitis and tuberculosis.[57] *P sidoides*, traditionally known as Umckaloabo, is rich in phenols and flavonoids, consisting of coumarins, tannins, diterpenes, and proanthocyanidins.[58–60] It has been standardized in Germany as an aqueous ethanolic extract of its root known as EPs 7630.

EPs 7630 has been shown to have significant antibacterial activity against multiresistant *Staphylococcus aureus* and antiviral effects against seasonal influenza A virus strains (H1N1, H3N2), respiratory syncytial virus, human coronavirus, parainfluenza virus, and Coxsackie virus.[58,61] Through its immunomodulatory effects, EPs 7630 has been demonstrated to specifically enhance human peripheral blood phagocyte activity as well as have antiadhesive effects through interaction with bacterial surface binding factors.[62–64]

A double-blind, randomized, multicenter trial conducted by Bachert and colleagues[65] enrolled 103 patients with radiographically and clinically confirmed acute RS and compared EPs 7630 (1:8–10; extraction solvent: ethanol 11% at a dosage of 60 drops 3 times daily for up to 22 days) with placebo. EPs 7630 was found to have superior efficacy and tolerance, based on changes in sinusitis severity scores. A Cochrane review concluded that *P sidoides* may be effective in alleviating symptoms, including headaches and nasal discharge, for acute RS and the common cold in adults.[66]

Bromelain
Bromelain, a mixture of proteolytic enzymes extracted from pineapples (*Ananas comosus*), has demonstrated antiinflammatory, antiedematous, antithrombotic, and fibrinolytic effects.[67] Three double-blind, randomized controlled trials were conducted in the 1960s on patients with acute and chronic RS, using similar protocols of 2 parallel treatment arms comparing bromelain with placebo, with each group also receiving conventional management consisting of antibiotics, decongestants, antihistamines, and analgesics.[68–70] A meta-analysis performed by Guo and colleagues[71] showed

a small but statistically significant difference in favor of adjunctive treatment with bromelain for nasal mucosal inflammation, nasal discomfort, breathing difficulty, and overall rating but not for nasal discharge.

A recent multicenter trial enrolling children less than 11 years of age with acute sinusitis had 3 treatment groups (bromelain vs bromelain + standard therapy vs standard therapy) and showed a statistically significant recovery time with bromelain monotherapy compared with other treatment groups.[72] Only one mild self-limiting allergic reaction was noted. The 1993 German Commission E monograph concluded that bromelain may be effective for "acute postoperative and post-traumatic swelling, especially of the nose and paranasal sinuses."[73]

Caution must be used when prescribing bromelain for patients already on anticoagulants because of the increased risk for bleeding as well as when prescribing various antibiotics, such as penicillin and tetracycline, because bromelain is also known to promote their absorption.[67] Moreover, bromelain strongly inhibits human cytochrome P450 2C9 (CYP2C9) activity and can, thereby, affect metabolism of its substrates.[74] Recommended dosages range from 500 to 2000 mg/d.[75]

Cineole

Cineole, or more specifically 1,8-cineole, is a monoterpene present in many plant-based essential oils and is commonly derived from *Eucalyptus globulus*; 1,8-cineole is also one of the main chemical ingredients identified in the Chinese herb *Flos magnoliae*.[76] It has been shown to enhance mucociliary clearance; block inflammation through inhibiting formation of cytokines, such as tumor necrosis factor (TNF)-alpha and interleukin-1beta; and activate antinociceptive properties, perhaps through a mechanism involving a nonopioid receptor.[77–79]

A prospective, randomized, double-blind study comparing cineole (200 mg 3 times per day) with placebo in 152 patients with acute nonpurulent RS showed a statistically significant difference in symptoms sum scores in the cineole group, in addition to a reduction in secondary symptoms, such as headache on bending, frontal headache, nasal obstruction, and nasal secretion.[80] Mild side effects, including heartburn and exanthema, were noted with cineole. The investigators concluded that cineole may serve as an integrative therapy during the first 4 days of acute RS, but antibiotics should be initiated if symptoms persist. In addition, another prospective, randomized, double-blind study demonstrated that cineole was more effective than an herbal preparation with 5 different components in the treatment of acute viral RS.[81]

Cod liver oil

Cod liver oil, which is rich in omega-3 fatty acids and vitamin D, was historically used as a remedy for rickets in the 1800s.[82] There is limited evidence for the use of cod liver oil for RS, including a 4-month, open-label study enrolling 4 children with recurrent chronic RS who were given escalating doses of cod liver oil and a multivitamin with selenium.[83,84] Three patients demonstrated a positive response with decreased sinus symptoms, fewer episodes of acute sinusitis, and fewer physician visits. The investigators concluded that cod liver oil in combination with a multivitamin containing selenium was an inexpensive, noninvasive adjunctive intervention that can be used for selected patients.

Manuka honey

Manuka honey is produced from the nectar of flowers native to Australia and New Zealand, particularly from the species of *Leptospermum*, and has potent antibacterial activity attributed to its high concentration of methylglyoxal, hyperosmolarity, hydrogen peroxide, and low pH.[85,86] It was found to have bactericidal activity against biofilms formed by *Pseudomonas aeruginosa* and *Staphylococcus aureus*, with significantly higher effects than commonly used antibiotics and may have implications for treating chronic RS.[87,88]

Thamboo and colleagues[89] studied the use of manuka honey in patients with allergic fungal RS. Thirty-four patients were treated with a topical combination of manuka honey and saline in one nostril daily for 30 days. Culture results from their ethmoid cavities were unchanged, as was their endoscopic staging. However, there was reported symptomatic improvement using the Sino-Nasal Outcome Test (SNOT)-20 as an outcome measure.

Herbal Supplements (Combination)

Sinupret

Sinupret (comprised of *Gentiana radix, Primula flos, Rumex herba, Sambucus flos,* and *Verbena herba*) is an herbal formula used widely in Germany for the treatment of respiratory infections. Approved by the German Commission E in 1994 for the treatment of acute and chronic inflammation of the paranasal sinuses, Sinupret is available as a coated tablet of 6 mg of *Gentiana radix* and 18 mg each of *Primula flos, Rumex herba, Sambucus flos,* and *Verbena herba* or as a water and alcohol extract in a proportion of 1:3:3:3:3.[73]

Sinupret has been shown to have antiviral activity in vitro against certain subtypes of viruses known to cause respiratory infections, including adenovirus, human rhinovirus, and respiratory syncytial virus and to strongly stimulate transepithelial Cl(-) secretion to maintain normal mucociliary clearance in sinonasal epithelium through the hydration of the airway surface liquid.[90,91]

Four randomized controlled trials (RCTs) evaluated Sinupret (either 2 tablets or 30 drops of liquid formula 3 times per day) as adjunctive therapy for acute RS (3 RCTs) and chronic RS (1 RCT) (Berghorn, Langer W, März RW, Bionorica GmbH, unpublished data, 1991).[92–94] A systematic review demonstrated that Sinupret may be effective as an adjunctive therapy in acute RS.[71] However, one study found no significant difference in olfactory function between patients treated with Sinupret versus placebo, although an initial therapy of oral prednisolone for 7 days had preceded the treatment intervention.[95]

Esberitox

Esberitox is an herbal extract containing *Thuja occidentalis* (white cedar), *Echinacea purpurea* and *pallida* (purple coneflower), and *Baptisia tinctoria* (wild indigo) with demonstrated immunomodulatory properties.[96]

A randomized, double-blind, placebo-controlled study showed a dose-dependent efficacy in the treatment of upper respiratory infections and, in particular, certain symptoms like rhinorrhea.[97] Another study that enrolled 90 patients with acute RS compared (1) Esberitox (3 tablets 3 times per day) and doxycycline, (2) Sinupret (5 tablets twice per day) and doxycycline, and (3) doxycycline alone and found that both groups with combination therapies had a significantly higher rate of response.[71,94] Reported adverse events included photosensitivity and gastrointestinal symptoms, such as nausea.

Myrtol

Myrtol is a standardized phytotherapeutic extract (Gelomyrtol/Gelomyrtol Forte) taken from *Pinus spp, Citrus aurantifolia,* and *Eucalyptus globulus*. It is mainly comprised of 3 monoterpenes: (+) alpha-pinene, D-limonene, and 1,8-cineole. It has been shown to inhibit 5-lipoxygenase activity as well as various mediators of the inflammatory and allergic response, including leukotriene C4 and prostaglandin E2.[98]

In a randomized, double-blind, multicenter trial, 330 patients with acute sinusitis were enrolled into one of 3 arms: (1) Myrtol extract (300 mg/d), (2) other unidentified essential oil, or (3) placebo.[99] Myrtol and the other essential oil groups both demonstrated superior efficacy to placebo based on the total symptom score of 7 items (headache, nasal secretion, nasal obstruction, pain on pressure, pain at bending over, general well-being, and fever), although there were insufficient statistical data to support this conclusion.[71] Mild to moderate adverse events that were mostly gastrointestinal in nature were reported.

Nasturtium and horseradish root

Nasturtium (*Tropaeoli majoris herba*) and horseradish root (*Armoraciae rusticanae radix*) have broad antibacterial activities against several gram-positive and gram-negative organisms, including *Haemophilus influenzae, Moraxella catarrhalis, Pseudomonas aeruginosa, Staphylococcus aureus*, and *Streptococcus pyogenes.*[100]

A prospective, multicenter, cohort study performed in children between 4 and 18 years of age with acute RS found that an herbal drug preparation, containing nasturtium and horseradish root, had similar efficacy and fewer adverse events compared with standard antibiotics.[101]

Nutrition: Ginger, Quercetin, and Epigallocatechin Gallate

Dietary polyphenols are widely available in food and well-known for their antiinflammatory effects. Both ginger and quercetin, a polyphenolic bioflavonoid commonly found in apples and onions, have potent antioxidant and antiinflammatory properties.[102,103] Mechanisms of action that have been elucidated for quercetin include suppression of the inflammatory mediator cyclooxygenase-2, inhibition of histamine release through downregulation of mast cell activity, and enhanced mucociliary clearance through augmented transepithelial chloride secretion via the cystic fibrosis transmembrane conductance regulator anion channel.[104–106]

A combination of ginger extract and green tea (*Camellia sinensis*), which is rich in epigallocatechin gallate (EGCG), showed significant antiallergy effects through the suppression of certain cytokines, such as TNF-alpha and MIP-1alpha (macrophage inflammatory protein).[107] The dietary polyphenols of [6]-gingerol, quercetin, and EGCG were found to effectively inhibit excess mucus secretion of respiratory epithelial cells while maintaining normal nasal ciliary movement.[108]

Homeopathy

Homeopathy, initially developed by German physician Samuel Christian Hahnemann at the end of the eighteenth century, is based on the principle of similars (like cures like) whereby therapeutic effects are achieved by stimulating the body's homeostatic healing response via substances that have been serially diluted and shaken. There is evidence from RCTs that homeopathy may be effective for the treatment of influenza and allergies.[109] In a recent prospective observational trial from Germany, 134 adult patients with treatment refractory chronic sinusitis were tried on different homeopathic remedies. Over the course of 8 years, the investigators found sustained improvements in quality-of-life outcomes (36-Item Short Form Health Survey) and decreased use of conventional medications, with the greatest change noted during the first 3 months of follow-up.[110]

Sinfrontal

Sinfrontal is a homeopathic remedy (containing *Cinnabaris* D4, *Ferrum phosphoricum* D3, *Mercurius solubilis* D6) that is commonly used in Germany for a variety of upper respiratory tract infections and has shown promise as a treatment for RS without the need for antibiotics. A prospective, randomized, double-blind, placebo-controlled, multicenter, clinical trial comparing Sinfrontal with placebo in 113 patients with radiography-confirmed acute maxillary sinusitis found that there was a significant difference in patients treated with Sinfrontal with no recurrence of symptoms 8 weeks after treatment.[111] Patients receiving Sinfrontal were instructed to take 1 tablet every hour until improvement was noted, with a maximum of 12 tablets per day, after which the dosing would change to 2 tablets 3 times per day. An economic analysis demonstrated that Sinfrontal can lead to substantial cost savings with markedly reduced absenteeism from work.[112]

Traditional Chinese Medicine

Traditional Chinese medicine (TCM) is a whole medical system that has been used for several millennia. The therapeutics used in TCM, such as Chinese herbal medicine and acupuncture, have grown in popularity with a parallel increase in scientific understanding and elucidation of mechanisms.[113] Specifically, the use of TCM for the treatment of disorders involving the ears, nose, and throat can be traced back as early as the fifth century BC, with several therapies that may be beneficial for RS.[114]

Acupuncture

The therapeutic effects of acupuncture primarily stem from reestablishing homeostasis of multiple physiologic cascades, whether through modulation of the immune system, inflammatory response, autonomic nervous system, neuroendocrine axis, limbic system, or pain pathway.[115–120] Although acupuncture may modulate many of these cascades during treatment of patients with RS, specific effects of improved mucociliary clearance and airway surface liquid have also been demonstrated.[121]

In a prospective randomized study, patients with nasal congestion and hypertrophic inferior turbinates were treated with acupuncture and found to have significant improvement on visual analog scale and in nasal airflow as measured by active anterior rhinomanometry.[122] Another study demonstrated a 60% reduction in sinus-related pain compared with only 30% in the placebo group.[123] Acupuncture also demonstrated beneficial results in the treatment of children with chronic maxillary sinusitis.[124]

A research team in Norway conducted 2 different studies using a similar protocol, whereby 65 patients with chronic RS were randomized into 3 arms: (1) traditional Chinese acupuncture, (2) sham acupuncture, or (3) conventional medical management with antibiotics, oral steroids, nasal saline irrigation, and local decongestants.[125,126] In both studies, there was improvement in health-related quality-of-life symptom scores in all 3 groups, although there was no overall statistically significant difference among them.

Chinese herbal medicine

Xanthii fructus (Chinese herbal name: Cang Er Zi) and *Flos magnoliae* (Chinese herbal name: Xin Yi Hua) are commonly used herbs in traditional Chinese medicine to treat RS. *Xanthii fructus* is also known as *Xanthium sibiricum* because the former is simply the fruit of the latter. From a TCM perspective, *Xanthii fructus* disperses wind and dampness and treats thick, viscous nasal discharge and sinus-related headaches, whereas *Flos magnoliae* is used to expel wind-cold and treat nasal discharge, hyposmia, sinus congestion, and headaches.[127] In fact, these two herbs are often combined and are key components of the Chinese herbal formula Cang Er Zi Wan or Cang Er Zi San, which are the pill and powder preparations, respectively.[128]

It is important to note that Chinese herbs should be used under the guidance of TCM theory. When Chinese herbs are not used according to TCM principles, severe adverse events can occur. One such example was the inappropriate use of Ephedra (Chinese name: Ma Huang) for weight loss, increased energy, and performance enhancement, when traditionally this is used only for upper respiratory infections for a short period of time, much like how pseudoephedrine is used only briefly for symptoms related to upper respiratory infections.[129]

Xanthii fructus (Chinese name: Cang Er Zi)

In a murine model, Xanthii fructus was found to exhibit (1) antiinflammatory effects through inhibiting interferon-gamma, TNF-alpha, and lipopolysaccharide-induced nitric oxide synthesis; (2) antiallergic effects through blocking mast cell–mediated histamine release; and (3) antioxidant effects through increased activities of catalase, superoxide dismutase, and glutathione peroxidase in the liver with enhanced radical scavenging and reducing activity.[130–132]

Sesquiterpene lactone and xanthatin, specific components of Xanthium sibiricum, displayed significant antibacterial activity against methicillin-resistant Staphylococcus aureus while also inhibiting other bacteria like Staphylococcus epidermidis, Klebsiella pneumoniae, Bacillus cereus, Pseudomonas aeruginosa, and Salmonella typhi.[133]

Zhao and colleagues[134,135] found that Xanthii fructus was able to modulate proinflammatory cytokines through inhibition of human mast cells and peripheral blood mononuclear cells and demonstrated that Shi-Bi-Lin, a modified version of the Chinese herbal formula Cang Er Zi San, ameliorated nasal symptoms, such as sneezing and nasal scratching, in a guinea pig model through reduced nasal thromboxane B2, eosinophil infiltration, and endothelial nitric oxide synthase activity. A double-blind, RCT enrolling 126 patients with allergic rhinitis with equal cohorts receiving Shi-Bi-Lin and placebo found that Shi-Bi-Lin significantly improved symptoms with a sustained response for at least 2 weeks after treatment.[136]

However, caution must be exercised when using either Xanthii fructus or Cang Er Zi Wan because they have been shown to lead to certain side effects like muscle spasm and hepatotoxicity and nephrotoxicity.[137,138]

Flos magnoliae (Chinese herbal name: Xin Yi Hua)

The primary bioactive components of Flos magnoliae include terpenoids, lignans, neolignans, epimagnolin, and fargesin.[139] Neolignans have been found to have antiinflammatory effects through mechanisms of action different from steroids, while epimagnolin and fargesin decrease production of nitric oxide, a potent mediator in inflammation, through inhibition of inducible nitric oxide synthase expression.[140,141] Flos magnoliae also demonstrates antiallergy activity via inhibition of immediate-type hypersensitivity reactions through blocking mast cell degranulation.[142] As an essential oil, its main chemical ingredients have been identified as 1,8-cineole, sabinene, beta-pinene, alpha-pinene, and transcaryophyllene.[76]

Chinese herbal supplements (postoperative)

Bi Yuan Shu is a Chinese herbal liquid mixture comprised of an unknown number of herbs but is reported to include at least Magnolia liliflora, Xanthium strumarium, Astragalus membranaceus, Angelica dahurica, and Scutellaria baicalensis. A multicenter RCT divided 340 postoperative patients with chronic RS and nasal polyps who had undergone endoscopic sinus surgery into 2 groups, with both groups receiving antibiotics and topical steroids; the test group was also treated with Bi Yuan Shu (10 mL 3 times per day).[143] Adjunctive treatment with Bi Yuan Shu was found to have significantly higher response rates on days 7, 14, 30, and 60 for purulent nasal discharge, breathing difficulty, pain, hyposmia, and halitosis, with positive trends noted for fever and cough.[71]

Table 1
Acupuncture point locations and indications

Name	Location	Purpose
Sinus Specific		
LI-4 (He Gu)	On the dorsum of the hand, at the midpoint of the second metacarpal bone, near its radial border	Nasal congestion, rhinorrhea, headache, wind-cold TCM pattern, neck pain, facial pain, stress
GB-20 (Feng Chi)	Near the base of skull, in the depression between the origins of the sternocleidomastoid and trapezius muscles	Nasal congestion, rhinorrhea, headache, wind-cold TCM pattern
ST-3 (Ju Liao)	Lateral to the nasolabial groove, level with the lower border of the ala nasi, directly inferior to the midpoint of the eye	Pain and swelling involving the maxillary sinus
LI-20 (Ying Xiang)	In the nasolabial groove, at the level of the midpoint of the lateral border of the ala nasi	Nasal congestion, rhinorrhea, anosmia
UB-2 (Zan Zhu)	Superior to the inner canthus, in a depression at the medial border of the eyebrow	Rhinitis, pain and swelling of the frontal sinus, frontal headache, wind TCM pattern
DU-23 (Shang Xing)	At the top of the head on the midline, 1 finger breadth posterior to the anterior hairline	Nasal obstruction and discharge, headache, rhinitis
Quality-of-Life Improvement		
LI-11 (Qu Chi)	With the elbow flexed, at the lateral end of the transverse cubital crease	Loss of voice, sore throat, heat TCM pattern
SJ-5 (Wai Guan)	Three finger breadths proximal to the wrist crease, on the radial side of the extensor digitorum communis tendons	Headache, neck pain, wind-heat TCM pattern
GB-21 (Jian Jing)	Midway between the spinous process of C7 and the tip of the acromion, at the highest point of the trapezius muscle	Neck pain, cough, phlegm
P-6 (Nei Guan)	Three finger breadths proximal to the wrist crease in between the tendons of the palmaris longus and flexor carpi radialis	Anxiety, pain of the head and neck, cough
ST-36 (Zu San Li)	With the knee extended, 4 finger breadths below the patella, just lateral to the tibia within the tibialis anterior muscle	Fatigue, vitality
LIV-3 (Tai Chong)	On the dorsum of the foot, in the depression distal to the junction of the first and second metatarsal bones	Headache, insomnia, stress, irritability

From Suh JD, Wu AW, Taw MB, et al. Treatment of recalcitrant chronic rhinosinusitis with integrative east-west medicine: a pilot study. Arch Otolaryngol Head Neck Surg 2012;138(3):294–300, with permission; and *Data from* Deadman P, Al-Khafaji M, Baker K. A manual of acupuncture. 2nd edition. Hove (England): Journal of Chinese Medicine Publications; 2001.

Another study assessing the efficacy of Chinese herbal medicine in the care of patients after undergoing endoscopic sinus surgery enrolled 97 patients into one of 3 treatment arms: (1) Tsang-Erh-San extract granules and Houttuynia extract powder, (2) oral amoxicillin, or (3) placebo. The study found no benefit of either treatment group over placebo.[144]

MULTI-MODAL APPROACHES

A multicenter, nonrandomized study of 63 patients with acute RS comparing multiple conventional (antibiotics, secretolytics and sympathomimetics) with combination complementary (Sinupret and homeopathic remedy, Cinnabaris 3X) therapies demonstrated similar effectiveness based on patients' self-assessment score, physicians' score, and HCG-5 questionnaire.[145] However, the only validated outcome parameter was the HCG-5 quality-of-life instrument. Other limitations with this study included a small sample size and lack of randomization and blinding.

Recently, a pilot study at the University of California, Los Angeles was conducted using integrative East-West medicine to treat patients with recalcitrant chronic RS.[146] Eleven patients underwent 8 weekly sessions of sequential acupuncture (**Table 1**) and therapeutic acupressure style massage and had received education consisting of dietary modification, lifestyle changes, and self-acupressure. Four items on the SNOT-20 (need to blow nose, runny nose, reduced concentration, and frustrated/restless/irritable) and 3 of 8 domains on the SF-36 (role physical, vitality, and social functioning) showed a statistically significant difference, whereas trends of improvement were noted in most other elements on both quality-of-life instruments. Although the data looks promising, this study was also limited by its small size and lack of randomization and control group.

PATIENT SELF-TREATMENTS

Lifestyle modifications can also be conducive toward achieving optimal sinus health and function. These modifications include regular aerobic exercise, adequate hydration, steam inhalation, stress management, and good-quality sleep. Minimizing exposure to pollution, smoke, and environmental toxins as well as incorporating nutritional changes, such as consuming an antiinflammatory diet and avoiding dairy products, refined sugars, and processed foods, are important.[147] A regular spiritual practice, such as prayer, is also beneficial, along with anger management and attitudes of forgiveness, gratitude, and optimism.[148] Self-acupressure of certain acupoints can also be helpful to reduce sinus-related symptoms (see **Table 1**).

SUMMARY

As we gain a greater understanding of the complex pathogenesis of RS, what is becoming apparent is a shift in philosophic paradigm. Our previous reductionist models of disease and health are being replaced by holism, systems biology, and complex, nonlinear dynamics.[149–151] Holism is a central philosophic underpinning of integrative medicine and many CIM modalities, such as TCM.

We now see this paradigm shift in our approach to RS. No longer is the medical community looking at the diagnosis of RS as solely an infectious process but rather as complex and multifactorial.[152] For example, Palmer[41] elegantly describes this transition whereby "generations of doctors and scientists were taught to envision bacteria as single cells that float or swim through some fluid … in fact, rhinologists continue to foster this view"; however, "structured community of cells enclosed in a matrix of polysaccharides, nucleic acids and proteins."[153] Biofilms demonstrate cell-to-cell signaling, a phenomenon known as "quorum sensing."[154] Such is an example of complexity science and holism.

The therapeutic repertoire, likewise, has broadened significantly from antibiotics alone as the mainstay of treatment to the use of multiple therapies to act on different pathophysiological facets of RS. Integrative medicine provides an expanded approach and armamentarium to help patients with RS, whether acute, chronic, or recalcitrant.

Summary box: recommendations for clinicians and algorithm for CIM treatment	
Dietary recommendations	• [6]-Gingerol: as ginger tea, soup, or food; consider as dietary supplement
	• Quercetin: as food (eg, apples, onions); consider as dietary supplement
	• EGCG: as green tea (*Camellia sinensis*); consider as dietary supplement
	• Horseradish: consider as a condiment to food
Medical treatments	• Intranasal or systemic steroids
	• Topical or oral antibiotics
	• Nasal saline irrigation
	• Topical or systemic decongestants
	• Antihistamines
	• Leukotriene antagonists
	• Mucolytics
	• Expectorants
	• Immunotherapy
	• Analgesics
If recalcitrant, consider	• Endoscopic sinus surgery
	• Antifungals
	• Proton-pump inhibitors
	• Bacterial lysates
	• Immunomodulators and immunostimulants
	• Long-term, low-dose macrolide therapy for antiinflammatory effects
Herbal supplements (starting with strongest evidence)	• *Pelargonium sidoides* EPs 7630: 60 drops 3 times daily, up to 3 weeks
	• Sinupret: either 2 tablets or 30 drops of liquid formula 3 times per day
	• Sinfrontal: 1 tablet every hour until improvement noted, after which change to 2 tablets 3 times per day (maximum of 12 tablets daily), up to 3 weeks
	• Bromelain: 500–2000 mg/d
	• Cineole: 200 mg 3 times per day (consider using during first 4 days of acute rhinosinusitis)

	• Esberitox: 3 tablets 3 times per day
	• Myrtol extract: 300 mg/d
	• Consider cod liver oil with multivitamin containing selenium for children with recurrent, chronic rhinosinusitis
	• Consider topical manuka honey
TCM	• Acupuncture: trial of 8 weekly sessions
	• Acupressure style massage
	• Consider Chinese herbal medicine
	○ *Xanthii fructus* (Chinese name: Cang Er Zi)
	○ *Flos magnoliae* (Chinese herbal name: Xin Yi Hua)
	• Postoperative (status-post endoscopic sinus surgery)
	○ Consider Bi Yuan Shu (10 mL 3 times per day) as adjunctive therapy
Lifestyle recommendations	• Minimize exposure to pollution, smoke, and environmental toxins
	• Adequate hydration
	• Steam inhalation
	• Avoidance of dairy products, refined sugars, and processed foods
	• Regular aerobic exercise
	• Stress management
	• Good-quality sleep
	• Regular spiritual practice, such as prayer
	• Expressing gratitude, forgiveness, and optimism
	• Anger management
	• Self-acupressure

REFERENCES

1. Lanza DC, Kennedy DW. Adult rhinosinusitis defined. Otolaryngol Head Neck Surg 1997;117(3 Pt 2):S1–7.
2. Rosenfeld RM, Andes D, Bhattacharyya N, et al. Clinical practice guideline: adult sinusitis [review]. Otolaryngol Head Neck Surg 2007;137(Suppl 3): S32–45.
3. Pleis JR, Lucas JW, Ward BW. Summary health statistics for U.S. adults: National Health Interview Survey, 2008. National Center for Health Statistics. Vital Health Stat 10 2009;(242):1–157.
4. Cherry DK, Hing E, Woodwell DA, et al. National Ambulatory Medical Care Survey: 2006 summary. National Center for Health Statistics. Natl Health Stat Report 2008;(3):1–29.
5. Cullen KA, Hall MJ, Golosinskiy A. Ambulatory surgery in the United States, 2006. National Health Statistics Report. Vital Health Stat 2009;(11):1–28.

6. Gliklich RE, Metson R. The health impact of chronic sinusitis in patients seeking otolaryngologic care. Otolaryngol Head Neck Surg 1995;113(1):104–9.
7. Senior BA, Glaze C, Benninger MS. Use of the Rhinosinusitis Disability Index (RSDI) in rhinologic disease. Am J Rhinol 2001;15(1):15–20.
8. Bhattacharyya N. Incremental health care utilization and expenditures for chronic rhinosinusitis in the United States. Ann Otol Rhinol Laryngol 2011; 120(7):423–7.
9. Anand VK. Epidemiology and economic impact of rhinosinusitis. Ann Otol Rhinol Laryngol Suppl 2004;193:3–5.
10. Anon JB, Jacobs MR, Poole MD, et al. Sinus and Allergy Health Partnership (SAHP). Antimicrobial treatment guidelines for acute bacterial rhinosinusitis. Otolaryngol Head Neck Surg 2004;130(Suppl 1):1–45.
11. Ahovuo-Saloranta A, Borisenko OV, Kovanen N, et al. Antibiotics for acute maxillary sinusitis. Cochrane Database Syst Rev 2008;(2):CD000243.
12. Small CB, Bachert C, Lund VJ, et al. Judicious antibiotic use and intranasal corticosteroids in acute rhinosinusitis. Am J Med 2007;120(4):289–94.
13. Piromchai P, Thanaviratananich S, Laopaiboon M. Systemic antibiotics for chronic rhinosinusitis without nasal polyps in adults. Cochrane Database Syst Rev 2011;(5):CD008233.
14. Ip S, Fu L, Balk E, et al. Update on acute bacterial rhinosinusitis. Evidence report/technology assessment No. 124. AHRQ Publication No. 05-E020-2. Rockville (MD): Agency for Healthcare Research and Quality; 2005.
15. Poole MD. Acute bacterial rhinosinusitis: clinical impact of resistance and susceptibility. Am J Med 2004;117(Suppl 3A):29S–38S.
16. Kunin CM. Resistance to antimicrobial drugs–a worldwide calamity. Ann Intern Med 1993;118(7):557–61.
17. Smith TL, Litvack JR, Hwang PH, et al. Determinants of outcomes of sinus surgery: a multi-institutional prospective cohort study. Otolaryngol Head Neck Surg 2010;142(1):55–63.
18. Brandsted R, Sindwani R. Impact of depression on disease-specific symptoms and quality of life in patients with chronic rhinosinusitis. Am J Rhinol 2007;21(1): 50–4.
19. Davis GE, Yueh B, Walker E, et al. Psychiatric distress amplifies symptoms after surgery for chronic rhinosinusitis. Otolaryngol Head Neck Surg 2005;132(2): 189–96.
20. Bhattacharyya N. Clinical and symptom criteria for the accurate diagnosis of chronic rhinosinusitis. Laryngoscope 2006;116(7 Pt 2 Suppl 110):1–22.
21. Eisenberg DM, Davis RB, Ettner S, et al. Trends in alternative medicine use in the United States, 1990-1997: results of a follow-up national survey. JAMA 1998;280(18):1569–75.
22. Eisenberg DM, Kessler RC, Foster C, et al. Unconventional medicine in the United States. Prevalence, costs, and patterns of use. N Engl J Med 1993; 328(4):246–52.
23. Tindle HA, Davis RB, Phillips RS, et al. Trends in use of complementary and alternative medicine by US adults: 1997-2002. Altern Ther Health Med 2005; 11(1):42–9.
24. Barnes PM, Powell-Griner E. Complementary and alternative medicine use among adults: United States, 2002. Adv Data. Vital Health Stat 2004;(343):1–19.
25. Krouse JH, Krouse HJ. Patient use of traditional and complementary therapies in treating rhinosinusitis before consulting an otolaryngologist. Laryngoscope 1999;109(8):1223–7.

26. Asher BF, Seidman M, Snyderman C. Complementary and alternative medicine in otolaryngology. Laryngoscope 2001;111(8):1383–9.
27. Pletcher SD, Goldberg AN, Lee J, et al. Use of acupuncture in the treatment of sinus and nasal symptoms: results of a practitioner survey. Am J Rhinol 2006; 20(2):235–7.
28. Blanc PD, Trupin L, Earnest G, et al. Alternative therapies among adults with a reported diagnosis of asthma or rhinosinusitis: data from a population-based survey. Chest 2001;120(5):1461–7.
29. Rotenberg BW, Bertens KA. Use of complementary and alternative medical therapies for chronic rhinosinusitis: a Canadian perspective. J Otolaryngol Head Neck Surg 2010;39(5):586–93.
30. Newton JR, Santangeli L, Shakeel M, et al. Use of complementary and alternative medicine by patients attending a rhinology outpatient clinic. Am J Rhinol Allergy 2009;23(1):59–63.
31. Yakirevitch A, Bedrin L, Migirov L, et al. Use of alternative medicine in Israeli chronic rhinosinusitis patients. J Otolaryngol Head Neck Surg 2009;38(4):517–20.
32. Report of the Rhinosinusitis Task Force Committee Meeting. Alexandria, Virginia, August 17, 1996. Otolaryngol Head Neck Surg 1997;117(3 Pt 2):S1–68.
33. Fokkens W, Lund V, Mullol J. European position paper on rhinosinusitis and nasal polyps 2007. Rhinol Suppl 2007;(20):1–136.
34. Benninger MS, Ferguson BJ, Hadley JA, et al. Adult chronic rhinosinusitis: definitions, diagnosis, epidemiology and pathophysiology. Otolaryngol Head Neck Surg 2003;129(Suppl 3):S1–32.
35. Meltzer EO, Hamilos DL, Hadley JA, et al. Rhinosinusitis: establishing definitions for clinical research and patient care. Otolaryngol Head Neck Surg 2004; 131(Suppl 6):S1–62.
36. Hilding AC. The role of the respiratory mucosa in health and disease. Minn Med 1967;50(6):915–9.
37. Loehrl TA. Autonomic function and dysfunction of the nose and sinuses. Otolaryngol Clin North Am 2005;38(6):1155–61.
38. Grossan M. The saccharin test of nasal mucociliary function. Eye Ear Nose Throat Mon 1975;54(11):415–7.
39. Kennedy DW. Pathogenesis of chronic rhinosinusitis. Ann Otol Rhinol Laryngol Suppl 2004;193:6–9.
40. Van Crombruggen K, Zhang N, Gevaert P, et al. Pathogenesis of chronic rhinosinusitis: inflammation. J Allergy Clin Immunol 2011;128(4):728–32.
41. Palmer JN. Bacterial biofilms: do they play a role in chronic sinusitis? Otolaryngol Clin North Am 2005;38(6):1193–201, viii.
42. Ponikau JU, Sherris DA, Kern EB, et al. The diagnosis and incidence of allergic fungal sinusitis. Mayo Clin Proc 1999;74(9):877–84.
43. Luong A, Marple B. The role of fungi in chronic rhinosinusitis. Otolaryngol Clin North Am 2005;38(6):1203–13.
44. Chiu AG. Osteitis in chronic rhinosinusitis. Otolaryngol Clin North Am 2005; 38(6):1237–42.
45. Seiberling KA, Grammer L, Kern RC. Chronic rhinosinusitis and superantigens. Otolaryngol Clin North Am 2005;38(6):1215–36, ix.
46. Bachert C, Gevaert P, Holtappels G, et al. Total and specific IgE in nasal polyps is related to local eosinophilic inflammation. J Allergy Clin Immunol 2001;107(4): 607–14.
47. Ferguson BJ, Otto BA, Pant H. When surgery, antibiotics, and steroids fail to resolve chronic rhinosinusitis. Immunol Allergy Clin North Am 2009;29(4):719–32.

48. Lacroix JS, Ricchetti A, Lew D, et al. Symptoms and clinical and radiological signs predicting the presence of pathogenic bacteria in acute rhinosinusitis. Acta Otolaryngol 2002;122(2):192–6.
49. Desrosiers MY, Kilty SJ. Treatment alternatives for chronic rhinosinusitis persisting after ESS: what to do when antibiotics, steroids and surgery fail. Rhinology 2008;46(1):3–14.
50. Lund VJ. Maximal medical therapy for chronic rhinosinusitis. Otolaryngol Clin North Am 2005;38(6):1301–10, x.
51. Statham MM, Seiden A. Potential new avenues of treatment for chronic rhinosinusitis: an anti-inflammatory approach. Otolaryngol Clin North Am 2005;38(6):1351–65, xi.
52. Woodbury K, Ferguson BJ. Recalcitrant chronic rhinosinusitis: investigation and management. Curr Opin Otolaryngol Head Neck Surg 2011;19(1):1–5.
53. Suzuki H, Ikeda K. Mode of action of long-term low-dose macrolide therapy for chronic sinusitis in the light of neutrophil recruitment. Curr Drug Targets Inflamm Allergy 2002;1(1):117–26.
54. Cervin A, Wallwork B. Macrolide therapy of chronic rhinosinusitis. Rhinology 2007;45(4):259–67.
55. Tamaoki J, Kadota J. Takizawa. Clinical implications of the immunomodulatory effects of macrolides. Am J Med 2004;117(Suppl 9A):5S–11S.
56. Smith TL, Batra PS, Seiden AM, et al. Evidence supporting endoscopic sinus surgery in the management of adult chronic rhinosinusitis: a systematic review. Am J Rhinol 2005;19(6):537–43.
57. Bladt S, Wagner H. From the Zulu medicine to the European phytomedicine Umckaloabo. Phytomedicine 2007;14(Suppl 6):2.
58. Kolodziej H. Fascinating metabolic pools of Pelargonium sidoides and Pelargonium reniforme, traditional and phytomedicinal sources of the herbal medicine Umckaloabo. Phytomedicine 2007;14(Suppl 6):9–17.
59. Janecki A, Kolodziej H. Anti-adhesive activities of flavan-3-ols and proanthocyanidins in the interaction of group A-streptococci and human epithelial cells. Molecules 2010;15(10):7139–52.
60. Kolodziej H, Kayser O, Radtke OA, et al. Pharmacological profile of extracts of Pelargonium sidoides and their constituents. Phytomedicine 2003;10(Suppl 4):18–24.
61. Michaelis M, Doerr HW, Cinatl J Jr. Investigation of the influence of EPs® 7630, a herbal drug preparation from Pelargonium sidoides, on replication of a broad panel of respiratory viruses. Phytomedicine 2011;18(5):384–6.
62. Kayser O, Kolodziej H, Kiderlen AF. Immunomodulatory principles of Pelargonium sidoides. Phytother Res 2001;15(2):122–6.
63. Conrad A, Hansmann C, Engels I, et al. Extract of Pelargonium sidoides (EPs 7630) improves phagocytosis, oxidative burst, and intracellular killing of human peripheral blood phagocytes in vitro. Phytomedicine 2007;14(Suppl 6):46–51.
64. Janecki A, Conrad A, Engels I, et al. Evaluation of an aqueous-ethanolic extract from Pelargonium sidoides (EPs® 7630) for its activity against group A-streptococci adhesion to human HEp-2 epithelial cells. J Ethnopharmacol 2011;133(1):147–52.
65. Bachert C, Schapowal A, Funk P, et al. Treatment of acute rhinosinusitis with the preparation from Pelargonium sidoides EPs 7630: a randomized, double-blind, placebo-controlled trial. Rhinology 2009;47(1):51–8.
66. Timmer A, Günther J, Rücker G, et al. Pelargonium sidoides extract for acute respiratory tract infections. Cochrane Database Syst Rev 2008;(3):CD006323.

67. Maurer HR. Bromelain: biochemistry, pharmacology and medical use. Cell Mol Life Sci 2001;58(9):1234–45.
68. Seltzer AP. Adjunctive use of bromelains in sinusitis: a controlled study. Eye Ear Nose Throat Mon 1967;46(10):1281–8.
69. Ryan RE. A double-blind clinical evaluation of bromelains in the treatment of acute sinusitis. Headache 1967;7(1):13–7.
70. Taub SJ. The use of bromelains in sinusitis: a double-blind clinical evaluation. Eye Ear Nose Throat Mon 1967;46(3):361–2.
71. Guo R, Canter PH, Ernst E. Herbal medicines for the treatment of rhinosinusitis: a systematic review. Otolaryngol Head Neck Surg 2006;135(4):496–506.
72. Braun JM, Schneider B, Beuth HJ. Therapeutic use, efficiency and safety of the proteolytic pineapple enzyme bromelain-POS in children with acute sinusitis in Germany. In Vivo 2005;19(2):417–21.
73. Schulz V, Hänsel R, Blumenthal M, et al. Rational phytotherapy: a physicians' guide to herbal medicine. 5th edition. Heidelberg (Germany): Springer; 2004.
74. Hidaka M, Nagata M, Kawano Y, et al. Inhibitory effects of fruit juices on cytochrome P450 2C9 activity in vitro. Biosci Biotechnol Biochem 2008;72(2):406–11.
75. Kelly GS. Bromelain: a literature review and discussion of its therapeutic applications. Alt Med Rev 1996;1(4):243–57.
76. Wu W. GC-MS analysis of chemical components in essential oil from Flos magnoliae. Zhong Yao Cai 2000;23(9):538–41 [in Chinese].
77. Dorow P, Weiss T, Felix R, et al. Effect of a secretolytic and a combination of pinene, limonene and cineole on mucociliary clearance in patients with chronic obstructive pulmonary disease. Arzneimittelforschung 1987;37(12):1378–81 [in German].
78. Juergens UR, Engelen T, Racké K, et al. Inhibitory activity of 1,8-cineol (eucalyptol) on cytokine production in cultured human lymphocytes and monocytes. Pulm Pharmacol Ther 2004;17(5):281–7.
79. Santos FA, Rao VS. Antiinflammatory and antinociceptive effects of 1,8-cineole a terpenoid oxide present in many plant essential oils. Phytother Res 2000; 14(4):240–4.
80. Kehrl W, Sonnemann U, Dethlefsen U. Therapy for acute nonpurulent rhinosinusitis with cineole: results of a double-blind, randomized, placebo-controlled trial. Laryngoscope 2004;114(4):738–42.
81. Tesche S, Metternich F, Sonnemann U, et al. The value of herbal medicines in the treatment of acute non-purulent rhinosinusitis. Results of a double-blind, randomised, controlled trial. Eur Arch Otorhinolaryngol 2008;265(11):1355–9.
82. Rajakumar K. Vitamin D, cod-liver oil, sunlight, and rickets: a historical perspective. Pediatrics 2003;112(2):e132–5.
83. Karkos PD, Leong SC, Arya AK, et al. 'Complementary ENT': a systematic review of commonly used supplements. J Laryngol Otol 2007;121(8):779–82.
84. Linday LA, Dolitsky JN, Shindledecker RD. Nutritional supplements as adjunctive therapy for children with chronic/recurrent sinusitis: pilot research. Int J Pediatr Otorhinolaryngol 2004;68(6):785–93.
85. Irish J, Blair S, Carter DA. The antibacterial activity of honey derived from Australian flora. PLoS One 2011;6(3):e18229.
86. Kwakman PH, Zaat SA. Antibacterial components of honey. IUBMB Life 2012; 64(1):48–55. http://dx.doi.org/10.1002/iub.578.
87. Alandejani T, Marsan J, Ferris W, et al. Effectiveness of honey on Staphylococcus aureus and Pseudomonas aeruginosa biofilms. Otolaryngol Head Neck Surg 2009;141(1):114–8.

88. Jervis-Bardy J, Foreman A, Bray S, et al. Methylglyoxal-infused honey mimics the anti-Staphylococcus aureus biofilm activity of manuka honey: potential implication in chronic rhinosinusitis. Laryngoscope 2011;121(5):1104–7.
89. Thamboo A, Thamboo A, Philpott C, et al. Single-blind study of manuka honey in allergic fungal rhinosinusitis. J Otolaryngol Head Neck Surg 2011;40(3):238–43.
90. Glatthaar-Saalmüller B, Rauchhaus U, Rode S, et al. Antiviral activity in vitro of two preparations of the herbal medicinal product Sinupret against viruses causing respiratory infections. Phytomedicine 2011;19(1):1–7.
91. Virgin F, Zhang S, Schuster D, et al. The bioflavonoid compound, Sinupret, stimulates transepithelial chloride transport in vitro and in vivo. Laryngoscope 2010; 120(5):1051–6.
92. Richstein A, Mann W. Treatment of chronic sinusitis with Sinupret. Therapie der Gegenwart 1980;119(9):1055–60 [in German].
93. Neubauer N, März RW. Placebo-controlled, randomized double-blind clinical trial with Sinupret sugar coated tablets on the basis of a therapy with antibiotics and decongestant nasal drops in acute sinusitis. Phytomedicine 1994;1:177–81.
94. Zimmer M. Gezielte konservative Therapie der akuten Sinusitis in der HNO-Praxis. Therapiewoche 1985;35:4042–408.
95. Reden J, El-Hifnawi DJ, Zahnert T, et al. The effect of a herbal combination of primrose, gentian root, vervain, elder flowers, and sorrel on olfactory function in patients with a sinonasal olfactory dysfunction. Rhinology 2011;49(3):342–6.
96. Wüstenberg P, Henneicke-von Zepelin HH, Köhler G, et al. Efficacy and mode of action of an immunomodulator herbal preparation containing Echinacea, wild indigo, and white cedar. Adv Ther 1999;16(1):51–70.
97. Naser B, Lund B, Henneicke-von Zepelin HH, et al. A randomized, double-blind, placebo-controlled, clinical dose-response trial of an extract of Baptisia, Echinacea and Thuja for the treatment of patients with common cold. Phytomedicine 2005;12(10):715–22.
98. Beuscher N, Kietzmann M, Bien E, et al. Interference of myrtol standardized with inflammatory and allergic mediators. Arzneimittelforschung 1998;48(10): 985–9.
99. Federspil P, Wulkow R, Zimmermann T. Effects of standardized Myrtol in therapy of acute sinusitis–results of a double-blind, randomized multicenter study compared with placebo. Laryngorhinootologie 1997;76(1):23–7 [in German].
100. Conrad A, Kolberg T, Engels I, et al. In vitro study to evaluate the antibacterial activity of a combination of the haulm of nasturtium (Tropaeoli majoris herba) and of the roots of horseradish (Armoraciae rusticanae radix). Arzneimittelforschung 2006;56(12):842–9 [in German].
101. Goos KH, Albrecht U, Schneider B. On-going investigations on efficacy and safety profile of a herbal drug containing nasturtium herb and horseradish root in acute sinusitis, acute bronchitis and acute urinary tract infection in children in comparison with other antibiotic treatments. Arzneimittelforschung 2007;57(4):238–46 [in German].
102. Dugasani S, Pichika MR, Nadarajah VD, et al. Comparative antioxidant and anti-inflammatory effects of [6]-gingerol, [8]-gingerol, [10]-gingerol and [6]-shogaol. J Ethnopharmacol 2010;127(2):515–20.
103. Chirumbolo S. The role of quercetin, flavonols and flavones in modulating inflammatory cell function. Inflamm Allergy Drug Targets 2010;9(4):263–85.
104. Xiao X, Shi D, Liu L, et al. Quercetin suppresses cyclooxygenase-2 expression and angiogenesis through inactivation of P300 signaling. PLoS One 2011;6(8): e22934.

105. Park HH, Lee S, Son HY, et al. Flavonoids inhibit histamine release and expression of proinflammatory cytokines in mast cells. Arch Pharm Res 2008;31(10):1303–11.
106. Zhang S, Smith N, Schuster D, et al. Quercetin increases cystic fibrosis transmembrane conductance regulator-mediated chloride transport and ciliary beat frequency: therapeutic implications for chronic rhinosinusitis. Am J Rhinol Allergy 2011;25(5):307–12.
107. Maeda-Yamamoto M, Ema K, Shibuichi I. In vitro and in vivo anti-allergic effects of 'benifuuki' green tea containing O-methylated catechin and ginger extract enhancement. Cytotechnology 2007;55(2–3):135–42.
108. Chang JH, Song KJ, Kim HJ, et al. Dietary polyphenols affect MUC5AC expression and ciliary movement in respiratory cells and nasal mucosa. Am J Rhinol Allergy 2010;24(2):e59–62.
109. Jonas WB, Kaptchuk TJ, Linde K. A critical overview of homeopathy. Ann Intern Med 2003;138(5):393–9.
110. Witt CM, Lüdtke R, Willich SN. Homeopathic treatment of patients with chronic sinusitis: a prospective observational study with 8 years follow-up. BMC Ear Nose Throat Disord 2009;9:7.
111. Zabolotnyi DI, Kneis KC, Richardson A, et al. Efficacy of a complex homeopathic medication (Sinfrontal) in patients with acute maxillary sinusitis: a prospective, randomized, double-blind, placebo-controlled, multicenter clinical trial. Explore 2007;3(2):98–109.
112. Kneis KC, Gandjour A. Economic evaluation of Sinfrontal in the treatment of acute maxillary sinusitis in adults. Appl Health Econ Health Policy 2009;7(3):181–91.
113. Kaptchuk TJ. Acupuncture: theory, efficacy, and practice. Ann Intern Med 2002;136(5):374–83.
114. Yap L, Pothula VB, Warner J, et al. The root and development of otorhinolaryngology in traditional Chinese medicine. Eur Arch Otorhinolaryngol 2009;266:1353–9.
115. Cabioğlu MT, Cetin BE. Acupuncture and immunomodulation. Am J Chin Med 2008;36(1):25–36.
116. Zijlstra FJ, van den Berg-de Lange I, Huygen FJ, et al. Anti-inflammatory actions of acupuncture. Mediators Inflamm 2003;12(2):59–69.
117. Carpenter RJ, Dillard J, Zion AS, et al. The acute effects of acupuncture upon autonomic balance in healthy subjects. Am J Chin Med 2010;38(5):839–47.
118. Zhou W, Longhurst JC. Neuroendocrine mechanisms of acupuncture in the treatment of hypertension. Evid Based Complement Alternat Med 2012;2012:878673.
119. Hui KK, Marina O, Liu J, et al. Acupuncture, the limbic system, and the anticorrelated networks of the brain. Auton Neurosci 2010;157(1–2):81–90.
120. Zhao ZQ. Neural mechanism underlying acupuncture analgesia. Prog Neurobiol 2008;85(4):355–7.
121. Tai S, Wang J, Sun F, et al. Effect of needle puncture and electro-acupuncture on mucociliary clearance in anesthetized quails. BMC Complement Altern Med 2006;6:4.
122. Sertel S, Bergmann Z, Ratzlaff K, et al. Acupuncture for nasal congestion: a prospective, randomized, double-blind, placebo-controlled clinical pilot study. Am J Rhinol Allergy 2009;23(6):e23–8.
123. Lundeberg T, Laurell G, Thomas M. Effect of acupuncture on sinus pain and experimentally induced pain. Ear Nose Throat J 1988;67(8):565–6, 571–2, 574–5.

124. Pothman R, Yeh HL. The effects of treatment with antibiotics, laser and acupuncture upon chronic maxillary sinusitis in children. Am J Chin Med 1982;10(1-4): 55-8.

125. Stavem K, Røssberg E, Larsson PG. Health-related quality of life in a trial of acupuncture, sham acupuncture and conventional treatment for chronic sinusitis. BMC Res Notes 2008;1:37.

126. Røssberg E, Larsson PG, Birkeflet O, et al. Comparison of traditional Chinese acupuncture, minimal acupuncture at non-acupoints and conventional treatment for chronic sinusitis. Complement Ther Med 2005;13(1):4-10.

127. Bensky D, Gamble A. Chinese herbal medicine: Materia Medica. Revised edition. Seattle (WA): Eastland Press; 1993.

128. Bensky D, Barolet R. Chinese herbal medicine: formulas & strategies. Seattle (WA): Eastland Press; 1990.

129. Haller CA, Benowitz NL. Adverse cardiovascular and central nervous system events associated with dietary supplements containing ephedra alkaloids. N Engl J Med 2000;343(25):1833-8.

130. An HJ, Jeong HJ, Lee EH, et al. Xanthii fructus inhibits inflammatory responses in LPS-stimulated mouse peritoneal macrophages. Inflammation 2004;28(5): 263-70.

131. Hong SH, Jeong HJ, Kim HM. Inhibitory effects of Xanthii fructus extract on mast cell-mediated allergic reaction in murine model. J Ethnopharmacol 2003; 88(2-3):229-34.

132. Huang MH, Wang BS, Chiu CS, et al. Antioxidant, antinociceptive, and anti-inflammatory activities of Xanthii Fructus extract. J Ethnopharmacol 2011; 135(2):545-52.

133. Sato Y, Oketani H, Yamada T, et al. A xanthanolide with potent antibacterial activity against methicillin-resistant Staphylococcus aureus. J Pharm Pharmacol 1997;49(10):1042-4.

134. Zhao Y, Yang H, Zheng YB, et al. The effects of Fructus Xanthii extract on cytokine release from human mast cell line (HMC-1) and peripheral blood mononuclear cells. Immunopharmacol Immunotoxicol 2008;30(3):543-52.

135. Zhao Y, van Hasselt CA, Woo JK, et al. Effect of a Chinese herbal formula, Shi-Bi-Lin, on an experimental model of allergic rhinitis. Ann Allergy Asthma Immunol 2006;96(6):844-50.

136. Zhao Y, Woo KS, Ma KH, et al. Treatment of perennial allergic rhinitis using Shi-Bi-Lin, a Chinese herbal formula. J Ethnopharmacol 2009;122(1):100-5.

137. West PL, Mckeown NJ, Hendrickson RG. Muscle spasm associated with therapeutic use of Cang Er Zi Wan. Clin Toxicol (Phila) 2010;48(4):380-4.

138. Zhang XM, Zhang ZH. The study of intoxication and toxicity of Fructus Xanthii. Zhong Xi Yi Jie He Xue Bao 2003;1(1):71-3 [in Chinese].

139. Shen Y, Li CG, Zhou SF, et al. Chemistry and bioactivity of Flos Magnoliae, a Chinese herb for rhinitis and sinusitis. Curr Med Chem 2008;15(16): 1616-27.

140. Baek JA, Lee YD, Lee CB, et al. Extracts of Magnoliae flos inhibit inducible nitric oxide synthase via ERK in human respiratory epithelial cells. Nitric Oxide 2009; 20(2):122-8.

141. Kimura M, Suzuki J, Yamada T, et al. Anti-inflammatory effect of neolignans newly isolated from the crude drug "Shin-i" (Flos magnoliae). Planta Med 1985;51(4):291-3.

142. Kim HM, Yi JM, Lim KS. Magnoliae flos inhibits mast cell-dependent immediate-type allergic reactions. Pharmacol Res 1999;39(2):107-11.

143. Liang CY, Wen P, Zhen Y, et al. Multi-centre randomized controlled trial of bi yuan shu liquid on patients with chronic nasal sinusitis or nasal polyp after endoscopic sinus surgery. Chin J Evid Based Med 2004;6:377–81 [in Chinese].

144. Liang KL, Su YC, Tsai CC, et al. Postoperative care with Chinese herbal medicine or amoxicillin after functional endoscopic sinus surgery: a randomized, double-blind, placebo-controlled study. Am J Rhinol Allergy 2011;25(3):170–5.

145. Weber U, Luedtke R, Friese KH, et al. A non-randomised pilot study to compare complementary and conventional treatments of acute sinusitis. Forsch Komplementarmed Klass Naturheilkd 2002;9(2):99–104.

146. Suh JD, Wu AW, Taw MB, et al. Treatment of recalcitrant chronic rhinosinusitis with integrative East-West medicine: a pilot study. Arch Otolaryngol Head Neck Surg 2012;138(3):294–300.

147. Helms S, Miller A. Natural treatment of chronic rhinosinusitis. Altern Med Rev 2006;11(3):196–207.

148. Ivker RS. Chronic sinusitis. In: Rakel: integrative medicine. 2nd edition. Philadelphia, Pa: Saunders Elsevier; 2007:chap 19.

149. Federoff HJ, Gostin LO. Evolving from reductionism to holism: is there a future for systems medicine? JAMA 2009;302(9):994–6.

150. Weston AD, Hood L. Systems biology, proteomics, and the future of health care: toward predictive, preventative, and personalized medicine. J Proteome Res 2004;3(2):179–96.

151. Goldberger AL, Peng CK, Lipsitz LA. What is physiologic complexity and how does it change with aging and disease? Neurobiol Aging 2002;23(1):23–6.

152. Ferguson BJ, Seiden A. Chronic rhinosinusitis: preface. Otolaryngol Clin North Am 2005;38(6):xiii–xv.

153. Costerton W, Veeh R, Shirtliff M, et al. The application of biofilm science to the study and control of chronic bacterial infections. J Clin Invest 2003;112(10):1466–77.

154. Platt TG, Fuqua C. What's in a name? The semantics of quorum sensing. Trends Microbiol 2010;18(9):383–7.

Complementary and Integrative Treatments Atypical Facial Pain

Chau T. Nguyen, MD[a],*, Marilene B. Wang, MD[b]

KEYWORDS

- Integrative • Atypical facial pain • Acupuncture • Holistic • Chronic pain
- Complementary therapy

KEY POINTS

- Atypical facial pain (AFP) is unilateral facial pain that lasts most of the day, is poorly localized and deep, is not associated with other physical signs or loss of sensation, and does not have an obvious anatomic or structural cause.
- The mainstay of medical treatment of persistent idiopathic facial pain is counseling.
- A key aspect of the integrative approach is to consider the patient's diet.
- Methods to engage the mind may play a useful role in crafting an individualized plan for pain management in patients with chronic facial pain.
- The role of religion and spirituality should be explored, as this may be a significant source of support for many patients with chronic pain.
- The best approach uses a multidisciplinary team.

OVERVIEW

In 1924, 2 neurosurgeons, Frazier and Russell, described a syndrome of pain along the territory of the trigeminal nerve that did not fit into the classically known cranial neuralgias (**Fig. 1**). This syndrome consisted of unilateral facial pain that lasted most of the day, was described as a severe ache, burning, or crushing sensation, and no autonomic abnormalities were noted. In fact, no abnormalities on examination or tests could be found. Today, this constellation of symptoms would fit into the diagnosis of persistent idiopathic facial pain (PIFP), or as it is more commonly called, atypical facial pain (AFP). AFP has an incidence of 1 in 100,000, affects mainly adults, and is

Funding Sources: None.
Conflict of Interest: None.
[a] Division of Otolaryngology-Head & Neck Surgery, Department of Surgery, Ventura County Medical Center, 3291 Loma Vista Road, Suite 401, Ventura, CA 93003, USA; [b] Department of Head & Neck Surgery, David Geffen School of Medicine at UCLA, University of California, Los Angeles, 10833 Le Conte Avenue, CHS 62-132, Los Angeles, CA 90095-1624, USA
* Corresponding author.
E-mail address: chau.nguyen@ventura.org

Otolaryngol Clin N Am 46 (2013) 367–382
http://dx.doi.org/10.1016/j.otc.2013.01.002
0030-6665/13/$ – see front matter © 2013 Elsevier Inc. All rights reserved.

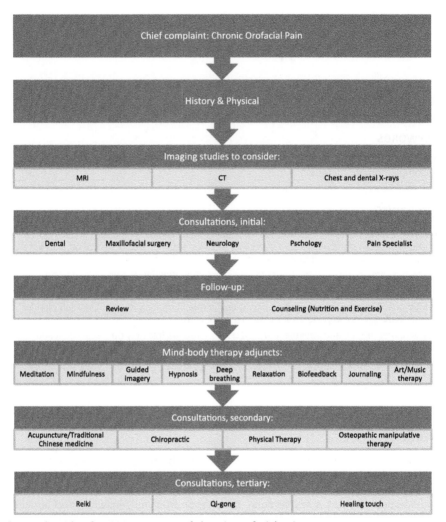

Fig. 1. Algorithm for CIM treatment of chronic orofacial pain.

equally distributed between men and women,[1] although women present more commonly for treatment, with postmenopausal women being more frequent.

The etiology of PIFP remains unknown. At one point, it was believed to be psychogenic.[2] Early reports of AFP suggested that more than two-thirds of patients had a comorbid psychiatric disorder.[3] A role for female hormones was postulated, as more women present with this condition. Today, different neuropathic mechanisms are hypothesized to be responsible.

PHYSIOLOGY AND ANATOMY

Sensation to the face is mediated by the trigeminal (Greek, "3 twins") nerve. It provides somatic sensory afferents from the skin of the face, forehead, anterior scalp, and tympanic membrane, as well as the mucous membranes of the nasal cavity, paranasal sinuses, and oral cavity, including the anterior two-thirds of the tongue, conjunctivae, and the dura of the anterior and middle cranial fossae. In addition, it also contains special visceral efferents that provide motor function to the muscles of mastication (temporalis, masseter, medial and lateral pterygoids), tensor tympani, tensor veli palatini, mylohyoid, and anterior belly of the digastric.

The nerve arises from the midsurface of the pons in the brainstem and travels to Meckel cave, a cerebrospinal fluid–filled space over the petrous portion of the temporal bone. Here, sensory neuron cell bodies are found that comprise the trigeminal or semilunar/Gasserian ganglion on the floor of the middle cranial fossa. It is posterior, inferior, and lateral to the cavernous sinus. The ganglion contains fibers from all divisions of the nerve, the ophthalmic (V1), maxillary (V2), and mandibular (V3) roots. From there, the sensory fibers of the ganglion enter the pons to terminate into 3 major nuclear complexes within the brainstem. These nuclei are the main sensory nucleus of the trigeminal nerve, the mesencephalic nucleus of the trigeminal, and the spinal nucleus of the trigeminal, which is the largest. The spinal nucleus contains 3 subnuclei, 2 of which are important in pain processing: the subnucleus interpolaris, which is associated with the transmission of tactile sense and dental pain, and the subnucleus caudalis, which is associated with nociception and thermal sensation from the head. There is no parasympathetic nucleus of the nerve, or parasympathetic ganglia, although the trigeminal nerve is associated with the parasympathetic ganglia of other cranial nerves (oculomotor, facial, and glossopharyngeal).

The trigeminal system also includes 3 tracts. The spinal tract of the trigeminal nerve carries first-order sensory fibers responsible for pain, touch, and temperature from the orofacial area to the spinal nucleus of the trigeminal. The tract also contains first-order sensory afferents from the facial, glossopharyngeal, and vagus nerves, which terminate in the spinal trigeminal nucleus. By way of the reticular formation, the thalamus receives indirect trigeminal nociceptive input (dull, aching).[4]

Half of the sensory fibers in the nerve are similar to the A (delta) and C (nociceptive) fibers found in the spinal nerves. Pain input is modulated in the nucleus by interneurons, and further processing occurs in the postcentral gyrus of the somatosensory cortex in the brain. Electrical stimulation of the midline periaqueductal gray matter, reticular nuclei, or medullary raphe nuclei, has an inhibitory effect on the nociceptive neurons. Substance P (a peptide found in the axon terminals of neurons involved in pain transmission) receptors and opiate receptors have been localized to the subnucleus caudalis, suggesting an endogenous opioid-mediated pain processing pathway, before integration into higher brain centers.[4]

The sensations of light touch and pain/temperature are mediated by the trigeminal nerve. Lesions proximal or at the trigeminal ganglion cause sensory dysfunction over the entire ipsilateral face and forehead. Those distal to the ganglion result in sensory loss, pain, and dysesthesia/paresthesia confined to a single division. Notably, if there is a dissociation between touch and pain/temperature, this differentiates causes affecting the principal sensory nucleus from lesions affecting the solitary tract and nucleus of the trigeminal nerve. Some injuries may not produce complete loss of sensation, but decreased sensation (hypesthesia), altered sensation (dysesthesia), abnormal sensation (paresthesia), or pain in the affected division.[5]

Transduction of painful stimuli occurs as a result of the interaction between molecules released after tissue injury (substance P, neuropeptide Y, histamine, bradykinin, glutamate, prostaglandins) and pain receptors located on free nerve endings. Peripheral sensitization of these free nerve endings produces increased excitability of the nerve, with spontaneous activity, a reduced activation threshold, and increased sensitivity to repeated stimulation. This may partly explain the findings of hyperalgesia, spontaneous pain, and allodynia in patients with chronic pain conditions. The altered activity of peripheral receptors may in turn cause functional alterations in central pain processing that further lead to chronic pain ("central sensitization"). Interestingly, recent research has uncovered gender differences in the peripheral molecular mechanisms of pain transduction, suggesting one reason why women may be predominantly affected in chronic pain conditions.[6]

SYMPTOMS

According to the International Headache Society's 2004 classification, PIFP is "Persistent facial pain that does not have the characteristics of the cranial neuralgias described above (**Table 1**) and is not attributed to another disorder."[7] The diagnosis therefore, is one of exclusion.

There are 4 criteria to be met for the diagnosis:

1. There is pain in the face present for most of the day or all day, and occurring daily.
2. Initially, the pain may be confined to a portion of the face, but is poorly localized and deep.
3. It is not associated with other physical signs or loss of sensation.
4. Workup in terms of imaging is unrevealing of an obvious anatomic or structural cause.

It may follow an operation or trauma to the face, teeth, or gums, but persists without a known local factor. Pain may start in the nasolabial crease or chin, and then spread to a wider region in the face and neck. One hypothesis for the etiology of the pain is a demyelination injury to the trigeminal nerve following trauma. In some cases, PIFP may be a precursor to trigeminal neuralgia, or the 2 may coexist and be difficult to differentiate.[8] In a large population study out of Germany, the lifetime prevalence of PIFP was estimated to be 0.03%.[9]

The key differential diagnoses are other causes of chronic orofacial pain, which may affect up to 10% of the adult population. This category includes temporomandibular joint disorders, atypical odontalgias, oral dysesthesias (including burning mouth syndrome), and atypical facial pain.[10] The cranial neuralgias, listed in **Table 1**, need to be considered, as does Eagle syndrome or stylohyoid complex syndrome,[11,12] first bite syndrome, postherpetic neuralgia (pain that persists 1–6 months following a herpes zoster infection), headache/migraine, and rare neurologic entities, such as Raeder syndrome (trigeminal ophthalmic branch distribution of a unilateral burning pain that may be associated with miosis, ptosis, and hyperesthesia and can be caused by a middle fossa tumor, sinusitis, or syphilis), and thalamic pain syndrome (severe burning, aching unilateral facial pain that may be associated with dysesthesias caused by a contralateral ventral-medial thalamic nuclei lesion). Neuralgia-inducing cavitational osteonecrosis has been hypothesized as a cause of chronic facial pain.[13] Lung cancer may also lead to referred facial pain, and sometimes the onset of facial pain precedes the onset of symptoms and signs due to lung cancer by several months.[14] Compression or invasion of the vagus nerve is implicated, and pain is usually temporal, along the ear or jaw, and described as a severe ache, either intermittent or continuous.[15] Multiple sclerosis, a demyelinating disease, should also be considered.

In patients with trigeminal neuralgia, the pain is excruciating but short lasting, and localized to a branch of the trigeminal nerve. Patients are typically older. There may be triggers as well. The cause is believed to be ephaptic transmission of the nerve, or "short-circuiting," from demyelination caused by nerve compression, such as from a vascular loop that envelops a nerve root.[4] This is in contrast to trigeminal

Table 1
IHS facial pain causation classification

IHS ICHD-II Code	WHO ICD-10NA Code	Diagnosis [and Etiological ICD-10 Code for Secondary Headache Disorders]
13.	[G44.847, G44.848 or G44.85]	Cranial neuralgias and central causes of facial pain
13.1	[G44.847]	Trigeminal neuralgia
13.1.1	[G44.847]	Classical trigeminal neuralgia [G50.00]
13.1.2	[G44.847]	Symptomatic trigeminal neuralgia [G53.80] + [code to specify etiology]
13.2	[G44.847]	Glossopharyngeal neuralgia
13.2.1	[G44.847]	Classical glossopharyngeal neuralgia [G52.10]
13.2.2	[G44.847]	Symptomatic glossopharyngeal neuralgia [G53.830] + [code to specify etiology]
13.3	[G44.847]	Nervus intermedius neuralgia [G51.80]
13.4	[G44.847]	Superior laryngeal neuralgia [G52.20]
13.5	[G44.847]	Nasociliary neuralgia [G52.80]
13.6	[G44.847]	Supraorbital neuralgia [G52.80]
13.7	[G44.847]	Other terminal branch neuralgias [G52.80]
13.8	[G44.847]	Occipital neuralgia [G52.80]
13.9	[G44.851]	Neck-tongue syndrome
13.10	[G44.801]	External compression headache
13.11	[G44.802]	Cold-stimulus headache
13.11.1	[G44.8020]	Headache attributed to external application of a cold stimulus
13.11.2	[G44.8021]	Headache attributed to ingestion or inhalation of a cold stimulus
13.12	[G44.848]	Constant pain caused by compression, irritation or distortion of cranial nerves or upper cervical roots by structural lesions [G53.8] + [code to specify etiology]
13.13	[G44.848]	Optic neuritis [H46]
13.14	[G44.848]	Ocular diabetic neuropathy [E10-E14]
13.15	[G44.881 or G44.847]	Head or facial pain attributed to herpes zoster
13.15.1	[G44.881]	Head or facial pain attributed to acute herpes zoster [B02.2]
13.15.2	[G44.847]	Post-herpetic neuralgia [B02.2]
13.16	[G44.850]	Tolosa-Hunt syndrome
13.17	[G43.80]	Ophthalmoplegic "migraine"
13.18	[G44.810 or G44.847]	Central causes of facial pain
13.18.1	[G44.847]	Anesthesia dolorosa [G52.800] + [code to specify etiology]
13.18.2	[G44.810]	Central post-stroke pain [G46.21]
13.18.3	[G44.847]	Facial pain attributed to multiple sclerosis [G35]
13.18.4	[G44.847]	Persistent idiopathic facial pain [G50.1]
13.18.5	[G44.847]	Burning mouth syndrome [code to specify etiology]
13.19	[G44.847]	Other cranial neuralgia or other centrally mediated facial pain [code to specify etiology]

Abbreviations: HIS, International Headache Society; ICD-10, International Classification of Diseases, 10th Revision; ICHD, International Headache Classification; WHO, World Health Organization.
Adapted from International Headache Society. Classification and WHO ICD-10NA Codes. Cephalalgia 2004;24(Suppl 1):16–22; with permission.

neuropathy, wherein injury to the trigeminal nerve, such as from facial trauma, dental trauma (most commonly), sinus trauma, or after destructive procedures (rhizotomies) used for treatment of trigeminal neuralgia is the root cause. Following injury, numbness may become associated with bothersome sensations or pain, sometimes called phantom pain or deafferentation pain. Pain is usually constant, aching, or burning, but may be worsened by exposure to triggers, such as wind and cold, and can start immediately or days to years following injury. The most extreme form, anesthesia dolorosa, presents with continuous severe pain in areas of complete numbness.[16]

MEDICAL TREATMENT APPROACHES AND OUTCOMES

The mainstay of medical treatment of PIFP is counseling.[6] Patients should be counseled about the chronic nature of the illness, and its nonmalignant nature. Their pain should be acknowledged, and they should feel that their concerns are being heard, and a plan for addressing them is forthcoming. Toward this end, a comprehensive multidisciplinary team approach is most helpful.[17] A short screening questionnaire for anxiety and/or depression (such as the Hospital Anxiety and Depression Scale[18]) or other surveys for common comorbidities in chronic pain may be administered, with appropriate referral to a psychologist/psychiatrist as necessary. A pain specialist may be able to initiate minimally invasive interventions, such as nerve blocks.[19,20] Neurologists may be better able to manage the nuances of antiepileptic therapy trials.

PHARMACOLOGIC TREATMENT
Tricyclic Antidepressants

The next line of therapy is pharmacologic. The tricyclic antidepressants have shown a moderate effect in several trials. They are postulated to work by altering the sensory discriminatory component of pain, in effect increasing the pain threshold. This effect is independent of their antidepressant action, as it is quicker in onset and observed even in nondepressed individuals, at lower dosages than those used for psychiatric use. Amitriptyline, one member of this class, has been shown to reduce the nociceptive discharges originating from myofascial tissues. Other drugs in this class are nortriptyline and duloxetine.[6] Typically, dosages of between 25 and 100 mg daily are used.

Because one mechanism of action of the tricyclic antidepressants is to inhibit serotonin reuptake, other drugs with similar mechanisms have been tried. Fluoxetine (Prozac 10–20 mg/day), a selective serotonin reuptake inhibitor, and venlafaxine (Effexor 50–75 mg/day), which inhibits serotonin, dopamine, and norepinephrine reuptake, have both been found to have modest results when used for alleviation of chronic facial pain.[21] Smaller doses initiated at nighttime and then titrated upward are recommended. In chronic neuropathic pain syndromes, the number of patients needed to treat (NNT) for antidepressants has been found to be 3, with NNT being an average of the number of patients who need to be treated for one to benefit compared with a control.[22]

Anticonvulsant Drugs

The anticonvulsant drugs, including gabapentin (Neurontin), topiramax (Topamax), carbamazepine (Tegretol), and pregabalin (Lyrica), are often tried in chronic neuropathic pain, and are thought to be indicated especially when the pain is lancinating or burning. Their molecular mechanisms are varied, but typically involve action at the level of cell membrane ion channels. They have narrow therapeutic indices and are therefore best applied by knowledgeable practitioners. A 2005 Cochrane Database review concluded that, "Although anticonvulsants are used widely in chronic pain surprisingly few trials show analgesic effectiveness...There is no evidence that anticonvulsants are effective for acute pain. In chronic pain syndromes other than trigeminal neuralgia, anticonvulsants should be withheld until other interventions have been tried."[23] Their use in chronic orofacial pain has been systematically reviewed, with the finding that a limited to modest benefit may be derived for some patients.[24]

Opioids

Interestingly, very few trials exist on the use of opioids for chronic facial pain.[10] The opioids are thought to be less effective in neuropathic pain conditions, and carry with them serious adverse effect profiles including respiratory depression, hypotension, seizures, paralytic ileus, and dependency.[25] Thus, their use is limited and requires careful monitoring.

Topical Anesthetic Agents

Topical anesthetic agents can be tested. Lidocaine patch (Lidoderm 5%) has been used in trigeminal neuralgia to decrease pain.[26] Capsaicin, a naturally occurring compound responsible for the spiciness of chili peppers, which induces a neurogenic inflammation via release of neuropeptides,[6] has also been studied. Amelioration of oral neuropathic pain symptoms was found in 60% of 24 patients in a small study from Vancouver, Canada.[27] As capsaicin used around the face and eyes may be extremely irritating, a preemptive application of EMLA (eutectic mixture of local anesthetics) cream may be given first.

Botox

Botulinum toxin A (Botox) has been suggested in cases in which masticatory hyperactivity is present. This functional disorder may be commonly associated with chronic facial pain and headache. A group of researchers in Germany reported encouraging results in a randomized, blinded, placebo-controlled study of 90 patients. Ninety percent of patients who received the botox injection improved by a mean of 3.2 on a visual analog scale (VAS), a significant difference compared with placebo.[28] In a similar vein, Italian researchers measured the electromyogram of the masseter and temporalis muscles in a group of patients with PIFP, at rest, during activation, and under kinesiography following transcutaneous electrical nerve stimulation (TENS). They used neuromuscular orthoses to correct identified discrepancies, which were found in all of their 21 patients. They found a net decrease in VAS pain score with a mean shift from 9.5 to 3.1.[29] In a review by the European Federation of Neurologic Societies Task Force on neurostimulation therapy for neuropathic pain, TENS was found to be better than placebo, but its level of evidence was weaker than that for electroacupuncture.[30]

Cannabis

Finally, cannabis, which is legal for medical purposes in several states including California but prohibited by federal law, has been studied for chronic pain. In a study from Canada, where medical marijuana use is allowed, a team from the department of anesthesia found that in patients with posttraumatic or postsurgical neuropathic pain, a single inhalation of 25 mg of 9.4% tetrahydrocannabinol herbal cannabis 3 times daily for 5 days reduced the intensity of pain, improved sleep, and was well tolerated.[31] Abrams and colleagues[32] at the University of California, San Francisco, studied vaporized cannabis for chronic pain. They reported that "vaporized cannabis augments the analgesic effects of opioids without significantly altering plasma opioid levels. The combination may allow for opioid treatment at lower doses with fewer side effects." Vaporized treatments are used to minimize the risks of smoke to the lungs.

SURGICAL TREATMENT APPROACHES AND OUTCOMES

At present, there is no role for surgical therapies in the management of PIFP, unlike in trigeminal neuralgia wherein a subset may be associated with a vascular loop syndrome, and are thereby ameliorated with vascular decompression therapies. In fact, Evans and Agostini state emphatically in the journal *Headache* in 2006, "Indeed, one of the main goals of a prompt diagnosis is to spare patients from futile and potentially harmful surgical treatments."[10] A study in 2005 from Lang and colleagues[33] is telling. Fourteen patients with PIFP were examined with quantitative sensory testing and magnetoencephalography of the somatotopy of the primary somatosensory cortex to tactile input from the pain area. They found that thresholds to light touch, pain, and temperature did not indicate a significant sensory deficit or hyperactivity in the pain area when compared with the asymptomatic side nor when compared with the values of healthy control subjects. They concluded that, "PIFP is maintained by mechanisms which do not involve somatosensory processing of stimuli from the pain area." This may be a clue as to why the treatment of this disorder is often elusive and unsatisfactory.

Experimental treatment options involving pulsed radiofrequency to the sphenopalatine ganglion[34] and low-energy level diode laser[35] have been described with some success in small patient cohorts.

INTEGRATIVE TREATMENT APPROACHES AND OUTCOMES

Because of the poor prognosis of PIFP with respect to treatment outcomes, patients afflicted with this condition have become fertile ground for studies involving complementary and alternative therapies. A better terminology may be "integrative medicine," which refers to the combination of trialing known and studied therapies, as well as those less studied and often underemphasized in the current medical paradigm, including nutrition, mind-body therapies, and spirituality. The emphasis is on the whole person and a "holistic" approach, in combination with evidence-based medicine.

In 1982, Dr Eric Cassel wrote the article "The nature of suffering and the goals of medicine," which was first published in the *New England Journal of Medicine*, and later became a book by the same name. In it he writes, "Suffering is experienced by persons, not merely by bodies, and has its source in challenges that threaten the intactness of the person as a complex social and psychological entity. Suffering can include physical pain but is by no means limited to it. The relief of suffering and the cure of disease must be seen as twin obligations of a medical profession that is truly dedicated to the care of the sick. Physicians' failure to understand the nature of suffering can result in medical intervention that (though technically adequate) not only fails to relieve suffering but becomes a source of suffering itself."[36] Perhaps nowhere else in medicine is the limitation of our current biomedical model more apparent than with chronic pain. Chronic pain is manifest not just physiologically, but shaped by one's experiences, culture, social norms, and expectations. It is known for example, that emotions, such as anger, fear, and anxiety, strongly influence pain perception. In fact, similar regions in the brain process pain, anger, and fear. Being positive, relaxed, and distracted can reduce pain sensitivity.[6] This more encompassing model of pain gives clinicians more targets to assess, then treat. One measure of success may be a "50% decrease in pain, a 50% increase in function and mobility, and a 50% decrease in medication with the elimination of agents with an addicting potential" according to McDonald and colleagues.[37] It is within this context that other less conventional avenues of treatment are considered.

In a recent review of complementary and integrative medicine (CIM) use by otolaryngology patients, a survey study from the United Kingdom found that 60% of patients had used some form of CIM, 35% within the past year.[38] Common nonherbal remedies were massage, acupuncture, and aromatherapy. Reasons cited for using CIM were for wellness, disease prevention, and immune-boosting effects.

Diet

One potential mediator in chronic pain states is inflammation.[39] Injury to muscle or deep tissue leads to changes in both central and peripheral pain pathways, leading to neuronal hyperresponsiveness, abnormal spontaneous discharge, and an increase in their receptive field. It is unclear if chronic inflammatory states render similar changes,[40] but researchers in Sweden have documented pain mediation through proinflammatory markers in chronic masseter muscle pain.[41]

A key aspect of the integrative approach is to consider the patient's diet. Hippocrates is attributed the quote, "Let food be thy medicine and medicine be thy food." The typical American diet is high in n-6 polyunsaturated fatty acids (PUFAS), which can contribute to an overall inflammatory state. The n-3 PUFAS, on the other hand, inhibit the generation of arachidonic acid and inflammatory eicosanoids. Examples of sources for the diet are ocean fish, kale, spinach, flaxseed oil. Shifting the patient's diet to a pattern of 4:1 or 1:1 n-6 to n-3 PUFAS may produce an anti-inflammatory effect, and aid in chronic inflammatory states, such as asthma, bronchitis, and rheumatoid arthritis. A diet low in saturated fat and promoting fruits, vegetables, and whole grains is recommended by the US Preventive Services Task Force for health promotion, as well as part of the 2005 Dietary Guidelines for Americans.[42]

Dietary supplementation with an omega-3 fatty acid, such as is commonly found in fish oil, may be required. In fact, a trial is currently under way examining this nutritional intervention strategy in chronic daily headache.[43] Because the anti-inflammatory effect of n-3 fatty acids tends to suppress T-cell function, the addition of a vitamin E supplement is useful to mitigate this effect.[42] A multivitamin may be worth considering, which is inclusive of the B vitamins, especially vitamin B 6 (neurotransmitter synthesis), vitamin B 12, folate, and thiamine (neuropathy if deficient), zinc and vitamin A (immune function), and vitamin C (neuroprotectant).[44] Numerous supplements have been found to be beneficial in cases of peripheral neuropathy, such as alpha-lipoic acid in diabetes, acetyl-L-carnitine in HIV, and L-glutamine, glutathione, and N-acetylcysteine in chemotherapy.[45] However, their roles in facial pain remains undefined.

Exercise

An emphasis should be placed on exercise, if feasible. A review in 2003 found evidence to support the role of therapeutic exercise in chronic pain. Different physical modalities yielded the same magnitude of effect on pain. Therefore, selection of an activity should be based on a patient's preferences, desired outcomes, and prior experiences. Certain patient characteristics portended a worse outcome: depression, anxiety, obesity, narcotic use, and an others locus of control.[46] Physical therapy, including use of cold packs, joint mobilization, massage, and an exercise program, has been used with some success in temporomandibular joint disorders (TMD).[47,48]

Osteopathic Manipulative Therapy

Osteopathic manipulative therapy (OMT), another manual medicine method taught in osteopathic schools of medicine, may likewise be considered. OMT was developed in approximately 1874 by an American physician, A.T. Still, who searched for a drug-free cure for disease. He developed a way to promote healing by manipulating bones to allow free circulation of blood and balanced functioning of nerves.[49] A randomized controlled trial published in the *Journal of Complementary and Alternative Medicine* in 2011 showed OMT to be effective in female patients with migraine. The study examined the well-known quality-of-life measure SF-36, finding significant improvement in 3 of 8 health-related quality-of-life domains, and pain intensity, disturbance in occupation due to migraine, and number of days of disablements also significantly reduced.[50]

Acupuncture

Acupuncture is increasingly being studied in many difficult to treat diseases. Its use in chronic facial pain was deemed to merit further study based on 8 trials reviewed in 2002.[51] Acupuncture is a part of Traditional Chinese Medicine (TCM), and has been in use for millennia in Asia. It involves the use of small needles placed superficially into any of more than 360 points on the body along 12 lines, called meridians, that are postulated to channel qi, or vital energy/life force. Disease occurs because of the blockage of qi in this paradigm. Acupuncture works by restoring these natural energetic flows.

In 2000, Novak[52] reported at the International Council of Medical Acupuncture and Related Techniques World Congress on 33 patients with facial pain using single-needle ear acupuncture. He found that in nearly half (15/33) of patients, sufficient pain relief was achieved up to the point of negating the need for concomitant medication. Five patients had no relief, and relapse occurred in 3. No side effects were reported other than minor bleeding from the site of needle removal. A study of more than 229,000 patients who underwent acupuncture in Germany concluded that physician-administered acupuncture is a relatively safe treatment.[53] In cases of intractable oral and facial pain, a combination of phenytoin and acupuncture was found to be effective in reducing the pain and its recurrence.[54] One acupoint studied for facial pain is stomach 36 (st36), located 10 mm distal to the knee joint. Workers in Brazil found that stimulation of this point provided pain relief in a rat model through opioid pathways, as the effect was attenuated by naloxone.[55] Another molecular mechanism elucidated for the antinociceptive property of acupuncture is via activation of adenosine A1 receptors.[56]

Cognitive Behavioral Therapy

Cognitive behavioral therapy (CBT), with its emphasis on effective coping strategies and acceptance of pain, is also recommended as adjunctive therapy for PIFP.[8] An evidence-based review of 4 CBT trials in TMD revealed 1 trial showing no effect, and 3 that showed both short-term and long-term improvement in outcomes.[57] Hypnosis, a deeply relaxed state of "inner absorption, concentration, and focused attention" according to the American Society of Clinical Hypnosis, is characterized by using the imagination, suggestibility, and the ability to explore the unconscious mind. It was compared with acupuncture in a single crossover study examining patients with facial pain. Both modalities were successful in relieving pain in this study of 25 patients, with an average pain relief of 4.2 units on a 10-point scale (with hypnosis reducing pain by a mean of 4.8 units, compared with 3.7 for acupuncture).

The study investigators found that patients with acute pain benefited most from acupuncture treatment, whereas patients with psychogenic pain were more likely to benefit from hypnosis. Participants with chronic pain experienced more variability in their responses.[58]

The Mind

Special consideration is afforded to the placebo response in pain. Greene and colleagues,[59] in a study looking at the placebo effect in TMD, write, "Present knowledge suggests that every treatment for pain contains a placebo component, which sometimes is as powerful as the so-called 'active' counterpart." They cite studies from functional brain imaging, showing placebo analgesia to be a real phenomenon, which can be pharmacologically blocked and whose effect is similar to that of known analgesic chemicals. The mind is a very powerful tool in pain management, whether focused, relaxed, or distracted. Therefore, methods to engage it, from meditation to biofeedback,[60] through journaling,[61] and art[62]/music therapy,[63] are additional tools that may play a useful role in crafting an individualized plan for pain management in patients with chronic facial pain.

Religion and spirituality

The role of religion and spirituality should be explored, as this may be a significant source of support for many patients with chronic pain.[64] Research on patients' reliance on spirituality in chronic illness and pain has revealed positive outcomes with improved sense of well-being, resiliency, and decreased pain and anxiety. Prayer is one of the most commonly used complementary modalities, and religious coping a common strategy for dealing with pain.[65] One framework to begin the discussion may be the HOPE model developed by Anandarajah and Hight[66]: H, sources of hope, strength, comfort, meaning, peace, love, and connection; O, the role of organized religion for the patient; P, personal spirituality and practices; E, effects on medical care and end-of-life decisions. A research group based in Portland hypothesized that patients with TMD unresponsive to usual medical care would respond to shamanic healing, an ancient form of spiritual healing, because they shared characteristics of individuals who are "dispirited" (marked biologic responsiveness to external stressors and concomitant emotional and psychosocial difficulties). Of 23 women who began the treatment, only 4 were clinically diagnosed with TMD at the end of the study.[67]

In Jonathan Ellerby's book *Return to the Sacred*, he describes Native American healing traditions as inclusive of the entire community, and not just as an isolated interaction between healer and patient.[68] Newer work confirms the importance of a supportive social network in chronic pain, as satisfaction with social support was significantly correlated with pain intensity and depressed mood in a recent study.[69] Using the model of support groups for alcoholism and cancer, patients may be steered toward chronic pain support groups, which may be located through the American Chronic Pain Association Web site.[70] Thus, the role of the patient's environment is important and must be considered.

Energy healing therapies

Energy healing therapies have also been trialed and studied for pain. Ernst's group in the United Kingdom examined external qi gong, an energy healing intervention based on the concept of qi and TCM precepts, in pain conditions. They found in their meta-analysis that "evidence for the effectiveness of external qigong is encouraging, though further studies are warranted."[71] Other bio-field techniques, such as reiki and healing touch, have likewise been studied with promising results. A 2010 evidence-based review concluded that "Biofield therapies show strong evidence for reducing pain intensity in pain populations, and moderate evidence for reducing pain intensity [in] hospitalized and cancer populations."[72]

The breadth of available integrative modalities, which include (1) integrative medical systems (eg, TCM [including acupuncture], naturopathic medicine, ayurvedic medicine, and homeopathy); (2) biologic-based therapies (eg, herbal, special dietary, and individual biologic treatments); (3) energy therapies (eg, Reiki, therapeutic touch, magnet therapy, Qi Gong, and intercessory prayer); (4) manipulative and body-based systems (eg, chiropractic, osteopathy, and massage); and (5) mind-body interventions (eg, meditation, biofeedback, hypnotherapy, and the relaxation response),[73] have vastly increased our arsenal of tools to assist the patient with chronic pain in general, and facial pain specifically. Meanwhile, they have also increased our understanding and appreciation of the biopsychosocial, whole-person paradigm in the management of complex diseases such as pain. As research continues into elucidating the molecular mechanisms of their action, for example, by means of nitric oxide pathways in relaxation, the key for clinicians is to familiarize themselves with novel or nontraditional approaches for the great benefit of alleviation of pain and suffering of patients.

PATIENT CASE

A 45-year-old woman presented to the ear, nose, and throat clinic with a chief complaint of chronic facial pain. It began 14 years earlier following a motor vehicle accident. She remembered her head hitting the steering wheel. Her best friend died in the accident, and she was at fault for the collision. The pain is near constant, dull and aching, and left-sided. She has seen other physicians and had multiple examinations, imaging tests, and laboratory tests performed, which have all been negative. In the interim, she has been to therapy and tried acupuncture and hypnosis. Review of her most recent magnetic resonance imaging scan of the orbit, face, and brain is unremarkable, as is her computed tomography scan of the maxillofacial bones from 2 years prior.

This patient meets all the criteria for PIFP as outlined by the International Headache Society. It is worth noting that she probably suffered a whiplash-type injury, with her head hitting the steering wheel and likely rebounding. In a recent study from Sweden assessing the frequency of jaw-face pain in chronic whiplash-associated disorders, 88% of patients who had experienced a whiplash injury reported jaw-face pain, as well as general symptoms, such as balance problems, stress, and sleep disturbances.[74] As this patient had undergone multiple prior workups, her office visit focused on counseling. Her previous trials of therapy were noted, and new avenues were explored, such as diet, different breathing exercises, exercise in general, mindfulness, journaling, and osteopathic treatment.

SUMMARY

Persistent idiopathic facial pain represents a challenging diagnostic and treatment entity. The best approach uses a multidisciplinary team. Therapy typically is a combination of agents and modalities that address not just the physical body, but also the psychosocial, emotional, behavioral, and spiritual components as they relate to the whole person. In this manner, patients may not be cured, but healed in a way that restores part of their humanity and integrity.

FEATURES: DATA TABLES: EVIDENCE, OUTCOME COMPARISONS

Because of the overall rarity of the symptom complex, there is a paucity of published data. Most studies to date have been small cohorts of patients in retrospective trials. As this pattern is unlikely to change given the disease incidence, systematic reviews and comparisons to diseases with similar profiles will continue to form much of the evidence base for treatment.

REFERENCES

1. Krolczyk SJ, Kalidas K, Myers MA. Persistent idiopathic facial pain. 2010. Available at: http://emedicine.medscape.com/article/1142187-overview. Accessed January 11, 2012.
2. Reik L. Atypical facial pain: a reappraisal. Headache 1985;25:30–2.
3. Remick RA, Blasberg B, Campos PE, et al. Psychiatric disorders associated with atypical facial pain. Can J Psychiatry 1983;28(3):178–81.
4. Patestas MA, Gartner LP. Cranial nerves, a textbook of neuroanatomy. Chapter 15. Blackwell Publishing; 2006. p. 253–81.
5. Devin K, Binder D, Sonne C, et al. Cranial nerves: anatomy, pathology, imaging. New York: Thieme Medical Publishers, Inc; 2010.
6. Sardella A, Demarosi F, Barbieri C, et al. An up-to-date view on persistent idiopathic facial pain. Minerva Stomatol 2009;58(6):289–99.
7. Olesen J. The international classification of Headache Disorders, Second edition. Cephalalgia 2004;24(Suppl 1):1–160.
8. Obermann M, Holle D, Katsarava Z. Trigeminal neuralgia and persistent idiopathic facial pain. Expert Rev Neurother 2011;11(11):1619–29.
9. Mueller D, Obermann M, Yoon MS, et al. Prevalence of trigeminal neuralgia and persistent idiopathic facial pain: a population-based study. Cephalalgia 2011; 31(15):1542–8.
10. Evans RW, Agostini E. Persistent idiopathic facial pain. Headache 2006;46: 1298–300.
11. Casale M, Rinaldi V, Quattrocchi C, et al. Atypical chronic head and neck pain: don't forget Eagle's syndrome. Eur Rev Med Pharmacol Sci 2008;12(2): 131–3.
12. Colby CC, Del Gaudio JM. Stylohyoid complex syndrome: a new diagnostic classification. Arch Otolaryngol Head Neck Surg 2011;137(3):248–52.
13. Bouquot JE, Roberts AM, Person P, et al. Neuralgia-inducing cavitational osteonecrosis (NICO). Osteomyelitis in 224 jawbone samples from patients with facial neuralgia. Oral Surg Oral Med Oral Pathol 1992;73(3):307–19 [discussion: 319–20].
14. Ruffatti S, Zanchin G, Maggioni F. A case of intractable facial pain secondary to metastatic lung cancer. Neurol Sci 2008;29(2):117–9.
15. Sarlani E, Schwartz AH, Greenspan JD, et al. Facial pain as first manifestation of lung cancer: a case of lung cancer-related cluster headache and a review of the literature. J Orofac Pain 2003;17(3):262–7.
16. Kaufmann AM, Patel M. Types of trigeminal neuralgia and their causes. 2001. Available at: http://www.umanitoba.ca/cranial_nerves/trigeminal_neuralgia/manuscript/types.html. Accessed January 18, 2012.
17. Madland G, Feinmann C. Chronic facial pain: a multidisciplinary problem. J Neurol Neurosurg Psychiatry 2001;71(6):716–9.
18. Zigmond AS, Snaith RP. The hospital anxiety and depression scale. Acta Psychiatr Scand 1983;67(6):361–70.

19. Ilfeld BM. Continuous peripheral nerve blocks: a review of the published evidence. Anesth Analg 2011;113(4):904–25.
20. Carron H. Control of pain in the head and neck. Otolaryngol Clin North Am 1981; 14(3):631–52.
21. Cornelissen P, van Kleef M, Mekhail N, et al. Evidence-based interventional pain medicine according to clinical diagnoses. 3. Persistent idiopathic facial pain. Pain Pract 2009;9(6):443–8.
22. Saarto T, Wiffen PJ. Antidepressants for neuropathic pain. Cochrane Database Syst Rev 2007;(4):CD005454.
23. Wiffen P, Collins S, McQuay H, et al. Anticonvulsant drugs for acute and chronic pain. Cochrane Database Syst Rev 2005;(3):CD001133.
24. Martin WJ, Forouzanfar T. The efficacy of anticonvulsants on orofacial pain: a systematic review. Oral Surg Oral Med Oral Pathol Oral Radiol Endod 2011; 111(5):627–33.
25. Ganzberg S. Pain management part II: pharmacologic management of chronic orofacial pain. Anesth Prog 2010;57(3):114–8 [quiz: 119].
26. Zakrzewska JM. Medical management of trigeminal neuropathic pains. Expert Opin Pharmacother 2010;11(8):1239–54.
27. Epstein JB, Marcoe JH. Topical application of capsaicin for treatment of oral neuropathic pain and trigeminal neuralgia. Oral Surg Oral Med Oral Pathol 1994;77(2):135–40.
28. von Lindern JJ, Niederhagen B, Bergé S, et al. Type A botulinum toxin in the treatment of chronic facial pain associated with masticatory hyperactivity. J Oral Maxillofac Surg 2003;61(7):774–8.
29. Didier H, Marchetti C, Borromeo G, et al. Persistent idiopathic facial pain: multidisciplinary approach and assumption of comorbidity. Neurol Sci 2010; 31(Suppl 1):S189–95.
30. Cruccu G, Aziz TZ, Garcia-Larrea L. EFNS guidelines on neurostimulation therapy for neuropathic pain. Eur J Neurol 2007;14(9):952–70.
31. Ware MA, Wang T, Shapiro S, et al. Smoked cannabis for chronic neuropathic pain: a randomized controlled trial. CMAJ 2010;182(14):E694–701.
32. Abrams DI, Couey P, Shade SB, et al. Cannabinoid-opioid interaction in chronic pain. Clin Pharmacol Ther 2011;90(6):844–51.
33. Lang E, Kaltenhäuser M, Seidler S, et al. Persistent idiopathic facial pain exists independent of somatosensory input from the painful region: findings from quantitative sensory functions and somatotopy of the primary somatosensory cortex. Pain 2005;118(1–2):80–91.
34. Bayer E, Racz GB, Miles D, et al. Sphenopalatine ganglion pulsed radiofrequency treatment in 30 patients suffering from chronic face and head pain. Pain Pract 2005;5(3):223–7.
35. Yang HW, Huang YF. Treatment of persistent idiopathic facial pain (PIFP) with a low-level energy diode laser. Photomed Laser Surg 2011;29(10):707–10.
36. Cassel EJ. The nature of suffering and the goals of medicine. N Engl J Med 1982; 306(11):639–45.
37. McDonald JS, Pensak ML, Phero JC. Thoughts on the management of chronic facial, head, and neck pain. Am J Otol 1990;11(5):378–82.
38. Shakeel M, Trinidade A, Ah-See KW. Complementary and alternative medicine use by otolaryngology patients: a paradigm for practitioners in all surgical specialties. Eur Arch Otorhinolaryngol 2010;267(6):961–71.
39. Sessle BJ. Peripheral and central mechanisms of orofacial inflammatory pain. Int Rev Neurobiol 2011;97:179–206.

40. Bennett GJ, Sessle BJ. Basic science issues related to improved diagnoses for chronic orofacial pain. Anesth Prog 1990;37(2–3):108–12.

41. Hedenberg-Magnusson B, Ernberg M, Alstergren P, et al. Pain mediation by prostaglandin E2 and leukotriene B4 in the human masseter muscle. Acta Odontol Scand 2001;59(6):348–55.

42. Katz DL, Friedman R. Nutrition in clinical practice. Philadelphia: Lippincott Williams & Wilkins; 2008.

43. Ramsden CE, Mann JD, Faurot KR, et al. Low omega-6 vs. low omega-6 plus high omega-3 dietary intervention for chronic daily headache: protocol for a randomized clinical trial. Trials 2011;12:97.

44. Shetreat-Klein M, Low Dog T. Introduction to integrative neurology. 2011. Available at: http://integrativemedicine.arizona.edu/program/2011w/introduction_to_integrative_neurology/key_supplements/1.html. Accessed January 25, 2012.

45. Head KA. Peripheral neuropathy: pathogenic mechanisms and alternative therapies. Altern Med Rev 2006;11(4):294–329.

46. Rakel B, Barr JO. Physical modalities in chronic pain management. Nurs Clin North Am 2003;38(3):477–94.

47. Murphy GJ. Physical medicine modalities and trigger point injections in the management of temporomandibular disorders and assessing treatment outcome. Oral Surg Oral Med Oral Pathol Oral Radiol Endod 1997;83(1):118–22.

48. Feine JS, Widmer CG, Lund JP. Physical therapy: a critique. Oral Surg Oral Med Oral Pathol Oral Radiol Endod 1997;83(1):123–7.

49. Clawson D. Manual medicine. 2011. Available at: http://integrativemedicine.arizona.edu/program/2011w/manual_medicine/osteopathy/2.html. Accessed January 25, 2012.

50. Voigt K, Liebnitzky J, Burmeister U, et al. Efficacy of osteopathic manipulative treatment of female patients with migraine: results of a randomized controlled trial. J Altern Complement Med 2011;17(3):225–30.

51. Myers CD, White BA, Heft MW. A review of complementary and alternative medicine use for treating chronic facial pain. J Am Dent Assoc 2002;133(9):1189–96 [quiz: 1259–60].

52. Novak HF. Treatment of facial pain syndromes with single needle ear acupuncture: preliminary results of an open pilot study. Poster session presented at: ICMART 2000. 9th World Congress on Medical Acupuncture and Related Techniques. Vienna (Austria), May 11–14, 2000.

53. Witt CM, Pach D, Brinkhaus B, et al. Safety of acupuncture: results of a prospective observational study with 229,230 patients and introduction of a medical information and consent form. Forsch Komplementmed 2009;16(2):91–7.

54. Lu DP, Lu WI, Lu GP. Phenytoin (Dilantin) and acupuncture therapy in the treatment of intractable oral and facial pain. Acupunct Electrother Res 2011;36(1–2):65–84.

55. Almeida RT, Perez AC, Francischi JN, et al. Opioidergic orofacial antinociception induced by electroacupuncture at acupoint St36. Braz J Med Biol Res 2008;41(7):621–6.

56. Goldman N, Chen M, Fujita T. Adenosine A1 receptors mediate local antinociceptive effects of acupuncture. Nat Neurosci 2010;13(7):883–8.

57. Aggarwal VR, Tickle M, Javidi H, et al. Reviewing the evidence: can cognitive behavioral therapy improve outcomes for patients with chronic orofacial pain? J Orofac Pain 2010;24(2):163–71.

58. Lu DP, Lu GP, Kleinman L. Acupuncture and clinical hypnosis for facial and head and neck pain: a single crossover comparison. Am J Clin Hypn 2001;44(2):141–8.

59. Greene CS, Goddard G, Macaluso GM, et al. Topical review: placebo responses and therapeutic responses. How are they related? J Orofac Pain 2009;23(2):93–107.
60. Stefano GB, Esch T. Integrative medical therapy: examination of meditation's therapeutic and global medicinal outcomes via nitric oxide (review). Int J Mol Med 2005;16(4):621–30.
61. Snyder M, Wieland J. Complementary and alternative therapies: what is their place in the management of chronic pain? Nurs Clin North Am 2003;38(3): 495–508.
62. Pratt RR. Art, dance, and music therapy. Phys Med Rehabil Clin N Am 2004; 15(4):827–41, vi–vii.
63. Kemper KJ, Danhauer SC. Music as therapy. South Med J 2005;98(3):282–8.
64. Boudreaux ED, O'Hea E, Chasuk R. Spiritual role in healing. An alternative way of thinking. Prim Care 2002;29(2):439–54, viii.
65. Moreira-Almeida A, Koenig HG. Religiousness and spirituality in fibromyalgia and chronic pain patients. Curr Pain Headache Rep 2008;12(5):327–32.
66. Anandarajah G, Hight E. Spirituality and medical practice: using the HOPE questions as a practical tool for spiritual assessment. Am Fam Physician 2001;63(1): 81–9.
67. Vuckovic NH, Gullion CM, Williams LA, et al. Feasibility and short-term outcomes of a shamanic treatment for temporomandibular joint disorders. Altern Ther Health Med 2007;13(6):18–29.
68. Ellerby J. Return to the sacred. Carlsbad (CA): Hay House, Inc; 2009.
69. López-Martínez AE, Esteve-Zarazaga R, Ramírez-Maestre C. Perceived social support and coping responses are independent variables explaining pain adjustment among chronic pain patients. J Pain 2008;9(4):373–9.
70. American Chronic Pain Association. 2012. Available at: http://www.theacpa.org/33/SupportGroups.aspx. Accessed February 3, 2012.
71. Lee MS, Pittler MH, Ernst E. External qigong for pain conditions: a systematic review of randomized clinical trials. J Pain 2007;8(11):827–31.
72. Jain S, Mills PJ. Biofield therapies: helpful or full of hype? A best evidence synthesis. Int J Behav Med 2010;17(1):1–16.
73. Staud R. Effectiveness of CAM therapy: understanding the evidence. Rheum Dis Clin North Am 2011;37(1):9–17.
74. Häggman-Henrikson B, Grönqvist J, Eriksson PO. Frequent jaw-face pain in chronic whiplash-associated disorders. Swed Dent J 2011;35(3):123–31.

Complementary and Integrative Treatments Managing Obstructive Sleep Apnea

Kathleen R. Billings, MD*, John Maddalozzo, MD

KEYWORDS

- Obstructive sleep apnea syndrome
- Complementary and alternative health care approaches • Integrative medicine

KEY POINTS

- Obstructive sleep apnea syndrome (OSAS) is a common disorder characterized by reduced airflow during sleep resulting in gas exchange abnormalities and disrupted sleep.
- The goal of any treatment is reduction in sleep disruption and the apnea-hypopnea index (AHI).
- Continuous positive airway pressure (CPAP) is recommended for the treatment of moderate to severe OSAS.
- There is a lack of existing evidence showing long-term benefits of acupuncture and auricular plaster therapy, although they may help to improve the comfort and quality of life of patients.
- It seems that there are no alternatives to the conventional treatment of OSAS that provide the same positive outcomes as CPAP, surgical interventions, or oral appliances when used appropriately for selected patients.

OVERVIEW

Obstructive sleep apnea syndrome (OSAS) is a common disorder affecting children and adults. The disorder is characterized by reduced airflow during sleep resulting in gas exchange abnormalities and disrupted sleep. This can lead to serious cardiovascular compromise; neurobehavioral alterations; hypertension; and in children, growth retardation. OSAS occurs more commonly in men than in women, and predisposing risk factors include obesity, adenotonsillar hypertrophy, retrognathia, hypothyroidism, nasal obstruction, and evening alcohol ingestion.[1] The gold standard for documenting severity of OSAS is overnight polysomnography (PSG). Once

Funding Sources and Conflict of Interest: None.
Division of Otolaryngology-Head and Neck Surgery, Ann and Robert H. Lurie Children's Hospital of Chicago, and the Northwestern Feinberg School of Medicine, Box 25, Chicago, Illinois 60611-2605, USA
* Corresponding author.
E-mail address: kbillings@luriechildrens.org

Otolaryngol Clin N Am 46 (2013) 383–388
http://dx.doi.org/10.1016/j.otc.2013.02.003
0030-6665/13/$ – see front matter © 2013 Elsevier Inc. All rights reserved.

diagnosed, treatment may include continuous positive airway pressure (CPAP) devices, weight loss, oral appliances, and surgical options. The goal of any treatment is reduction in sleep disruption and the apnea-hypopnea index (AHI), with resultant improved overall health and quality of life.

MEDICAL TREATMENT APPROACHES AND OUTCOMES FOR OSAS
CPAP

The diagnosis of OSAS must be established by PSG before instituting CPAP. CPAP is recommended for the treatment of moderate to severe OSAS, because it has been shown to significantly reduce sleep-related respiratory events and is the most uniformly effective therapy. Once initiated, full-night, attended studies in the laboratory are recommended for titration to the optimal pressure. CPAP is effective for the treatment of OSAS, but regular follow-up is recommended yearly to assess mask, machine, and usage issues.[2] Baltzan and colleagues[3] found that 17 of 101 patients undergoing PSG while using CPAP had an AHI higher than 10. Persistent apnea was found to be associated with high body mass index, higher prescribed pressures, and unresolved mask leak. Unresolved or unsuspected apnea, and the resultant daytime somnolence and neurobehavioral changes, may be an impetus for some to look at integrative treatment approaches.

Medical Approaches to OSAS

A variety of medical approaches for the treatment of OSAS have been assessed as additional modes of therapy. Weight loss in particular is shown to result in a substantial improvement in OSAS if sufficient weight is lost. In one study, a 10% weight reduction predicted a reduction in AHI by 26%.[4,5] Bariatric surgery can be an adjunct to the treatment of OSAS in patients who are obese, although there are reports suggesting a recurrence of OSAS after several years even without gaining weight.[5]

Oxygen supplementation has not been recommended as a primary treatment of OSAS, because the effect on apneas, hypopneas, and sleepiness is inconsistent.

Pharmacologic approaches to treatment have been investigated in several studies, such as serotonergic agents, REM sleep suppressant therapy, and ventilator stimulants. When evaluating these studies, Veasey and colleagues[4] stated that few conclusions could be drawn because of design limitations and insufficient knowledge of neurochemical mechanisms through which sleep places the upper airway at risk for collapse.

Sleep positional therapies, which keep the patient in a nonsupine position during sleep, can be a supplement to primary treatments in select patients.

Oral appliances are another approach to the treatment of OSAS. Mandibular advancement devices actively reposition and support the mandible in a more anterior and open position than the physiologic resting position of the mandible.[6,7] The American Academy of Sleep Medicine suggests that although oral appliances may not be as efficacious as CPAP, they are indicated for use in patients with mild to moderate OSAS who prefer oral appliances to CPAP, or who fail attempts with CPAP or behavioral methods, such as weight loss or sleep position changes. Patients fitted with an oral appliance should undergo PSG with the appliance in place after final adjustments to the fit have been performed. Regular dental visits are recommended to assess overall dental health and occlusion while the appliance is being used.[8] Upper airway surgery may supersede use of oral appliances in those deemed to have a high potential for benefit.

SURGICAL TREATMENT APPROACHES AND OUTCOMES FOR SLEEP APNEA

Surgical options include tonsillectomy, adenoidectomy, palate reduction procedures, tongue reduction procedures, mandible advancement, and tracheostomy. Surgical options are selected based on area of pharyngeal narrowing or collapse. For example, uvulopalatopharyngoplasty enlarges the retropalatal airway, whereas a midline glossectomy widens the retrolingual airway. The American Academy of Sleep Medicine suggests that a stepwise approach to surgical treatment is acceptable if the patient is advised about the likelihood of success, and the need for possible additional surgery before instituting treatment. Tracheostomy is the only operation shown to be consistently effective as a sole procedure in successfully treating obstructive sleep apnea.[1] Clearly, this option is considered on a limited basis for those with no other recourse. For those whose symptoms persist despite surgical intervention or for those who have compliance issues with their therapy, such as CPAP or oral appliances, complementary and integrative medicine (CIM) approaches to treatment may be sought.

INTEGRATIVE TREATMENT APPROACHES AND OUTCOMES FOR SLEEP APNEA

CIM is defined as a group of diverse medical and health care systems, practices, and products that are not presently considered to be part of conventional medicine.[9] The five subgroups of CIM therapies are

1. Integrative medical systems
2. Mind-body interventions, such as meditation
3. Biologically based therapies, such as herbal supplements
4. Manipulative and body-based methods
5. Energy therapies

Complementary interventions are used along with conventional treatments, whereas alternative approaches are used instead of conventional medicine. People who choose CIM approaches are potentially seeking ways to improve their health and well-being, or to relieve symptoms associated with chronic illnesses or the side effects of conventional treatments. In the United States, increased use of acupuncture, deep breathing exercises, massage therapy, naturopathy, and yoga was seen in adults between the years 2002 and 2007.[10]

Integrative Therapies for OSAS

Those with OSAS may seek these treatments for chronic fatigue and fragmented sleep. Patients with undiagnosed OSAS in particular, may seek relief from CIM for their symptoms without realizing there are conventional approaches. For those with known OSAS, conventional approaches may be dissatisfying, and compliance with treatment modalities poor. The impact of conventional therapy on daytime sleepiness, neurobehavioral performance, quality of life, and cardiovascular morbidity may not be complete. Again, this may lead patients to look at CIM for potential benefits. For example, in their study, Sood and colleagues[9] looked at the number of patients with OSAS who had reported previous or current use of CIM therapies. They found that 20% of the 406 patients evaluated had used CIM therapy at some point to improve sleep, and 7% were currently using CIM therapies. Fifty-eight percent of their patients expressed an interest in future CIM use. Women expressed more interest than men in exploring CIM options, such as massage, relaxation therapy, herbal sleep aids, and stress management. The authors suggested that, given the high popularity of CIM and the small risk of adverse effects with some of the interventions, even modest efficacy might translate to clinically relevant effectiveness.[9]

Herbal and Dietary Supplements for OSAS and Sleep Disturbance

The most common biologic products used by patients in the previously mentioned study included herbal tea, melatonin, chamomile, St. John's wort, lavender, and valerian. Melatonin is a natural hormone produced and secreted by the pineal gland causing an increase in hypothalamus aminobutyric and serotonin. Increased secretion occurs during dark hours. Melatonin has been shown to help regulate the circadian rhythm, and has been studied for treatment of delayed sleep phase syndrome and insomnia. Caution with use is recommended because of several drug interactions.[11] Melatonin, chamomile, lavender, and valerian have a sedative effect, and are not specifically recommended for the treatment of OSAS.

The efficacy of oral dietary supplements has largely been based on subjective reports, and safety is assumed based on lack of reported adverse effects. Meoli and colleagues[12] describe a study evaluating the efficacy of a herbal lubricating nasal spray. No significant objective difference in snoring intensity or frequency was seen, but bed-partners reported a lessening in snoring intensity in 65% of patients. Physicians should question their patients about the use of these products, given the lack of published scientific evidence of objective benefits for these treatments in managing OSAS. Patients should be counseled as to their potential risks and benefits, and the role of these remedies as a complement to conventional therapies not as an alternative should be reinforced.

Acupuncture for OSAS and Sleep Disturbance

Acupuncture originated in China thousands of years ago and has been used to treat a large number of maladies. Even today, it is one of the potential treatment options for those with chronic pain who are seen by the pain management services at many institutions. Evidence has shown that the effects of acupuncture include the release of serotonin from the caudal raphe nucleus and endogenous opioid systems.[13]

Given the lack of evidence that many CIM therapies provide a lowering of the AHI, Freire and colleagues[13] designed a randomized, placebo-controlled trial looking at the efficacy of treating moderate OSAS with acupuncture. The authors noted that investigations have shown signs of sensory nerve damage in the upper airway of patients with OSAS, and a reduction of the excitatory drive from the caudal raphe serotonergic neurons responsible for exciting the upper airway muscles. This can lead to aggravated pharyngeal collapse. Patients enrolled in the study received acupuncture or sham acupuncture once a week for 10 weeks. A control group received no acupuncture. The sham group was stimulated with the same number of needles, but not in regions related to any acupoints, and the needles were not manipulated. The AHI and the number of respiratory events decreased significantly in the acupuncture group but not in the sham group. The sham group did not differ from the control group in any of the posttreatment PSG measurements. All the acupuncture patients did have improved mental health scores on the posttreatment Epworth and SF-36 questionnaires, and the authors noted the potential of acupuncture for a profound placebo effect.

Although the previously mentioned study demonstrated a potential role for a CIM therapy for the treatment of OSAS in a small number of patients (N = 26), it did not determine if there would be a long-term benefit to acupuncture in lowering the AHI. Similarly, a Chinese study assessing 30 patients with documented OSAS on PSG showed improvements in the hypoventilation index, the respiratory disturbance index, and sleeping parameters in those patients receiving auricular plaster therapy compared with control subjects.[14] In this type of therapy, specific points on the auricle are punctured or pressed, activating meridians and collaterals. This helps regulate the Qi and blood and helps achieve a balance between Yin and Yang status of internal organs, thereby treating a variety of disorders of the body.

Again, the long-term impact on OSAS was not explored in the study. Given the lack of existing evidence showing a long-term benefit to these therapies, they cannot be recommended as a primary treatment of OSAS. As an adjunct to improving the comfort and quality of life of the patients, they are an intriguing option.

Manipulative and Body-based Therapies for OSAS

Other potential CIM therapies that some may seek out for the treatment of OSAS include massage, relaxation, stress management, meditation, chiropractic, hypnosis, biofeedback, and tai chi.[9] Scientific studies assessing their benefits in lowering the AHI and raising the oxyhemoglobin saturation are lacking. Their use and benefits seem to be targeted at the neurobehavioral sequellae of OSAS, including the daytime somnolence, attention, and focus.

SUMMARY

It seems that there are no alternatives to the conventional treatment of OSAS that provide the same positive outcomes as CPAP, surgical interventions, or oral appliances when used appropriately for selected patients. Their complementary role in improving sleep disturbance and quality of life should be the focus of their use until better scientific evidence is available. As more and more patients seek these treatments, physicians need to be aware of their implications in the treatment of this potential serious health concern.

REFERENCES

1. Standards of Practice Committee of the American Sleep Disorders Association. Practice parameters for the treatment of obstructive sleep apnea in adults: the efficacy of surgical modifications of the upper airway. Sleep 1996;19(2):152–5.
2. Kushida CA, Littner MR, Hirshkowitz M, et al. Practice parameters for the use of continuous and bilevel positive airway pressure devices to treat adult patients with sleep related breathing disorders. Sleep 2006;29(3):375–80.
3. Baltzan MA, Kassissia I, Elkholi O, et al. Prevalence of persistent sleep apnea in patient treated with continuous positive airway pressure. Sleep 2006;29(4):557–63.
4. Veasey SC, Guilleminault C, Strohl KP, et al. Medical therapy for obstructive sleep apnea: a review by the medical therapy for obstructive sleep apnea task force for the standards of practice committee of the American Academy of Sleep Medicine. Sleep 2006;29(8):1036–44.
5. Peppard PE, Young MP, Dempsey J, et al. Longitudinal study of moderate weight change and sleep disordered breathing. JAMA 2000;248:3015–21.
6. Morgenthaler TI, Kapen S, Teofilo LC, et al. Practice parameters for the medical therapy of obstructive sleep apnea. Sleep 2006;29(8):1031–5.
7. Moses AJ, Bedoya JA, Learreta JA. Case study of the anatomic changes effected by a mandibular advancement device in a sleep apnea patient. Sleep Diag Therapy 2010;5(1):30–4.

8. Kushida CA, Morgenthaler TI, Littner MR, et al. Practice parameters for the treatment of snoring and obstructive sleep apnea with oral appliances: an update for 2005. Sleep 2006;29(2):240–3.

9. Sood A, Narayanan S, Wahner-Roedler DL, et al. Use of complementary and alternative medicine treatments by patients with obstructive sleep apnea hypopnea syndrome. J Clin Sleep Med 2007;3(6):575–9.

10. Barnes PM, Bloom B, Nahin RL. Complementary and alternative medicine use among adult and children: United States, 2007. Natl Health Stat Report 2008;(12):1–23.

11. Natural Standard Research Collaboration. Sleep disorders. Natural Standard Monogragh 2011;1–14.

12. Meoli AL, Rosen CL, Kristo D, et al. Nonprescription treatments of snoring or obstructive sleep apnea: an evaluation of products with limited scientific evidence. Sleep 2003;26(5):619–24.

13. Freire AO, Sugal GC, Chrispin FS, et al. Treatment of moderate sleep apnea syndrome with acupuncture: a randomized, placebo-controlled pilot trial. Sleep Med 2007;8(1):43–50.

14. Wang X, Xiao L, Wang B, et al. Influence of auricular plaster therapy on sleeping structure in OSAS patients. J Tradit Chin Med 2009;29:3–5.

Complementary and Integrative Treatments
Tinnitus

Gregory S. Smith, MD[a], Massi Romanelli-Gobbi, BM[b],
Elizabeth Gray-Karagrigoriou, Au.D[a], Gregory J. Artz, MD[a,*]

KEYWORDS

- Tinnitus • Complementary medicine • Transcranial magnetic stimulation
- Herbal supplements

KEY POINTS

- Tinnitus is defined as the perception of sound within the central nervous system (classical auditory pathway) without an external source.
- Data suggest that tinnitus can also be processed through nonclassical pathways in the amygdala and limbic structures, which are areas of the brain thought to be responsible for some affective disorders.
- There are several types of sound therapy for tinnitus that studies suggest can be successful, including maskers, hearing aids, Neuromonics, and Sound Cure. The common denominator in all of these treatment modalities is professional counseling by an experienced audiologist.
- Tinnitus studies with transcranial magnetic stimulation (TMS) have shown mixed results concerning the effect on tinnitus duration and responsiveness to TMS, but do show significant reduction of tinnitus loudness and perception with higher-frequency stimulation (10–25 Hz).
- Agents such as anesthetics, anticonvulsants, benzodiazepines, and antidepressant medications have all been used in the treatment of tinnitus, with some positive effects.
- Many herbal and traditional medicines are used as a means to treat tinnitus, including gingko biloba, zinc, melatonin, vitamin B_{12}, garlic, and others; however, evidence-based medicine is severely lacking for almost all of these treatment modalities, and clinicians rely on patient testimonials.

OVERVIEW

Giving tinnitus patients the respect and time they deserve to properly diagnose and treat their symptoms requires an integrative approach. Too often physicians tell patients with classic, nonpulsatile subjective tinnitus, "there is nothing you can do

[a] Department of Otolaryngology–Head and Neck Surgery, Thomas Jefferson University Hospitals, 925 Chestnut Street 6th floor, Philadelphia, PA 19107, USA; [b] Jefferson Medical College of Thomas Jefferson University, 1025 Walnut Street, Philadelphia, PA 19107, USA
* Corresponding author.
E-mail address: gregory.artz@jefferson.edu

Otolaryngol Clin N Am 46 (2013) 389–408
http://dx.doi.org/10.1016/j.otc.2013.02.005
0030-6665/13/$ – see front matter © 2013 Elsevier Inc. All rights reserved.

oto.theclinics.com

for your problem, you are going to have to learn to live with it." This answer is not the one most tinnitus patients are looking for. Patients want a physician to listen to their symptoms, give them an explanation for their symptoms, and provide potential treatment options, other than "to live with it."

Tinnitus symptoms can be divided into pulsatile and nonpulsatile, with nonpulsatile symptoms present in the overwhelming majority of patients. This article briefly covers the less common pulsatile tinnitus, its etiology, workup, and treatment options; however, most of the article discusses the treatment of patients with nonpulsatile tinnitus, as these patients benefit most from the integrative treatment approach.

The authors are proud of their approach to the treatment of tinnitus patients because at the end of the patient evaluation they are extremely satisfied with the time, effort, and respect given to them. The authors use a team approach involving a nurse/nurse practitioner, physician, and audiologist. Once the history and physical examination have been performed, and all testing and studies have been reviewed, a long discussion is undertaken with the patient regarding diagnosis, the etiology of symptoms, and a sweeping overview of treatment options, including conventional allopathic, alternative, and holistic options. A standardized tinnitus informational packet with information about tinnitus and various treatment options is given to the patients. The most important part of this packet is a series of 3 questionnaires used to establish a baseline severity of symptoms, which include a tinnitus handicap index and quality-of-life questionnaires.

The last step of this team approach is an optional 1.5-hour consultation appointment with an audiologist who has specific training and a special interest in treating patients with tinnitus. The physician may recommend behavioral modifications (masking), medication, or supplements on a patient-by-patient basis; the audiologist is responsible for helping the patient decide if any other options are worth pursuing, including hearing aids, other forms of masking, sound therapy (ie, Neuromonics or Sound Cure), or even an evaluation with a psychologist if severe anxiety or depression are thought to be major contributing factors.

Since the authors started using this approach, it has resulted in an extremely high rate of patient satisfaction. There are so many treatment options for tinnitus because there is very little evidence-based research to validate their effectiveness or lack thereof. However, of the many treatments available the authors are able to confidently tell patients that one of the various options discussed will offer some degree of relief.

DEFINING TINNITUS

Tinnitus is defined as the perception of sound without an external source. Historically it has been broken down into 2 categories: objective or subjective. Subjective tinnitus represents the vast majority of cases; the sound perception reported by patients can be continuous, intermittent, or pulsatile. It is often described as a hissing, ringing, whooshing, or static-like noise. The tinnitus, whether constant or pulsatile, cannot be heard by the examiner. Objective tinnitus that is reported by a patient can be detected by an examiner using an ear-canal microphone or stethoscope. It is always pulsatile and is extremely uncommon. For the purposes of this discussion of current theories and evolving evaluation and treatment, subjective, nonpulsatile tinnitus is the main focus.

Tinnitus affects nearly 30 million Americans. These estimates may be slightly low, considering that most tinnitus is benign and often underreported; those affected do not always seek medical attention. Of those affected, approximately 3% to 5% are estimated to suffer from severe disturbing tinnitus causing disability and disruption in daily functioning.[1] What makes one patient consider their symptoms debilitating, and another with the same complaints not debilitating? Methods to quantify the intensity and character of tinnitus have typically led to poor results in trying to correlate sound intensity with the disability caused by tinnitus. Patients with severe disabling tinnitus often give the intensity of their tinnitus a rating similar to that of someone with benign tinnitus.[2] Masking and matching studies found that 75% of unilateral tinnitus patients matched their tinnitus in the unaffected ear to sounds that are at a 10-dB sensation level or less,[3] and a large study evaluating masking levels found the average level required to mask tinnitus to be only 23.8 dB.[4] The volume of the tinnitus that patients experience may be low, but the disturbance it causes can be high in some patients. This type of data suggests that different pathways exist for the neural signaling and processing involved in tinnitus, as opposed to normal external sound processing by the auditory pathways.

PHYSIOLOGY AND ANATOMY

The classical auditory pathway responsible for how we hear involves input to the primary auditory cortex by way of neural impulses generated by mechanical displacement of kinocilium on the cochlear hair cells. Tinnitus, along with the emotional reactions patients have to their symptoms, is processed through nonclassical pathways of the amygdala and limbic structures, which are areas of the brain thought to be responsible for some affective disorders such as depression and anxiety.[5] Similar to our other senses, such as olfaction and vision, evidence favors the idea that these accessory or nonclassical pathways may play some role in the creation of abnormalities.[6] A recent study using single-photon emission computed tomography (SPECT) and magnetic resonance fusion imaging demonstrated altered uptake in the medial temporal, inferotemporal, and temporoparietal areas in 55 patients with chronic tinnitus, suggesting that these associative auditory cortices are more involved with tinnitus generation than the primary auditory cortex.[7]

A common theory in the generation of tinnitus involves the mechanism of neural plasticity. Neuroplasticity is a term referring to the ability of the brain and nervous system to change structure and functionally as a result of input from the environment.[8,9] For example, parallels can be drawn between the causes of tinnitus and phantom limb syndrome. The phenomenon of phantom limb syndrome is defined by continued sensation of the presence of an absent limb after an amputation.[9] The disturbance caused from amputation has been shown to be worsened in unexpected as opposed to planned amputations.[10] Acute transient tinnitus is almost universal in those affected by acoustic trauma with explosives, gunfire, or excessively loud noise, just as phantom limb sensation is after traumatic amputation.[11] About 30% of those inflicted with acute tinnitus after acoustic trauma will develop chronicity, as suggested in several military studies.[12,13] It is unknown whether acoustic trauma–induced tinnitus and noise-induced hearing loss (NIHL) associated with tinnitus share the same pathogenesis, but studies have found that 50% to 70% of those with noise-induced hearing loss experience chronic tinnitus.[14,15] The mechanism of hair-cell and neural injury is likely related to the idea that intense sound exposure causes a reduction of blood flow, which triggers inflammatory mediators and resultant cell death within the cochlea.[16,17] The overall hypothesis is that hearing loss decreases the afferent stream of neural input from the cochlea to the auditory cortex. Injury to the auditory pathway alters activity in the brainstem and subcortical regions, which may lead to reorganization of the auditory cortex and result in subjective tinnitus.[18–20]

An alternative theory concerning tinnitus pathology is linked to the somatic tinnitus hypothesis, which suggests that the reduction of afferent inputs from the cochlea may allow for inappropriate upregulation of inputs from somatosensory fibers to the auditory brainstem.[21–23] Nonclassical auditory pathways help explain why some patients experience relief from their tinnitus with electrical stimulation of the trigeminal and median nerves.[24,25]

The exact mechanism of tinnitus is not known, although it is agreed that a change in normal neural code leads to the pathogenesis of tinnitus. Dividing subjective tinnitus into subtypes based on common causes (traumatic, noise-induced, postinflammatory, presbycusis, anxiety, and so forth) can be useful in diagnosing and treating tinnitus, because treatments that are effective in one group of tinnitus patients may be ineffective in another group because of differing causes of their symptoms.[26] Treating all tinnitus patients in the same way will lead to poor results. Each case must be addressed on an individual basis, which is why intensive counseling with both an experienced physician and audiologist is crucial to patient satisfaction and success.

Pulsatile Tinnitus

In establishing a treatment algorithm for tinnitus it is recommended that the definition of tinnitus be broadened to include both subjective and objective tinnitus, to encompass those patients referred with pulsatile complaints.[27] Pulsatile tinnitus has a broad differential diagnosis (**Box 1**). It can be a result of normal anatomic variations, such as a right dominant or dehiscent sigmoid sinus or a dehiscent carotid artery in the middle ear. Other pathologic causes include glomus (tympanicum or jugulare) tumors, superior canal dehiscence, patulous eustachian tube, otitis media, or intracranial vascular aneurysms or vascular malformations. Atherosclerotic carotid artery disease, hypertension, and tortuous vessels (anterior inferior cerebellar artery loop) can be seen in patients complaining of pulsatile tinnitus.[28] Some recent literature presented cases of benign intracranial hypertension or pseudotumor cerebri as a causative agent behind pulsatile tinnitus.[29,30] Because this form of tinnitus may involve both otologic

---

Box 1
Differential diagnosis of pulsatile tinnitus

Benign intracranial hypertension/pseudotumor cerebri

Chiari malformation

Dehiscent carotid artery in the middle ear

Dominant sigmoid sinus (usually right-sided)

Dehiscent sigmoid sinus into mastoid air cells

Glomus tumor (tympanicum, jugulare)

Intracranial vascular malformation (aneurysm, arteriovenous malformation)

Menière disease

Otitis media

Patulous eustachian tube

Persistent stapedial artery

Petrous apex lesion

Sigmoid sinus diverticulum

Superior canal dehiscence syndrome

Vascular compression syndrome of the cochleovestibular nerve

and nonotologic sources, it is imperative to make the distinction and refer these patients onward for further medical workup before considering the treatment options outlined here.

After a detailed history and physical examination that includes auscultating with a standard and an otologic stethoscope to evaluate for objective pulsatile tinnitus, basic pulsatile tinnitus diagnostic workup includes a noncontrast computed tomography (CT) scan of the temporal bone, magnetic resonance imaging (MRI), magnetic resonance angiography, magnetic resonance venography, and a fundoscopic evaluation by an ophthalmologist to assess for papilledema, which can be a sign of pseudotumor cerebri. Rarely, imaging can miss subtle vascular findings. An angiogram is considered the gold standard for vascular malformation; however, with modern imaging techniques a CT angiogram can provide a less invasive alternative to an angiogram, and provide excellent resolution of the intracranial vascular system. Even after an exhaustive search and thorough diagnostic workup, many patients will be diagnosed with idiopathic pulsatile tinnitus for which the main treatment is reassurance.

Nonpulsatile Tinnitus

Subjective tinnitus is a challenging chronic condition that is predominantly managed symptomatically because little evidence-based research exists concerning the pathogenesis behind the condition.[31] The initial workup for patients with subjective tinnitus should include a comprehensive audiometric evaluation including audiogram with tinnitus matching, tympanograms, testing for hyperacusis, and tests of central auditory processing when indicated.[32] Acoustic reflex testing is a simple addition to most audiologic evaluations and is especially useful if there is suspicion of tensor tympani or stapedius myoclonus. However, in the authors' office reflexes are rarely performed on tinnitus patients, owing to the high prevalence of hyperacusis and the risk or exacerbating a patient's symptoms and eroding patient trust. A contrast-enhanced MRI of the brain is the most useful radiologic test and can reveal acoustic neuromas, multiple sclerosis, ischemic microvascular disease, temporomandibular joint disorder, and Chiari malformations as well.[33,34] Performing other audiometric tests such as otoacoustic emissions, electrocochleography, auditory brainstem response, and vestibular evoked myogenic potential is determined based on the clinical picture.[35,36] Finally, blood work including antinuclear antibodies, vitamin B_{12}, erythrocyte sedimentation rate, fluorescent treponemal antigen, 20-channel serum multiple analysis, complete blood count, hemoglobin A_{1c}, fasting glucose, thyroid-stimulating hormone, and antimicrosomal antibodies can assist in a workup looking for metabolic, syphilis-related, or autoimmune causes of tinnitus.

All patients seen in the authors' office fill out a Tinnitus Handicap Inventory (THI) questionnaire. The THI is a validated measure that is helpful in the quantification of tinnitus and how it affects daily living. The questionnaire can be used at a patient's initial evaluation and after treatment to measure progress.[37] A questionnaire such as the THI allows for a standardized, validated evaluation for physicians and audiologists to better understand how incapacitating the disease process may be and to help in treatment planning.

MEDICAL TREATMENT APPROACHES AND OUTCOMES
Sound Therapy: Masking, Tinnitus Retraining Therapy, Hearing Aid, and Modulated Sound Therapy

There are several types of sound therapy for tinnitus. The common denominator in all of these modalities is counseling by an experienced audiologist to personalize the treatment plan. Tinnitus retraining therapy (TRT) and hearing aids have been around for decades, while commercially available devices that provide acoustic desensitization through sound modulation such as Neuromonics and Sound Cure are more recent additions the menu of treatment options. However, without counseling by an experienced audiologist, patients will not achieve optimal results.

Sound therapy to help patients cope with tinnitus is one of the easiest recommendations. There are few to no side effects, and the presence of sound can provide adequate coverage to prevent awareness of the tinnitus. Whereas some patients may become fixated on the tinnitus so that even very loud masking sounds cannot cover it, many patients will learn to habituate to the tinnitus with time. Sound therapy can help them cope with the tinnitus and reduce the time to habituation. Sound therapy is most effective when combined with counseling to help patients better understand the tinnitus and their reaction to it.

Sound enrichment can be as simple and natural as sitting next to the ocean and listening to the waves crash on the shoreline, or as complex as a surround-sound speaker array with a multitude of acoustic stimuli presented. Careful questioning of the patient often leads to 1 or 2 sounds that either completely or partially mask the tinnitus. Inexpensive sound machines are available that create an array of musical or nature sounds; these can serve as maskers and deliver soothing sound to promote relaxation. Although these sounds provide only short-term relief, they can be a basis for counseling and can be very successful in cases of normal hearing to moderately severe hearing loss. In cases of binaural severe or profound hearing loss, sound enrichment can be very difficult. Cochlear implantation may be an option to improve hearing, with the potential benefit of tinnitus reduction in patients who meet cochlear implantation criteria.

In today's world, technology is at many patients' finger tips. The availability of tinnitus sound applications on many smartphones allows patients to try a variety of different sounds at a very low price. Patients can also plug their phone or MP3 player into a speaker that is embedded in a pillow to allow sound to reach the better hearing ear, especially if they are a stomach or side sleeper.

Maskers and Tinnitus Retraining Therapy

Maskers, which have been in use since the early 1970s, can be worn at the ear level with appearance similar to that of hearing aids, or be table side. Maskers can provide white noise (broad-band), pink noise (less high-frequency emphasis), or even notched noise (sound centered on a specific frequency). Many patients find that they experience a temporary reduction in their tinnitus after they stop listening to the masker. This phenomenon is termed residual inhibition. Ear-level maskers are used with TRT, developed by Pawel Jasterbowf in the 1990s. His theory of a neurophysiologic model of tinnitus is used in counseling along with a low level of broad-band noise to help patients habituate to the tinnitus. A concise outline of this theory can be found at http://www.tinnitus-pjj.com. Therapy can take 12 to 18 months to complete, and has been found to be successful. Bauer and Brozoski[38] report that TRT shows moderate improvement for adults with moderate to severe tinnitus without significant hearing loss, depression, or hyperacusis. One drawback to TRT is the amount of time patients spend in active therapy, and many drop out before completion of their therapy.

Hearing Aids

Brief mention should be made regarding the benefit of hearing aids for tinnitus. With the advent of advanced digital signal processing, modern hearing aids are able to fit a precipitously sloping high-frequency hearing loss with an open ear canal style of fit. In the past this configuration of hearing loss made amplification difficult to fit without causing acoustic feedback from the hearing aid. As many patients with tinnitus have an accompanying hearing loss in the high frequencies, appropriately fit hearing aids should be tried in such cases. Parazzini and colleagues[39] reported that open-fit hearing aids were equally as effective as sound generators in TRT therapy for the treatment of tinnitus.

Other areas of advancement in hearing-aid technology arise from combination devices. Masking noise can be modulated by frequency shaping, intensity, speed of modulation, and degree of modulation in combination with sound amplification.[40] This type of masking sound can lead to habituation of tinnitus more quickly and comfortably. Another approach is with integrated musical tone therapy described as fractal tone, again delivered through the hearing aid. Sweetow and Sabes[41] reported success in clinically reducing the annoyance of tinnitus through the combination of amplification with fractal tones.

Modulated Sound Therapy

Neuromonics uses a strict protocol whereby the patient spends 2 to 4 hours per day listening to spectrally modified music based on the patient's hearing loss and tinnitus profile. The course of therapy is completed in a minimum of 6 months. During the first phase of therapy, the music is accompanied by a masking sound; this provides many patients with excellent relief from their tinnitus. Once they have achieved a degree of relief and have habituated to the music, the second phase removes the masking sound. The patient is now intermittently exposed to the tinnitus during the pauses in the music. Intermittent exposure helps desensitize the brain from engaging the limbic system to alert the individual to the tinnitus. Not all patients with tinnitus are good candidates for Neuromonics, and continuing tinnitus education and counseling are keys to a better outcome.

Newman and Sandrige[42] did a cost analysis of Neuromonics versus a traditional ear-level masker in patients with normal hearing sensitivity, and found at the 6-month mark that the overall cost-effectiveness per unit of decrease on the Tinnitus Reaction Questionnaire was less with the ear-level masker. The strict protocol and clinical support provided by Neuromonics can assure patients of outcomes similar to those reported in the literature because of the standardization; however, experienced audiologists with a long-established practice with tinnitus patients may find equivalent results to Neuromonics using a more flexible program with an ear-level masker at a fraction of the cost. Each clinic should compile its own clinical data and critically evaluate its outcomes to best serve its patient population.

Another newer sound therapy to recently gain approval from the Food and Drug Administration is Sound Cure. This modulated sound therapy is delivered via headphones with independent volume controls for each ear. It is not programmed specifically for each patient, and unlike Neuromonics it has no formal clinical protocol. The basis for the therapy is S-tones, a phenomenon that was first reported in the electrical domain with cochlear-implant patients and inhibition of tinnitus, but was also found to be effective in the auditory domain.[43] This novel approach may be helpful for patients who are not as greatly disturbed by their tinnitus, because it can be used as much or as little as the patient would like. Clinical outcome data with which to compare the efficacy of Sound Cure with that of other similar sound-modulating products are not yet available.

Transcranial Magnetic Stimulation

Transcranial magnetic stimulation (TMS) is a newer method for both evaluation and treatment of tinnitus. TMS uses an electrical current to induce a magnetic field in the brain, thereby temporarily disrupting normal cortical neuronal activity.[44] Depending on the frequency and length of TMS, the amount of cortical excitability can be increased or decreased, thus allowing for tailored treatment regimens that can lead to altered cortical plasticity.[45] When combined with functional imaging such as functional MRI and positron emission tomography (PET), TMS can be directed toward specific brain structures, which may be beneficial both in the initial treatment of tinnitus and in future research. Tinnitus studies with TMS have shown mixed results concerning the effect of tinnitus duration on responsiveness to TMS, but do show significant reduction of tinnitus loudness and perception with higher-frequency stimulation (10–25 Hz).[46,47] When combined with PET imaging, the areas shown to be correlated with tinnitus were located in the sensory association or nonclassical pathway associated with the limbic system, such as the temporal cortex, the right gyrus angularis, and the posterior cingulum.

Electrical Stimulation/Cochlear Implantation

Treatment of tinnitus using electrical stimulation has been an evolving therapy for centuries. Most recently, cochlear implantation has shown statistical significance in studies measuring its effect on the improvement of tinnitus. One study found that about two-thirds of patients with tinnitus noticed suppression of their symptoms on initial stimulation, and 93% found relief after a 2-month period of stimulation.[48] The benefit of cochlear implantation is said to come from the decrease in spontaneous activity and increase in correlated firing in auditory nerve fibers achieved with direct stimulation.[49] One theory in the pathogenesis of tinnitus involves deprivation of cochlear inputs, leading to plastic changes within auditory pathways. Stimulation from one cochlear implant has been shown to decrease the perception of tinnitus in the ipsilateral as well as the contralateral side, because the input from the auditory nerve to brainstem nuclei is bilateral.[48]

Pharmacologic Treatment of Tinnitus

When applying an integrative approach to tinnitus, using traditional techniques of Western medicine can be a helpful adjunct for patients. Moderate success can be achieved in some patients by improving their sleeping habits, stress levels, anxiety, or depression. Correcting medical disorders such as hyperthyroidism or hypercholesterolemia can also provide patient relief. Many of the medications used to help tinnitus sufferers can have side effects, and interactions with other medications should be considered. Management in conjunction with a patient's primary care physicians or mental health professionals is strongly recommended.

Initial efforts with pharmacologic intervention for tinnitus were directed toward neural inhibition, assuming symptoms were related to an imbalance in the spontaneous neural activity in the auditory system. Receptor-targeted therapy toward the glutamate system (excitatory neurotransmitter), the γ-aminobutyric acid (GABA) system (inhibitory neurotransmitter), and the dopamine and serotonin neuromodulators have been the main targets of pharmacologic treatment in hopes to treat the neural dysfunction that results in tinnitus.[50–52]

Agents such as anesthetics (lidocaine, tocainide, mexilitine), anticonvulsants (carbamazepine, dilantin), benzodiazepines, and antidepressant medications (selective serotonin reuptake inhibitors [SSRIs]) have all been used in the treatment of tinnitus, with some positive effects. Studies on the effects of these inhibitory and modulatory agents on tinnitus have been unsuccessful as a whole in the treatment of a heterogeneous group of tinnitus patients. Clinical evidence from other treatment modalities suggests that tinnitus is a heterogeneous disorder, therefore testing such a group with a drug having a single mechanism of action is unlikely to yield high significance in studies.[52]

Klonopin, a benzodiazepine with known antiseizure activity, has been reported in various case reports to give relief of symptoms to some tinnitus patients. Benzodiazepines alter the $GABA_A$ inhibitory receptor and increase the effectiveness of GABA's ability to open chloride channels and inhibit neural activity. In animal studies the benzodiazepines have reduced the signs of neural hyperactivity and restored temporal integration via the GABA receptor (inhibitory neural transmitter).[53] Shulman and colleagues[54] proposed that a benzodiazepine deficiency syndrome is thought to be involved in some patients with subjective idiopathic tinnitus. Subsequent SPECT studies involving a benzodiazepine ligand identified diminished benzodiazepine-binding sites in the medial temporal cortex of those with severe tinnitus, and are the basis of multiple pharmacologic interventions.[55,56] Klonopin arguably assists the emotional components of tinnitus reported by many clinicians by treating anxiety that can exacerbate tinnitus and improve sleep hygiene. Klonopin, or any medication for that matter, gives patients some control over their symptoms, which can help them psychologically and may benefit by creating a placebo effect. No randomized controlled trials exist that demonstrate a significant benefit of benzodiazepines for tinnitus severity and loudness.

Gabapentin, a drug with a highly debated mechanism of action initially created to mimic the neurotransmitter GABA, has been used with altering efficacy. Its initial uses were for neuropathic pain and antiseizure treatment, and it was proposed to affect tinnitus by increasing neural inhibition. The drug was first introduced for tinnitus users in the early 1990s.[57] Shulman and colleagues[54] report long-term tinnitus relief with gabapentin supplemented with Klonopin, as shown by improvement in Tinnitus Intensity Index, Tinnitus Annoyance Index, and Tinnitus Stress Test scores. No statistical significance, however, was seen in the THI. In randomized controlled trials, gabapentin alone has failed to demonstrate statistical significance in tinnitus by measures in loudness score and Tinnitus Severity Index values.

The anesthetic medications are limited in utility by their side-effect profiles because most drugs used in tinnitus treatment require lifelong administration. Lidocaine infusion was originally introduced in 1980; however, the short duration of relief made it impractical as a treatment option.[58] A study published in 2005 reproduced the statistical significance of lidocaine infusion affecting tinnitus loudness and distress.[59] This study also demonstrated the short-lasting effect of lidocaine by the lack of statistical significance shortly after (20 minutes) drug administration, thus highlighting its shortfall as a realistic treatment modality.

Recent pharmacologic intervention using antidepressants for tinnitus has become extensively prescribed. Not only is there a well-documented association between mood disorders and tinnitus, but there is also a wealth of knowledge in the neuroscience literature indicating that serotonin and other neurotransmitters affect sensory and cognitive centers.[60] It is hypothesized that serotonin may play a role in the behavioral conditioning and neuroplasticity within the auditory cortex.

Antidepressant medications were originally tried for tinnitus relief based on the hypothesis that depression can coincide with chronic tinnitus. Initial studies and case reports showed some efficacy in treatment with SSRIs and other serotonin and dopamine modulators.[61] A Cochrane review of 5 trials found insufficient evidence to show that antidepressant medications improve tinnitus directly. Instead, improvement of tinnitus symptoms by SSRIs as measured by the THI may indeed be secondary to an improvement of coinciding depressive symptoms.

For many otologic disorders intratympanic injection of topical medications has been successful, particularly for sudden sensorineural hearing loss and episodic vertigo, such as Menière disease. There has been a recent attempt to apply this wealth of clinical data to tinnitus patients, and the results have been disappointing. Initial studies suggested a benefit of intratympanic steroid injection in treating subjective nonpulsatile tinnitus; however, several follow-up randomized controlled studies have not revealed any statistical significance to suggest benefit of intratympanic steroids over placebo.[62–66] The one exception to these data is a recent prospective, double-blind study treating acute subjective tinnitus. Shim and colleagues[67] reported that for acute subjective idiopathic tinnitus, the combination of alprazolam and intratympanic dexamethasone injections resulted in a significantly higher tinnitus improvement rate (75%) than treatment with alprazolam alone (50%). Few studies have been performed using intratympanic steroids; however, the low-risk profile and relative ease of administration make it a viable treatment option in the acute setting, and one more option to offer patients who can often be severely affected by tinnitus, particularly in the acute-phase.

INTEGRATIVE TREATMENT APPROACHES AND OUTCOMES

This final section discusses the major supplements and herbs that claim to benefit tinnitus patients or have been part of research evaluating positive effects for tinnitus. Also briefly discussed are acupuncture and its role in tinnitus treatment.

Many herbal and traditional medicines are used as a means to treat tinnitus by attempting to decrease free-radical damage to the cochlea or increase blood flow, and theoretically improve the health of the inner ear. The traditional Chinese medicinal practice of acupuncture uses centuries-old techniques to improve energy flow through distinct meridians in the body, and to promote stress relief and improve overall health and well-being with the hope of improving the symptoms of tinnitus. Evidence-based medicine (EBM) is severely lacking for almost all of these treatment modalities, and clinicians must rely on patient testimonials. Because of the lack of EBM, the authors remind patients to temper their expectations for success; however, most options are safe and have a low side-effect profile. The authors encourage patients to seek out these options because their risk profile is low. Many patients do claim that these products work, and until better studies are performed clinicians will continue to wonder whether the effect is placebo or a result of the product's active ingredients.

Herbal Supplementation

Ginkgo biloba

Ginkgo biloba leaf extract is the most widely sold phytomedicine in Europe,[68,69] where it is used to treat the symptoms of early-stage Alzheimer disease, vascular dementia, peripheral claudication, and tinnitus of vascular origin.[69] It also is 1 of the 10 best-selling herbal medications in the United States.[68] The 2 main active ingredients in ginkgo, flavonoids and terpenoids, account for a wide range of pharmacologic effects. These constituents act as free-radical scavengers, neuroprotective agents, antioxidants, membrane stabilizers, and inhibitors of platelet-activating factor via the terpene ginkgolide B.[69,70] A lot of today's current research using ginkgo biloba studies the possible effects on cognitive function, with the hope that it will play a future role in the treatment of dementia. In addition, there is a body of evidence suggesting that ginkgo biloba may play a role in the treatment of tinnitus. All of the studies concluding that ginkgo is effective used ginkgo biloba extract EGb761.[71–75] Given that ginkgo biloba is thought to cause an improvement in overall cognitive function, a positive effect on tinnitus may be real but nonspecific. Because ginkgo is showing promising results in improving cognitive function, it may have its most potent effect in the subgroup of elderly patients with tinnitus. Ginkgo is also well known to have effects on platelet-activating factor and possibly on endothelium relaxation.[76,77] Based on this research, ginkgo biloba has the potential to benefit patients with tinnitus of ischemic etiology, owing to ginkgo's ability to increase blood flow to the inner ear.

Physicians should be aware of the inhibiting effects of ginkgo on platelet-activating factor because this can lead to potential interactions when used in conjunction with aspirin, warfarin, or any other antiplatelet agent. Gingko also slows liver enzymes; thus, it may interact with medications processed by the liver's cytochrome P450, among which are the antiseizure medications (phenytoin, phenobarbital, carbamazepine, and valproate).

Zinc

Zinc is an essential trace element present in all organs, tissues, fluids, and secretions of the body, and is widely distributed in the central nervous system, including the auditory pathway in synapses of the eighth cranial nerve and in the cochlea.[78] Zinc is an essential component of Cu/Zn superoxide dismutase (SOD) and is important for the proper function of more than 300 enzymes, and the synthesis and stabilization of proteins, deoxyribonucleic acid (DNA), and ribonucleic acid (RNA). It also plays a structural role in the function of ribosomes and membranes. Otolaryngology-related research studies have been conducted to investigate the effects of abnormal zinc levels as a cause for anosmia[79] and burning mouth syndrome.[80] Three possible mechanisms have linked zinc to tinnitus[81]: cochlear Cu/Zn SOD activity, synaptic transmission, and depression. Literature suggests prevalence rates of zinc deficiency in individuals with tinnitus to range from 2% to 69%, affecting elderly individuals more frequently.[81,82] Small studies indicate that administration of zinc has a beneficial effect on tinnitus,[78,82,83] although not all studies have shown clinically significant results.[84,85] It may be possible to classify patients with tinnitus by measuring serum zinc level, which would lead to improvement of the overall treatment effect.

Melatonin

Melatonin is a hormone produced mainly by the pineal gland at night. Its main function seems to be the regulation of the sleep/wake cycle. However, not all of its effects have been fully described.[86] It is readily available as an over-the-counter remedy and is widely used to help patients with sleep disturbances. A few studies have looked at whether its use is associated with improvement of tinnitus. In 1998 Rosenberg and colleagues[87] conducted a randomized, prospective, double-blind, placebo-controlled trial on 23 patients, and reported that melatonin was useful in the treatment of subjective tinnitus. Patients with sleep disturbances were more likely to experience benefits. Other studies have shown similar results, and no short-term side effects have been reported.[88–91]

Vitamin B_{12}

There have been some reports suggesting a relationship between vitamin B_{12} deficiency and dysfunction of the auditory pathway. Shemesh and colleagues[92] observed that vitamin B_{12} replacement therapy led to improvement in tinnitus for some patients, and concluded that routine vitamin B_{12} serum levels should be determined when evaluating patients for chronic tinnitus. In a few cases of severe B_{12} deficiency, one possible mechanism is that the anemia caused by B_{12} deficiency leads to increased cardiac output and arterial pressure. This increased flow is perceived in the ear as tinnitus. Vitamin B_{12} deficiency is a potentially treatable cause of pulsatile tinnitus. Another possible mechanism is that vitamin B_{12} is essential for the activation of the enzyme methylmalonyl coenzyme A mutase, which is necessary for myelin synthesis.[93] Thus, cobalamin deficiency can lead to combined peripheral and central nervous system dysfunction.

Garlic

Garlic seems to be associated with some lipid-lowering effects, and a few studies have shown some potential for fibrinolytic activity and lowering of blood pressure.[94] Its main effects on tinnitus are believed to derive from its potential to improve blood flow to the cochlear artery by decreasing plaque buildup, stabilizing blood pressure, and improving antioxidant capabilities of the blood. This effect is only theoretical, and no scientific studies have been conducted to investigate the possible effects of garlic on tinnitus.

Medicinal Herbal Mixtures

The variety of herbal treatments and the lack of standardization in their preparation make it almost impossible to draw any meaningful conclusions about their effectiveness. No studies with a scientific methodology have been conducted to date, and any claim about their benefits is only anecdotal.

Traditional Korean medicine and traditional Chinese medicine

The use of bojungikgitang and banhabaekchulchonmatang herbal medicines for tinnitus is based on the principles of traditional Korean medicine, according to which tinnitus is thought to usually result from irregularities in bowel and visceral functioning. Bojungikgitang is used to treat qi-deficiency and banhabaekchulchonmatang is used to treat the gallbladder deficiency thought to be linked with tinnitus. These 2 remedies are very common in Korea and are approved by the Korea Food and Drug Administration as herbal remedies for the treatment of tinnitus in adults. Kim and colleagues[95] are actively conducting a randomized, double-blind, 3-arm, placebo-controlled study to investigate the efficacy and safety of these 2 remedies.

There are anecdotal reports that traditional Chinese medicine has been successful in alleviating tinnitus, although no scientifically sound studies have been conducted. Er Ming Fang (EMF01) is a Chinese medicinal herbal concoction that contains several different herbs. Research studies have not shown any benefit in salicylate-induced tinnitus in rats.[96] Yoku-kan-san is a Japanese traditional herbal remedy that is believed to be an effective treatment for tinnitus in undifferentiated somatoform disorder complicated with headache and insomnia. However, no EBM studies exist.[97]

Arches Tinnitus Formula

Arches Tinnitus Formula is a commercially available product that contains 3 primary ingredients thought to have beneficial effects for tinnitus patients (see earlier discussion):

- pharmaceutical-grade ginkgo biloba extract
- zinc picolinate
- deodorized garlic

Clear Tinnitus

Clear Tinnitus contains "active" ingredients of:

- calcarea carbonica
- cinchona officinalis

- chininum sulphuricum
- graphites
- kali carbonicum
- kali iodium
- lycopodium
- salicylicum acidum

Other ingredients (herbal extracts) include:

- pueraria root
- platycodon root
- angelica root
- liguistici root
- peony root
- coix seed
- magnolia flower
- notopterygii root
- scutallaria root
- tangerine peel
- cinnamon bark
- ginger root
- licorice root

Ring Stop

Ring Stop contains "active" ingredients of:

- calcarea carbonica
- carbo vegetabilis
- chininum sulphuricum
- cimicifuga racemose
- cinchona officinalis
- coffea cruda
- graphites
- kali carbonicum
- lycopodium
- natrum salicylicum
- salicylicum acidum

Other ingredients include:

- α-lipoic acid
- black sesame (Hei Zhi Ma) (seed)
- butchers broom extract (leaf)
- cassia (Gui Zhi)
- CoEnzyme Q10
- cyanocobalamin
- folic acid
- garlic (bulb) (odor-controlled)
- gelatin
- ginger (root)
- ginkgo biloba extract (leaf)
- glycerin
- inositol hexaniacinate
- Job's tears (Yi Yi Ren) (seed)

- kelp extract
- L-arginine hydrochloride
- *Ligusticum wallichii* (Chuan Xiong) (root)
- magnesium amino acid chelate
- methylcobalamin
- *N*-acetylcarnitine HCl
- *N*-acetylcysteine
- peony (Chi Shao) (root)
- pueraria (Ge Gen) (root)
- pyridoxine HCl
- riboflavin
- thiamine HCl
- titanium dioxide (natural mineral capsule color)
- vinpocetine
- vitamin A acetate
- zinc amino acid chelate

Quisetus
Ingredients include:

- *Apis mellifica*
- *Matricaria chamomilla*
- *Lachesis mutus*
- *Aristolochia clematis*
- salicylic acid
- *Thuja occidentalis*
- *Calendula officinalis*
- *Kalium phosphoricum*

It should be noted that aspirin is known to induce tinnitus, and it is curious to see the use of salicylic acid as one of the main ingredients in the aforementioned remedies Clear Tinnitus, Ring Stop, and Quietus.

Acupuncture

Several studies have been conducted to assess the effectiveness of acupuncture in relieving tinnitus symptoms. In 2006, Okada and colleagues[98] performed a prospective, randomized, double-blind study on 76 patients. In the study group, needles were applied to the cochleovestibular area in scalp acupuncture. A 0- to 10-point visual analog scale was used by the patients to rate their symptoms. The investigators concluded that there was a significant reduction in noise in both groups, but bigger in the study group. Average duration of symptom relief was 72.3 hours for the placebo group and 106.9 hours for the study group. Tan and colleagues[99] compared acupuncture at cervical Jiaji (EX-B 2) with modified Buzhong Yiqi decoction (decocted in water) and Western medical intervention (Dextran 40, bandazol, Danshen, and vitamin B_{12}). The acupuncture was found to be more beneficial than both the Chinese herbal compound and the Western medical intervention.

On the other hand, other studies have shown no difference between the placebo and study groups. In particular, Park and colleagues[100] conducted a systematic review of controlled trials, and concluded that "acupuncture has not been demonstrated to be efficacious as a treatment for tinnitus on the evidence of rigorous randomized controlled trials." The investigators recommended further research using the highest methodological standards.

Complications of acupuncture, which are extremely rare, are usually caused by mistakes made by the acupuncturist, and include infections attributable to nonsterile handling of needles, bruising, fainting, muscle spasms, bleeding, nerve damage, and accidental injury to organs, with the most common major organ injury being a pneumothorax.

It should be briefly mentioned that there are many sources claiming the positive effects of chiropractic maneuvers, particularly manipulation of the cervical spine. However, there are no scientific studies to support these claims. Present evidence consists of few case reports of patients concurrently afflicted by other cervical or temporomandibular joint disorders.[101,102] In 2004, Hulse and Holzl[103] did not find a correlation between cervical spine manipulation and tinnitus resolution.

SUMMARY

Tinnitus therapy is an area of intense investigation and refinement. Gone are the days of telling a patient to "go home and learn to live with it." Patients with tinnitus should be reassured that there are many options available to help with their problem. By implementing an integrative approach combined with medical acumen, counseling by a qualified otolaryngologist and audiologist, and using alternative therapies, patients can take control of their problem and help lessen or even eliminate the impact of their symptoms on their everyday life.

REFERENCES

1. Cooper JC Jr. Health and Nutrition Examination Survey of 1971-75: part II. Tinnitus, subjective hearing loss, and well-being. J Am Acad Audiol 1994; 5(1):37–43.
2. Reed GF. An audiometric study of two hundred cases of subjective tinnitus. AMA Arch Otolaryngol 1960;71:84–94.
3. Vernon J. The history of masking as applied to tinnitus. J Laryngol Otol Suppl 1981;(4):76–9.
4. Schleuning AJ, Johnson RM, Vernon JA. Evaluation of a tinnitus masking program: a follow-up study of 598 patients. Ear Hear 1980;1(2):71–4.
5. Moller AR. Similarities between severe tinnitus and chronic pain. J Am Acad Audiol 2000;11(3):115–24.
6. Moller AR. Pathophysiology of tinnitus. Otolaryngol Clin North Am 2003;36(2): 249–66, v–vi.
7. Farhadi M, Mahmoudian S, Saddadi F, et al. Functional brain abnormalities localized in 55 chronic tinnitus patients: fusion of SPECT coincidence imaging and MRI. J Cereb Blood Flow Metab 2010;30(4):864–70.
8. Moller AR. The role of neural plasticity in tinnitus. Prog Brain Res 2007;166: 37–45.
9. Ramachandran VS, Hirstein W. The perception of phantom limbs. The D.O. Hebb lecture. Brain 1998;121(Pt 9):1603–30.
10. Simmel ML. Phantom experiences following amputation in childhood. J Neurol Neurosurg Psychiatry 1962;25:69–78.
11. Norena AJ, Eggermont JJ. Changes in spontaneous neural activity immediately after an acoustic trauma: implications for neural correlates of tinnitus. Hear Res 2003;183(1–2):137–53.
12. Barney R, Bohnker BK. Hearing thresholds for U.S. Marines: comparison of aviation, combat arms, and other personnel. Aviat Space Environ Med 2006; 77(1):53–6.

13. Helfer TM, Jordan NN, Lee RB. Postdeployment hearing loss in U.S. Army soldiers seen at audiology clinics from April 1, 2003, through March 31, 2004. Am J Audiol 2005;14(2):161–8.
14. Axelsson A, Sandh A. Tinnitus in noise-induced hearing loss. Br J Audiol 1985; 19(4):271–6.
15. Axelsson A, Jerson T, Lindberg U, et al. Early noise-induced hearing loss in teenage boys. Scand Audiol 1981;10(2):91–6.
16. Le Prell CG, Hughes LF, Miller JM. Free radical scavengers vitamins A, C, and E plus magnesium reduce noise trauma. Free Radic Biol Med 2007;42(9):1454–63.
17. Attias J, Weisz G, Almog S, et al. Oral magnesium intake reduces permanent hearing loss induced by noise exposure. Am J Otolaryngol 1994;15(1):26–32.
18. Moller AR, Rollins PR. The non-classical auditory pathways are involved in hearing in children but not in adults. Neurosci Lett 2002;319(1):41–4.
19. Moller AR. Vascular compression of cranial nerves. I. History of the microvascular decompression operation. Neurol Res 1998;20(8):727–31.
20. De Ridder D, De Mulder G, Verstraeten E, et al. Somatosensory cortex stimulation for deafferentation pain. Acta Neurochir Suppl 2007;97(Pt 2):67–74.
21. Gerken GM, Saunders SS, Paul RE. Hypersensitivity to electrical stimulation of auditory nuclei follows hearing loss in cats. Hear Res 1984;13(3):249–59.
22. Møller AR. Sensory systems: anatomy and physiology. San Diego, CA: Academic Press; 2003.
23. Levine RA. Somatic (craniocervical) tinnitus and the dorsal cochlear nucleus hypothesis. Am J Otolaryngol 1999;20(6):351–62.
24. Sanchez TG, da Silva Lima A, Brandão AL, et al. Somatic modulation of tinnitus: test reliability and results after repetitive muscle contraction training. Ann Otol Rhinol Laryngol 2007;116(1):30–5.
25. Herraiz C, Toledano A, Diges I. Trans-electrical nerve stimulation (TENS) for somatic tinnitus. Prog Brain Res 2007;166:389–94.
26. Hoare DJ, Kowalkowski VL, Kang S, et al. Systematic review and meta-analyses of randomized controlled trials examining tinnitus management. Laryngoscope 2011;121(7):1555–64.
27. Henry JA, Dennis KC, Schechter MA. General review of tinnitus: prevalence, mechanisms, effects, and management. J Speech Lang Hear Res 2005;48(5): 1204–35.
28. Sismanis A, Smoker WR. Pulsatile tinnitus: recent advances in diagnosis. Laryngoscope 1994;104(6 Pt 1):681–8.
29. Sismanis A, Butts FM, Hughes GB. Objective tinnitus in benign intracranial hypertension: an update. Laryngoscope 1990;100:33–6.
30. Sismanis A, Hughes GB, Abedi E, et al. Otologic symptoms and findings of the pseudotumor cerebri syndrome: a preliminary report. Otolaryngol Head Neck Surg 1985;93(3):398–402.
31. Hoare DJ, Hall DA. Clinical guidelines and practice: a commentary on the complexity of tinnitus management. Eval Health Prof 2011;34(4):413–20.
32. Seabra JC, Diamantino H, Faria EA. Neurootological evaluation of tinnitus. Int Tinnitus J 1995;1(2):93–7.
33. Branstetter BF, Weissman JL. The radiologic evaluation of tinnitus. Eur Radiol 2006;16(12):2792–802.
34. Ikner CL, Hassen AH. The effect of tinnitus on ABR latencies. Ear Hear 1990; 11(1):16–20.
35. Ceranic BJ, Prasher DK, Luxon LM. Tinnitus and otoacoustic emissions. Clin Otolaryngol Allied Sci 1995;20(3):192–200.

36. de Azevedo AA, Langguth B, de Oliveira PM, et al. Tinnitus treatment with piribedil guided by electrocochleography and acoustic otoemissions. Otol Neurotol 2009;30(5):676–80.

37. Newman CW, Sandridge SA, Jacobson GP. Psychometric adequacy of the Tinnitus Handicap Inventory (THI) for evaluating treatment outcome. J Am Acad Audiol 1998;9(2):153–60.

38. Bauer CA, Brozoski TJ. Effect of tinnitus retraining therapy on the loudness and annoyance of tinnitus: a controlled trial. Ear Hear 2011;32(2):145–55.

39. Parazzini M, Del Bo L, Jastreboff M, et al. Open ear hearing aids in tinnitus therapy: an efficacy comparison with sound generators. Int J Audiol 2011;50(8):548–53.

40. Pisckosz MK, S. Resound Live TS: an innovative tinnitus sound generator device to assist in tinnitus management. 2012.

41. Sweetow RW, Sabes JH. Effects of acoustical stimuli delivered through hearing aids on tinnitus. J Am Acad Audiol 2010;21(7):461–73.

42. Newman CW, Sandridge SA. A comparison of benefit and economic value between two sound therapy tinnitus management options. J Am Acad Audiol 2012;23(2):126–38.

43. Reavis KM, Chang JE, Zeng FG. Patterned sound therapy for the treatment of tinnitus. Hear J 2010;63(11):21–4.

44. Pascual-Leone A, Valls-Solé J, Wassermann EM, et al. Responses to rapid-rate transcranial magnetic stimulation of the human motor cortex. Brain 1994;117(Pt 4):847–58.

45. Bestmann S, Ruff CC, Blakemore C, et al. Spatial attention changes excitability of human visual cortex to direct stimulation. Curr Biol 2007;17(2):134–9.

46. Langguth B, de Ridder D, Dornhoffer JL, et al. Controversy: does repetitive transcranial magnetic stimulation/transcranial direct current stimulation show efficacy in treating tinnitus patients? Brain Stimul 2008;1(3):192–205.

47. Khedr EM, Rothwell JC, Ahmed MA, et al. Effect of daily repetitive transcranial magnetic stimulation for treatment of tinnitus: comparison of different stimulus frequencies. J Neurol Neurosurg Psychiatry 2008;79(2):212–5.

48. Quaranta N, Wagstaff S, Baguley DM. Tinnitus and cochlear implantation. Int J Audiol 2004;43(5):245–51.

49. Brackmann DE. Reduction of tinnitus in cochlear-implant patients. J Laryngol Otol Suppl 1981;(4):163–5.

50. Stephens SD. The treatment of tinnitus—a historical perspective. J Laryngol Otol 1984;98(10):963–72.

51. Bauer CA, Brozoski TJ, Myers K. Primary afferent dendrite degeneration as a cause of tinnitus. J Neurosci Res 2007;85(7):1489–98.

52. Bauer CA. Mechanisms of tinnitus generation. Curr Opin Otolaryngol Head Neck Surg 2004;12(5):413–7.

53. Brozoski TJ, Spires TJ, Bauer CA. Vigabatrin, a GABA transaminase inhibitor, reversibly eliminates tinnitus in an animal model. J Assoc Res Otolaryngol 2007;8(1):105–18.

54. Shulman A, Strashun AM, Seibyl JP, et al. Benzodiazepine receptor deficiency and tinnitus. Int Tinnitus J 2000;6(2):98–111.

55. Millet P, Graf C, Moulin M, et al. SPECT quantification of benzodiazepine receptor concentration using a dual-ligand approach. J Nucl Med 2006;47(5):783–92.

56. Shulman A, Strashun AM, Afriyie M, et al. SPECT imaging of brain and tinnitus-neurotologic/neurologic implications. Int Tinnitus J 1995;1(1):13–29.

57. Piccirillo JF, Finnell J, Vlahiotis A, et al. Relief of idiopathic subjective tinnitus: is gabapentin effective? Arch Otolaryngol Head Neck Surg 2007;133(4):390–7.

58. Otsuka K, Pulec JL, Suzuki M. Assessment of intravenous lidocaine for the treatment of subjective tinnitus. Ear Nose Throat J 2003;82(10):781–4.
59. Baguley DM, Jones S, Wilkins I, et al. The inhibitory effect of intravenous lidocaine infusion on tinnitus after translabyrinthine removal of vestibular schwannoma: a double-blind, placebo-controlled, crossover study. Otol Neurotol 2005;26(2): 169–76.
60. Thompson GC, Thompson AM, Garrett KM, et al. Serotonin and serotonin receptors in the central auditory system. Otolaryngol Head Neck Surg 1994;110(1): 93–102.
61. Dobie RA. A review of randomized clinical trials in tinnitus. Laryngoscope 1999; 109(8):1202–11.
62. Silverstein H, Choo D, Rosenberg SI, et al. Intratympanic steroid treatment of inner ear disease and tinnitus (preliminary report). Ear Nose Throat J 1996;75(8): 468–71, 474, 476 passim.
63. Shulman A, Goldstein B. Intratympanic drug therapy with steroids for tinnitus control: a preliminary report. Int Tinnitus J 2000;6(1):10–20.
64. Araujo MF, Oliveira CA, Bahmad FM Jr. Intratympanic dexamethasone injections as a treatment for severe, disabling tinnitus: does it work? Arch Otolaryngol Head Neck Surg 2005;131(2):113–7.
65. Topak M, Sahin-Yilmaz A, Ozdoganoglu T, et al. Intratympanic methylprednisolone injections for subjective tinnitus. J Laryngol Otol 2009;123(11):1221–5.
66. She W, Dai Y, Du X, et al. Treatment of subjective tinnitus: a comparative clinical study of intratympanic steroid injection vs. oral carbamazepine. Med Sci Monit 2009;15(6):PI35–9.
67. Shim HJ, Song SJ, Choy AY, et al. Comparison of various treatment modalities for acute tinnitus. Laryngoscope 2011;121(12):2619–25.
68. Drew S, Davies E. Effectiveness of Ginkgo biloba in treating tinnitus: double blind, placebo controlled trial. BMJ 2001;322(7278):73.
69. Sierpina VS, Wollschlaeger B, Blumenthal M. Ginkgo biloba. Am Fam Physician 2003;68(5):923–6.
70. Karkos PD, Leong SC, Arya AK, et al. 'Complementary ENT': a systematic review of commonly used supplements. J Laryngol Otol 2007;121(8):779–82.
71. Meyer B. Multicenter randomized double-blind drug vs. placebo study of the treatment of tinnitus with Ginkgo biloba extract. Presse Med 1986;15(31): 1562–4 [in French].
72. von Boetticher A. Ginkgo biloba extract in the treatment of tinnitus: a systematic review. Neuropsychiatr Dis Treat 2011;7:441–7.
73. Holstein N. Ginkgo special extract EGb 761 in tinnitus therapy. An overview of results of completed clinical trials. Fortschr Med Orig 2001;118(4):157–64 [in German].
74. Morgenstern C, Biermann E. The efficacy of Ginkgo special extract EGb 761 in patients with tinnitus. Int J Clin Pharmacol Ther 2002;40(5):188–97.
75. Jastreboff PJ, Zhou S, Jastreboff MM, et al. Attenuation of salicylate-induced tinnitus by Ginkgo biloba extract in rats. Audiol Neurootol 1997;2(4):197–212.
76. Rejali D, Sivakumar A, Balaji N. Ginkgo biloba does not benefit patients with tinnitus: a randomized placebo-controlled double-blind trial and meta-analysis of randomized trials. Clin Otolaryngol Allied Sci 2004;29(3):226–31.
77. Ernst E, Stevinson C. Ginkgo biloba for tinnitus: a review. Clin Otolaryngol Allied Sci 1999;24(3):164–7.
78. Shambaugh GE Jr. Zinc for tinnitus, imbalance, and hearing loss in the elderly. Am J Otol 1986;7(6):476–7.

79. Alexander TH, Davidson TM. Intranasal zinc and anosmia: the zinc-induced anosmia syndrome. Laryngoscope 2006;116(2):217–20.
80. Cho GS, Han MW, Lee B, et al. Zinc deficiency may be a cause of burning mouth syndrome as zinc replacement therapy has therapeutic effects. J Oral Pathol Med 2010;39(9):722–7.
81. Coelho CB, Tyler R, Hansen M. Zinc as a possible treatment for tinnitus. Prog Brain Res 2007;166:279–85.
82. Arda HN, Tuncel U, Akdogan O, et al. The role of zinc in the treatment of tinnitus. Otol Neurotol 2003;24(1):86–9.
83. Ochi K, Ohashi T, Kinoshita H, et al. The serum zinc level in patients with tinnitus and the effect of zinc treatment. Nihon Jibiinkoka Gakkai Kaiho 1997;100(9): 915–9 [in Japanese].
84. Paaske PB, Pedersen CB, Kiems G, et al. Zinc in the management of tinnitus. Placebo-controlled trial. Ann Otol Rhinol Laryngol 1991;100(8):647–9.
85. Yetiser S, Tosun F, Satar B, et al. The role of zinc in management of tinnitus. Auris Nasus Larynx 2002;29(4):329–33.
86. Pirodda A, Raimondi MC, Ferri GG. Exploring the reasons why melatonin can improve tinnitus. Med Hypotheses 2010;75(2):190–1.
87. Rosenberg SI, Silverstein H, Rowan PT, et al. Effect of melatonin on tinnitus. Laryngoscope 1998;108(3):305–10.
88. Hurtuk A, Dome C, Holloman CH, et al. Melatonin: can it stop the ringing? Ann Otol Rhinol Laryngol 2011;120(7):433–40.
89. Lopez-Gonzalez MA, Santiago AM, Esteban-Ortega F. Sulpiride and melatonin decrease tinnitus perception modulating the auditolimbic dopaminergic pathway. J Otolaryngol 2007;36(4):213–9.
90. Megwalu UC, Finnell JE, Piccirillo JF. The effects of melatonin on tinnitus and sleep. Otolaryngol Head Neck Surg 2006;134(2):210–3.
91. Seabra ML, Bignotto M, Pinto LR Jr, et al. Randomized, double-blind clinical trial, controlled with placebo, of the toxicology of chronic melatonin treatment. J Pineal Res 2000;29(4):193–200.
92. Shemesh Z, Attias J, Ornan M, et al. Vitamin B12 deficiency in patients with chronic-tinnitus and noise-induced hearing loss. Am J Otolaryngol 1993;14(2):94–9.
93. Seidman MD, Babu S. Alternative medications and other treatments for tinnitus: facts from fiction. Otolaryngol Clin North Am 2003;36(2):359–81.
94. Linde K, ter Riet G, Hondras M, et al. Systematic reviews of complementary therapies—an annotated bibliography. Part 2: herbal medicine. BMC Complement Altern Med 2001;1:5.
95. Kim NK, Lee DH, Lee JH, et al. Bojungikgitang and banhabaekchulchonmatang in adult patients with tinnitus, a randomized, double-blind, three-arm, placebo-controlled trial—study protocol. Trials 2010;11:34.
96. Zheng Y, Vagal S, Zhu XX, et al. The effects of the Chinese herbal medicine EMF01 on salicylate-induced tinnitus in rats. J Ethnopharmacol 2010;128(2):545–8.
97. Okamoto H, Okami T, Ikeda M, et al. Effects of Yoku-kan-san on undifferentiated somatoform disorder with tinnitus. Eur Psychiatry 2005;20(1):74–5.
98. Okada DM, Onishi ET, Chami FL, et al. Acupuncture for tinnitus immediate relief. Braz J Otorhinolaryngol 2006;72(2):182–6.
99. Tan KQ, Zhang C, Liu MX, et al. Comparative study on therapeutic effects of acupuncture, Chinese herbs and Western medicine on nervous tinnitus. Zhongguo Zhen Jiu 2007;27(4):249–51 [in Chinese].
100. Park J, White AR, Ernst E. Efficacy of acupuncture as a treatment for tinnitus: a systematic review. Arch Otolaryngol Head Neck Surg 2000;126(4):489–92.

101. Whedon J. Reduction of tinnitus by spinal manipulation in a patient with presumptive rotational vertebral artery occlusion syndrome: a case report. Altern Ther Health Med 2006;12(3):14–7.

102. Alcantara J, Plaugher G, Klemp DD, et al. Chiropractic care of a patient with temporomandibular disorder and atlas subluxation. J Manipulative Physiol Ther 2002;25(1):63–70.

103. Hulse M, Holzl M. The efficiency of spinal manipulation in otorhinolaryngology. A retrospective long-term study. HNO 2004;52(3):227–34 [in German].

Complementary and Integrative Treatments Balance Disorders

Chau T. Nguyen, MD[a],*, Malcolm B. Taw, MD[b],
Marilene B. Wang, MD[c]

KEYWORDS

- Integrative • Balance disorder • Acupuncture • Holistic • Vertigo
- Complementary therapy

KEY POINTS

- Antihistamines, benzodiazepines, anticholinergics, calcium channel blockers, neuroleptics, and antidepressants all may achieve reduction in the length and severity of dizzy spells. Their use is not recommended long-term.
- Vestibular rehabilitation therapy is a program of physical therapy designed to habituate symptoms and promote adaptation to various deficits engendered by an array of balance disorders.
- Several essential micronutrients are vital for proper balance; therefore identification and supplementation of deficiencies are crucial for patients with symptoms of balance disorders.
- Acupuncture may be used for patients with Menière disease and for relief of vertigo.
- Tai chi has been studied as an aid to improving balance, and studies suggest that it can reduce falls or risk of falls.
- Osteopathic manipulative therapy has been described for disorders of dizziness and balance.
- Cognitive-behavioral therapy, with its emphasis on challenging distorted thinking to change maladaptive behavior, has been recommended as an adjunct to vestibular rehabilitation. Dialectical behavior therapy, which incorporates mindfulness, has been helpful in difficult or treatment-resistant cases.

Funding Sources: None.
Conflict of Interest: None.
[a] Division of Otolaryngology-Head & Neck Surgery, Department of Surgery, Ventura County Medical Center, 3291 Loma Vista Road, Suite 401, Ventura, CA 93003, USA; [b] Department of Medicine, UCLA Center for East-West Medicine, 2428 Santa Monica Boulevard, Suite 208, Santa Monica, CA 90404, USA; [c] Department of Head and Neck Surgery, David Geffen School of Medicine at UCLA, 10833 Le Conte Avenue, CHS 62-132, Los Angeles, CA 90095-1624, USA
* Corresponding author.
E-mail address: chau.nguyen@ventura.org

Otolaryngol Clin N Am 46 (2013) 409–422
http://dx.doi.org/10.1016/j.otc.2013.02.006
0030-6665/13/$ – see front matter © 2013 Elsevier Inc. All rights reserved.

OVERVIEW

Balance disorders are the ninth most common reason that patients seek medical care from their primary care doctors, and result in 2 million office visits annually.[1] The balance system is complex, integrating the functions of the vestibular, visual, and proprioceptive systems. A dysfunction in any of these may result in imbalance.[2] Imbalance disproportionately affects elderly individuals, and dizzy complaints are the chief reason why persons older than 75 years seek medical attention. Falls are the leading cause of serious injury and death in those older than 65 years.[3] New research points out that changes in gait and balance may be the earliest signs of Alzheimer disease or incidental dementia.[4]

PHYSIOLOGY AND ANATOMY

Balance is defined as the ability of the body to maintain its center of mass over its base. Its ability to do so also encompasses being able to judge direction and speed of movement and orientation with respect to gravity. It allows us to see clearly when we are moving and make adjustments in our posture, resulting in stability in a variety of environments.

In humans, the balance system comprises 3 parts:

- a peripheral sensory apparatus
- a central processor
- a motor output mechanism

Peripheral sensors include the vestibular organs as well as the eyes and the muscles and joints. The vestibular labyrinth contains 2 types of sensors: the semicircular canals and the otolith organs. There are 3 paired semicircular canals:

- the horizontal
- superior
- posterior

They are roughly orthogonal to one another and sense angular velocity of the head in their respective planes. For example, lateral motion of the head stimulates the horizontal canals, whereas up and down motion stimulates the vertically oriented canals. The canals are housed in the dense bony labyrinth of the temporal bone and contain perilymph, which has a composition similar to cerebrospinal fluid (CSF) with a high sodium/potassium ratio. Perilymph is in communication with CSF via the cochlear aqueduct, and therefore disorders of CSF pressure may affect inner ear function.

Inside the bony labyrinth and suspended in the perilymph is the membranous labyrinth, which is filled with endolymph and has an opposite composition to CSF, with a high potassium/sodium ratio. An enlarged area within each canal, the ampulla, contains a gelatinous cupula matrix, which completely seals the canal. Movements of the head trigger deformation of the matrix material and cause underlying specialized hair cells to activate, sending signals to the vestibular nerve. The otolith organs (the utricle and saccule) are similarly housed. They sense linear acceleration in a left and right orientation and up and down, respectively. Maculae are the sensory transduction means in these organs. An otolithic membrane contains tiny crystals of calcium carbonate, or otoconia, overlying hair cells. Deformation of this membrane by linear acceleration or change of orientation with respect to gravity induces electrical changes within the hair cells, which leads to signaling through the vestibular nerve. These otoconia are constantly being reformed and absorbed by the macular supporting cells and dark cells, and this process is likely important in the development of benign paroxysmal positional vertigo (BPPV).[5]

The blood supply to the vestibular organs is from the labyrinthine artery, usually a branch of the anterior inferior cerebellar artery. Because no collateral anastomotic network exists to supply the vestibular apparatus, it is extremely sensitive to ischemia; 15 seconds of cessation of blood flow may halt vestibulocochlear nerve excitability.[6]

The nerve supply to the semicircular canals and otolith organs derives from the vestibular nerve, which are afferent projections from the bipolar neurons of the Scarpa ganglion. The vestibular nerve travels from the peripheral sensory organs through the internal auditory canal of the petrous temporal bone to the pontomedullary junction of the brainstem in the posterior fossa. Here, it synapses with cells in the vestibular nucleus as well as the cerebellum. Vestibular neurons are unique among sensory neurons in the body in terms of having a resting discharge rate, making them sensitive, capable of bidirectional responses (inhibitory or excitatory), and able to continuously monitor head motion.[5]

The paired vestibular nuclei are connected by commissures that are mutually inhibitory, allowing sharing and integration of information from the vestibular organs in a push-pull format.[7,8] For example, with the head turned to the right, the right vestibular nerve and nuclei activity are increased, whereas the left vestibular nerve and nuclei activity are decreased. Asymmetric neural activity is therefore interpreted by the central nervous system (CNS) as movement, even when such asymmetry may result from disease.[5]

Ascending pathways from the vestibular nuclei to higher brain centers is important for processing of the vestibulo-ocular reflex (VOR) and vestibular sensations. Descending pathways are significant for vestibulospinal reflexes. Two white matter tracts go to the ocular motor nuclei:

- the ascending tract of Dieter to the ipsilateral abducens nucleus
- the medial longitudinal fasciculus (MLF) to all other ocular motor nuclei

Because the MLF is often implicated in multiple sclerosis, this explains the central vestibular symptoms seen in this disease.[6] Other projections go to the vestibuloautonomic system, leading to nausea and vomiting with vestibular imbalance. The vestibular nucleus also receives sensory input from visual, auditory, proprioceptive, and tactile sources. Because of this multimodal input, patients may have difficulty describing their dizzy complaints.[5]

The cerebellum receives key input from the vestibular nuclei and is essential in the VOR and trunk stability. Lesions in the cerebellum, ranging from tumors and degeneration to Arnold-Chiari malformation and alcoholism with thiamine deficiency, may lead to nystagmus and ataxia, which mimic a peripheral vestibular insult.

Reflex pathway arcs form an important basis in the vestibular system, including the VOR, to maintain stable vision during head motion, to assist in balance and stability. The vestibulospinal reflex helps maintain body stability. Cervical reflexes like the vestibulocollic and cervicocollic reflexes work on neck muscles to stabilize the head.[6]

Proprioceptive information comes from skin, muscle, and joint receptors in the body that are sensitive to stretch or pressure. Sensory input from the neck indicates the direction in which the neck is turned, and cues from the ankles help the brain evaluate the sway or movement of the body with respect to the ground, as well as the quality of the ground: flat, hard, uneven, or slippery. This additional information is useful when conflicting information is being processed, for example, in car sickness. The body is still and appropriate sensors convey this, although the vestibular input suggests movement.

It is up to higher cognitive centers in the brain, including memory, to sort this information out. Learning in the brain involves synaptic reorganization and underlies basic human activity such as balance when learning to walk. Through a process of facilitation, nerve impulses that are repeated down a motor output pathway become easier. This process also explains why practice is useful to athletes.[9,10]

SYMPTOMS

Patients with imbalance may be unsteady when walking, or tend to veer to 1 side. They may describe dizziness, as if spinning, floating, or moving, even when still or lying down. Associated ear symptoms can include hearing loss and tinnitus. Vegetative symptoms of nausea or vomiting may be present. Headache may or may not be present. Visual changes such as diplopia, blurriness, or jumpy vision can occur. Oscillopsia is the blurring of vision with head movement; a walking form occurs wherein patients describe their surroundings as bouncing or bobbing.[11] These episodes may last variably and be chronic. There may be associated triggers like a change in head or body position, walking into a dark room, disembarking from a moving vehicle, foods, stress, diving, exercise, loud noise, alcohol, and heat.[12,13]

A thorough history should elicit all these factors, and include a full review of systems focusing on the cardiovascular, musculoskeletal, and neurologic systems. Pertinent positives may also be recorded in the endocrine, visual, and psychological system reviews.

Falling may be the result of imbalance. Falls account for up to 50% of accidental deaths in elderly individuals. The annual cost of treating fall-related injuries is projected to cost close to $55 billion dollars by the year 2020.[3]

Several rating scales exist to help quantify the degree of disability experienced by patients as a result of their disequilibrium. These measures include the Dizziness Handicap Inventory and the Activities-Specific Balance Confidence Scale. These tools may give a fuller picture of the impact on patients' quality of life.

MEDICAL TREATMENT APPROACHES

Pharmacotherapy provides symptom relief of dizziness via central mechanisms affecting vestibular suppression. Antihistamines, benzodiazepines, anticholinergics, calcium channel blockers, neuroleptics, and antidepressants all may achieve reduction in the length and severity of dizzy spells. However, none of the medications works to prevent an episode, and many can be addictive and cause drowsiness (ie, benzodiazepines). Thus, their use is not recommended long-term, and using them may prove counterproductive to brain adaptation.[14,15]

A cornerstone of therapy for imbalance is vestibular rehabilitation therapy (VRT). VRT is a program of physical therapy designed to habituate symptoms and promote adaptation to various deficits engendered by an array of balance disorders, among the most serious of which is falls. VRT has been shown to be effective in improving functional deficits and subjective symptoms resulting from vestibular disorders and central balance disorders.[3] It is also effective for children. Studies have shown a customized program to be superior to generic exercise.

VRT uses specialized exercises to enable gaze and gait stabilization. Many of these exercises use head movement, because this is essential in stimulating and retraining the vestibular system. The basis of VRT is existing neural mechanisms that allow for adaptation, plasticity, and compensation. Because of this situation, patient selection criteria are crucial. Optimal candidates are highly motivated, and have intact cognitive, cerebellar, visual, and proprioceptive systems. For example, studies show that VRT offers little benefit to patients with cerebellar dysfunction.[3]

Typically, patients are referred if symptoms persist for greater than 2 to 3 months. This is the time period it takes the brain to recover from a vestibular injury. However, recent reports suggest that VRT may be efficacious even for acute vertigo, lessening the need for medicine and shortening the duration of symptoms.[16] After vestibular schwannoma resection, early VRT offered to patients resulted in improved outcomes when compared with a control group.[17]

VRT uses the following strategies:

- substitution
- adaptation
- habituation

Substitution strategies involve several techniques, applying alternate senses to replace lost vestibular function by biasing away from the dysfunctional vestibular input.[3] An example is developing the cervico-ocular reflex to stabilize vision during head movements. Habituation involves desensitizing the vestibular system. Cawthorne head exercises, first described in the 1940s, use eye, head, and body movements in a provocative fashion to stimulate vestibular signs and symptoms and fatigue the vestibular response, forcing the CNS to compensate. Adaptation refers to long-term changes in neural pathways that seek to reestablish homeostasis within the vestibular system. Several VOR exercises help facilitate the gain, timing, and direction of the VOR response.

In addition to VOR exercises, ocular motor exercise, gait exercise, and balance exercise are prescribed. An obstacle course may be set up to simulate challenging environments that patients may face in the real world. Virtual reality computer technology is being used for oscillopsia[11] as well as for NASA (National Aeronautics and Space Administration) astronaut training to increase function in space and speed recovery when returning to gravity and a ground environment. Electrotactile vestibular substitution systems have been used for patients with bilateral vestibular loss, as in aminoglycoside toxicity.[3] A new twist on VRT is working with patients in a pool environment. Researchers in Brazil[18] using aquatic physiotherapy for patients with uncompensated unilateral vestibular loss found "improvement in quality of life, body balance and self-perception of dizziness intensity, regardless of age, time since symptom onset, and use of antivertigo medication."

SURGICAL TREATMENT APPROACHES

Surgery is reserved for individuals who have failed medical therapy. It is typically indicated in patients with Ménière disease with disabling features. Intervention is not indicated in cases of bilateral vestibular dysfunction. Surgical procedures include endolymphatic sac surgery, vestibular nerve section, and chemical labyrinthectomy.[14] Other potential surgical remedies include:

- perilymphatic fistula repair
- occlusion of the posterior semicircular canal in BPPV versus division of the singular nerve[19]
- middle cranial fossa versus transmastoid repair of superior semicircular canal dehiscence syndrome.[15]

Persistent disequilibrium, hearing loss, and CSF leak are potential complications from surgery.

PATIENT SELF-TREATMENTS

In the case of BPPV, particle repositioning maneuvers may be used by patients at home. These maneuvers include the Epley and Semont maneuvers, and Brandt-Daroff exercises. These activities attempt to remove wayward otoconia in the semicircular canals into a less sensitive location.[12,19] Although such maneuvers have a median efficacy of 80%, nearly a third of patients experience recurrent symptoms within a year.

A commercially available product, DizzyFix, is a plastic molded headband type device that may assist patients with getting into the correct position for particle repositioning maneuvers. Several small studies suggest it to be comparable with office-based procedures.[20]

INTEGRATIVE TREATMENT APPROACHES
Vitamin B₁₂ (Cyanocobalamin)

Several essential micronutrients are vital for proper balance; therefore, identification and supplementation of deficiencies are crucial for patients with symptoms of balance disorders. Vitamin B_{12}, or cyanocobalamin, is a critical micronutrient for vestibular health. Deficiency causes damage to the myelin sheath of neurons and can lead to numbness and tingling of the legs, difficulty walking, and disorientation. Neurologic symptoms may be predominant in 25% of individuals deficient in vitamin B_{12}. It is estimated that 10% to 15% of adults older than 60 years suffer from such a deficiency. One reason is that the incidence of atrophic gastritis in the elderly population is between 10% and 30%.[21] Gastric parietal cells secrete intrinsic factor, which is needed to bind to vitamin B_{12} for its absorption in the small intestine. Anti-intrinsic factor antibodies may be present in pernicious anemia, an autoimmune inflammation of the stomach lining. Also, the widespread use of gastric acid–suppressive drugs may play a similar role in leading to decreased food-based absorption, because acid is required to free the vitamin B_{12} found in foods.

The US recommended dietary allowance (RDA) for vitamin B_{12} in adults is 2.4 μg/d. No upper limit is set on the daily intake. It is found in animal products, and therefore vegetarians need supplemental sources. Oral and injectable forms are readily available.

Vitamin B₁ (Thiamine)

In Wernicke-Korsakoff syndrome, patients experience nystagmus, gait abnormality, and confusion. This syndrome is brought on by a lack of vitamin B_1 or thiamine. It is usually caused by a poor diet associated with alcoholism.[22] Treatment involves thiamine supplementation, although the dose, duration, frequency, and route of administration are unclear.[23] The US RDA for thiamine is 1.2 mg/d in adult men and 1.1 mg/d in women. Vitamin B_1 is found in legumes, nuts, and whole grain cereals.

Vitamin D

Vitamin D, in conjunction with calcium and sodium fluoride, showed promise in the management of inner ear otosclerosis in some patients, from a report by Brookler and Glenn.[24] These investigators suggest that there are "patients with symptoms similar to those of Menière's disease who do not have Menière's disease and therefore do not respond to conventional medical or conservative surgical management. Some have subtle disorders of carbohydrate and lipid metabolism" and are remedied by dietary therapy.

Antioxidant Compounds

Antioxidant compounds have been studied for vertigo symptom relief. A study from Japan looked at vitamin C (600 mg/d), glutathione (300 mg/d), and rebamipide (300 mg/d) in patients with Menière disease who had failed conventional therapy. This small pilot study[25] found "marked improvement of vertigo" in 21 of 22 patients. These compounds act by limiting the free-radical damage to tissue, cell membranes, and DNA. Because glutathione is poorly absorbed, precursor compounds such as lipoic acid or N-acetylcysteine may be substituted.[26]

Ginkgo Biloba

Among herbal remedies, ginkgo biloba has been one of the most studied. Properties of ginkgo include being an efficient free-radical scavenger and inhibiting platelet activation factor. Researchers in Italy[27] examined the ginkgo biloba extract EGb761 in patients with vertigo of vascular origin. These investigators used a dose of 80 mg twice daily for 3 months. Neuro-otologic and balance examinations were performed at baseline and on study completion. "Considerable" improvement was found in oculomotor and visuovestibular function, although no change was noted in the overall equilibrium score.

A national committee tasked with studying the then known effects of popular herbal treatments in Germany published their findings as the German Commission E monograph in 1994. For ginkgo, they concluded that EGb761 "aids in the compensation of disturbed equilibrium, acting particularly at the level of the microcirculation."[28–30] The Commission recommended doses in the 120-mg to 240-mg range per day, divided in 2 or 3 separate doses, for vertigo or tinnitus of vascular or involutional origin. In a study carried out in Taiwan, researchers found that elderly patients with dizziness, vertigo, and findings of leukoaraiosis ("a diminution of density in the white matter, related to a specific type of cerebral ischemia, which has been identified as a low-density area on a computed tomographic scan or high signal intensity on a T2-weighted magnetic resonance imaging scan") who were treated with a plasma expander (hydroxyethyl starch) for 3 days, followed by ginkgo (40 mg), a daily multivitamin, and oxazolam twice daily, for 3 months, had improvement with their vertigo and balance.[31] Side effects from ginkgo extract taken over a 3-month period included nausea, headache, stomach problems, diarrhea, allergy, anxiety, and sleep disturbance in 1.69% of more than 10,000 patients evaluated.[28]

Vertigoheel

Homeopathic treatments use the principle of like treats like, such that compounds that may instigate a particular symptom are used in the treatment of that symptom in serially diluted quantities; 1:10 (X) or 1:100 (C) dilutions, or multiples thereof. One homeopathic remedy, Vertigoheel (Biologische Heilmittel Heel, Baden-Baden, Germany), consists of *Cocculus indicus* 4 × 210 mg, *Conium masculatum* 3 × 300 mg, and *Ambra grisea* 6 × 30 mg, petroleum 8 × 30 mg.[29] A randomized, double-blind trial was performed in 2005 of 170 elderly patients with atherosclerosis-related vertigo to assess the noninferiority of Vertigoheel versus ginkgo biloba.[32] After 6 weeks of treatment, both groups improved by approximately 10 points on a dizziness scale. Further corroborative tests, such as line walking and the Unterberg stepping test, confirmed physician and patient global assessment of improvement. A systematic review from 2007[33] found good levels of evidence for the use of Vertigoheel in the treatment of vertigo but larger trials are required.

Another popular homeopathic remedy for vertigo is *Bryonia alba*, although the evidence is scant. One scientific study referenced the key chemical, cucurbitacin R diglucoside, as a plant adaptogen, modulating the stress response.[34]

TRADITIONAL CHINESE MEDICINE

In traditional Chinese medicine (TCM), dizziness and vertigo are often caused by internal wind involving the liver, first described in the Yellow Emperor's *Classic of Internal Medicine*: "various types of wind disease [such as] dizziness belong to the Liver."[35] Liver wind usually develops from an underlying TCM pattern of either excess (liver-fire, liver-yang rising or turbid phlegm) or deficiency (kidney and liver-yin deficiency, kidney-essence deficiency or qi and blood deficiency).[36,37] A Chinese herbal formulation, Tian Ma Gou Teng Yin–*Gastrodia* and *Uncaria* decoction, is purported to be helpful to expel wind, extinguish internal wind, calm the liver-yang, invigorate the blood and tonify the liver and kidney.[38] It is composed of 11 herbs, including:

- *Gastrodia* rhizome
- stems of gambir vine
- *Uncaria* vine
- abalone shell
- jasmine fruit
- skullcap root
- Chinese motherwort
- *Eucommia* bark
- others

A usual recommended dose is between 5 and 7 pills daily, with results expected in 3 to 5 weeks. It is contraindicated for pregnant patients, and caution is advised in the setting of acute illness and in those with digestive disease.[39] Its mechanism of action may involve protein modulation, affecting neuroprotection and regeneration.[40]

Another cause of dizziness and vertigo is wind invasion, which enters the body through the ears, leading to accumulation of phlegm.[41] Two strategies to ameliorate this condition include protecting the ears against wind and reducing phlegm. The former may be as simple as covering up the ears on a windy day, and the latter can be accomplished through attention to diet. Highly refined and processed starches, sugar and sweets, alcohol, and greasy fried foods should be avoided because these promote phlegm. Examples of foods that are helpful in combating the ill effects of wind include:

- pine nuts
- basil
- chamomile tea
- celery
- flax oil

Acupuncture

Acupuncture has been used for patients with Menière disease and for relief of vertigo. An early report from 1983[42] evaluated a cohort of 34 patients with treatment-refractory Menière disease in a nonrandomized, unblinded study. Acupuncture afforded "great improvement" in their series, with the symptom of vertigo universally addressed. Bergamaschi and colleagues[43] looked at postural instability in elderly patients and whether laser acupuncture and auriculotherapy could provide benefit. In this small study, balance function as assessed on a force platform improved by 5% to 30% in the short-term. The investigators hypothesized that the mechanism of action of acupuncture could be reduction of nociceptive interference with proprioceptive signaling, leading to improved postural control.

Taiwanese researchers performed a controlled, randomized study of acupuncture in stroke patients.[44] The Baihui acupoint (GV 20), found at the vertex of the head along the midline, as well as 4 associated points on the scalp, were chosen for acupuncture with manual stimulation, which was achieved through twisting of the needles until patients experienced sensations of soreness, numbness, swelling, or heaviness. A control group underwent needling alone without manual stimulation. Balance testing included the time taken for a patient to stand vertically from a seated position, the time taken for a patient to walk a distance of 6 m, and muscle strength of both lower extremities. Both groups experienced a decrease in the time for the twin tasks of rising to a seated position and walking 6 m; although only the group that received acupuncture with manual stimulation showed an increase in lower extremity muscle strength. The investigators concluded that acupuncture with stimulation may improve balance function in stroke patients.

Tai Chi

Tai chi has been studied as an aid to improving balance and is a form of exercise believed to originate from the thirteenth century Ming dynasty in China, influenced by Taoism philosophy. It focuses on breathing with slow, flowing movement, complete relaxation, and a serene mind: "Once you begin to move, the entire body must be light and limber. Each part of your body should be connected to each other part...The internal energy should be vibrated, like the beat of a drum. The spirit should be condensed in toward the center of your body."[45] A study published in 2012 followed a group of elderly Vietnamese individuals. One group was randomized to their usual daily activity, whereas the other performed 6 months of tai chi. The investigators studied 3 end points:

- the Falls Efficacy Scale
- the Pittsburgh Sleep Quality Index
- the Trail Making Test, which assesses cognitive function

The study found a significant improvement in the tai chi group for cognitive performance, sleep, and balance compared with the control group.[46] This report echoes an earlier systematic review that found that "Tai Chi has the potential to reduce falls or risk of falls among the elderly, provided that they are relatively young and non-frail..."[47] However, in a separate meta-analysis by Leung and colleagues,[48] although tai chi was recommended as an alternative treatment to reduce falls, it was not found to be necessarily superior to other interventions.

OSTEOPATHIC MANIPULATIVE THERAPY

Osteopathic manipulative therapy (OMT) has been described for disorders of dizziness and balance. OMT is taught in schools of osteopathic medicine and is also practiced by physical therapists and physiatrists. Its origin dates back to the late nineteenth century and a physician, Dr A.T. Still, who searched for a cure for diseases without using drugs. He developed a system to promote healing by manipulating bones, theoretically allowing free circulation of blood and balanced nerve function.[49] Techniques used are:

- counterstrain
- myofascial release

- cranial osteopathy
- muscle energy
- high-velocity low-amplitude therapies

A pilot study showed that OMT, with an emphasis on cranial manipulation, could benefit the postural stability of healthy, elderly individuals. The measurement of balance in this small nonrandomized sample of 40 patients was change in sway values.[50] Fraix[51] looked at the outpatient treatment of vertigo in a university setting using OMT. He found significant improvement of Dizziness Handicap Inventory scores in all 16 of his patients. This study reported that 3 patients (16.7%) experienced an exacerbation of their vertigo, and 5 (27.8%) experienced muscle soreness after the session. These adverse effects were rated as mild and did not last longer than 24 hours.

Eustachian tube dysfunction leading to dizziness and tinnitus may also be treated with OMT. A case report in the *Journal of the American Osteopathic Association*[52] details the modified Muncie technique: using a gloved finger, the physician palpates the pharyngeal orifice of the Eustachian tube in a pumping fashion, effecting a lysis of adhesions or myofascial release.

MIND-BODY APPROACHES

Mind-body approaches to dizziness have also been developed. Researchers in Northern California investigated the effectiveness of an interdisciplinary program comprising mindfulness, cognitive-behavioral techniques, and vestibular rehabilitation for patients with dizziness seen in an outpatient neurotology clinic.[53] The investigators discussed in detail their rationale for and approach to vestibular dysfunction and noted that anxiety is common in patients with disequilibrium, and moreover, dizziness was frequently associated with anxiety disorders. A shared neural circuit exists between the vestibular system and pathways for the emotional processing of anxiety. Patients' anxiety about their vestibular handicap may lead to avoidance of triggering behaviors, which then prolongs recovery. Chronic anxiety, therefore, may perpetuate vestibular dysfunction.

Cognitive-behavioral therapy (CBT), with its emphasis on challenging distorted thinking to change maladaptive behavior, has been recommended as an adjunct to vestibular rehabilitation. Dialectical behavior therapy (DBT), which incorporates mindfulness, has been helpful in difficult or treatment-resistant cases. It provides skills to help patients regulate their emotions, and mindfulness is a form of meditative awareness, a moment-to-moment focus on the here and now, stressing acceptance of each moment.[54] The investigators combined these modalities (CBT, DBT, and mindfulness) along with vestibular rehabilitation, in an effort to improve balance and address underlying autonomic arousal induced by a constant state of anxiety. Their interdisciplinary model examined the effects of a structured program using these services on:

- vestibular function
- mood
- coping
- health care use

A total of 129 patients were selected for the trial, and data were collected retrospectively. Patients attended an all-day panel, with visits to a physical therapist, neurologist, neuropsychologist, neuro-otologist, and audiologist, and had 5 group sessions over 10 weeks. The patients completed surveys including the Beck Depression Inventory, Beck Anxiety Inventory (BAI), SF-12v2 Mental Coping and Physical Coping Scales, Dizziness Handicap Inventory-short form, and Functional Level Scale before and after treatment. The investigators reported that group treatment resulted in better mood, physical and mental health, functionality, and coping, and less impairment. Group treatment also decreased health care use for similar complaints in the 1-year period studied after the treatment protocol. Higher pretreatment rated depression, poorer mental or physical health, and a diagnosis of peripheral vestibulopathy were predictive of a better outcome in logistic regression analysis. Patients rated mindfulness, diaphragmatic breathing, and DBT as being more helpful than vestibular rehabilitation. Patients' self-reported anxiety as measured on the BAI also did not change.

SUMMARY

Balance problems are prevalent, especially among elderly individuals. A 2008 National Health Interview Survey of elderly Americans (older than 65 years, with a mean age of 74.4 years) found that approximately 1 in 5 elderly persons experience annual problems with dizziness or balance.[55] This finding included difficulty with unsteadiness (68.0%), walking on uneven surfaces (54.8%), and vertigo (30.1%). Women reported more problems than men. A significant number were disabled in terms of not being able to exercise (61.2%), drive (47.1%), or participate in social events (45.8%). Given the aging of the population, the importance of a thorough understanding of the complex balance system is paramount. Strategies for treatment necessarily encompass a broad range of beneficial modalities, as more research is accomplished and the lay public demands more choice, control, and effective solutions. Integrative techniques may be helpful, particularly for refractory cases.

REFERENCES

1. Vestibular Balance Disorders. Available at: http://www.medicinenet.com/vestibular_balance_disorders/los-angeles-ca_city.htm. Accessed June 13, 2012.
2. Balance disorder. Available at: http://en.wikipedia.org/wiki/Balance_disorder. Accessed June 13, 2012.
3. Zapanta PE. Vestibular rehabilitation. 2012. Available at: http://emedicine.medscape.com/article/883878-overview. Accessed July 2, 2012.
4. Wang L, Larson EB, Bowen JD, et al. Performance-based physical function and future dementia in older people. Arch Intern Med 2006;166(10):1115–20.
5. Furman JM, Cass SP, Whitney SL. Vestibular anatomy and physiology. In: Cass JM, Whitney SP, Furman SL, editors. Vestibular disorders: a case study approach to diagnosis and treatment. New York: Oxford University Press; 2010. p. 5–16.
6. Hain, TC, Helminski JO. "Anatomy and physiology of the normal vestibular system." In Vestibular rehabilitation, by S Herdman, 2–18. Philadelphia:2007.
7. Hain TC, Helminski JO. Anatomy and physiology of the normal vestibular system. In: Herdman S, editor. Vestibular rehabilitation. Philadelphia: F.A. Davis; 2007. p. 2–18.
8. Higdon J, Drake VJ, Blumberg J. Micronutrient information center–vitamin B12. 2007. Available at: http://lpi.oregonstate.edu/infocenter/vitamins/vitaminB12/. Accessed July 10, 2012.
9. The Vestibular Disorders Association. Watson (MA): Black FO, The human balance system. Available at: http://vestibular.org/understanding-vestibular-disorder/human-balance-system. Accessed June 27, 2012.
10. Vellas BJ, Wayne SJ, Romero L, et al. One-leg balance is an important predictor of injurious falls in older persons. J Am Geriatr Soc 1997;45(6):735–8.

11. Pothier DD, Hughes C, Dillon W, et al. The use of real-time image stabilization and augmented reality eyewear in the treatment of oscillopsia. Otolaryngol Head Neck Surg 2012;146(6):966–71.
12. Hain TC. Benign paroxysmal positional vertigo. 2012. Available at: http://www.dizziness-and-balance.com/disorders/bppv/bppv.html. Accessed July 6, 2012.
13. Otoneurology questionnaire. 2012. Available at: http://www.dizziness-and-balance.com/practice/resources/questcdh2007b.pdf. Accessed July 2, 2012.
14. Kaylie D, Garrison D, Tucci DL. Evaluation of the patient with recurrent vertigo. Arch Otolaryngol Head Neck Surg 2012;138(6):584–7.
15. Lee D. Superior semicircular canal dehiscence syndrome. 2011. Available at: http://otosurgery.org/sscd_definition.htm. Accessed July 6, 2012.
16. Venosa AR, Bittar RS. Vestibular rehabilitation exercises in acute vertigo. Laryngoscope 2007;117(8):1482–7.
17. Vereeck L, Wuyts FL, Truijen S, et al. The effect of early customized vestibular rehabilitation on balance after acoustic neuroma resection. Clin Rehabil 2008;22(8):698–713.
18. Gabilan YP, Perracini MR, Munhoz MS, et al. Aquatic physiotherapy for vestibular rehabilitation in patients with unilateral vestibular hypofunction: exploratory prospective study. J Vestib Res 2008;18(2–3):139–46.
19. Benign Paroxysmal Positional Vertigo (BPPV). 2012. Available at: http://www.umm.edu/otolaryngology/bppv.htm#surgery. Accessed July 6, 2012.
20. Bromwich M, Hughes B, Raymond M, et al. Efficacy of a new home treatment device for benign paroxysmal positional vertigo. Arch Otolaryngol Head Neck Surg 2010;136(7):682–5.
21. Higdon J, Drake VJ, Blumberg J. Micronutrient information center- Vitamin B12. August 2007. http://lpi.oregonstate.edu/infocenter/vitamins/vitaminB12. Accessed July 10, 2012.
22. Jasmin L, Zieve D. Pubmed Health A.D.A.M. Medical Encyclopedia. 2012. Available at: http://www.ncbi.nlm.nih.gov/pubmedhealth/PMH0001776/. Accessed July 10, 2012.
23. Day E, Bentham P, Callaghan R, et al. Thiamine for WernickeKrsakoff syndrome in people at risk from alcohol abuse. Cochrane Database Syst Rev 2004;(1):CD004033.
24. Brookler KH, Glenn MB. Ménière's syndrome: an approach to therapy. Ear Nose Throat J 1995;74(8):534–8, 540, 542.
25. Takumida M, Anniko M, Ohtani M. Radical scavengers for Ménière's disease after failure of conventional therapy: a pilot study. Acta Otolaryngol 2003;123(6):697–703.
26. Vertigo–maintaining a steady outlook. 2012. Available at: http://www.lef.org/protocols/eye_ear/vertigo_01.htm. Accessed July 11, 2012.
27. Cesarani A, Meloni F, Alpini D. Ginkgo biloba (EGb 761) in the treatment of equilibrium disorders. Adv Ther 1998;15(5):291–304.
28. Schulz V, Hansel R, Blumenthal M, et al. Rational phytotherapy: a reference guide for physicians and pharmacists. Berlin: Springer-Verlag; 2004.
29. Seidman M. Balance disorders (vertigo, lightheadedness, dizziness and dysequilibrium). 2007. Available at: http://secure.bodylanguagevitamin.com/balance.asp. Accessed July 18, 2012.
30. Shumway-Cook A, Brauer S, Woollacott M. Timed-up & go test. UB Physical Therapy. Available at: http://gsa.buffalo.edu/DPT/tug_0109.pdf. Accessed July 6, 2012.
31. Wu CC, Young YH. Association between leukoaraiosis and saccadic oscillation. Arch Otolaryngol Head Neck Surg 2007;133(3):245–9.

32. Issing W, Klein P, Weiser M. The homeopathic preparation Vertigoheel versus Ginkgo biloba in the treatment of vertigo in an elderly population: a double-blinded, randomized, controlled clinical trial. J Altern Complement Med 2005; 11(1):155–60.
33. Karkos PD, Leong SC, Arya AK, et al. Complementary ENT: a systematic review of commonly used supplements. J Laryngol Otol 2007;121(8):779–82.
34. Panossian A, Gabrielian E, Wagner H. On the mechanism of action of plant adaptogens with particular reference to cucurbitacin R diglucoside. Phytomedicine 1999;6(3):147–55.
35. Lu HC. A Complete Translation of Yellow Emperor's Classics of Internal Medicine (Nei-jing and Nan-jing). Vancouver: Academy of Oriental Heritage; 1990.
36. Maciocia G. The practice of Chinese medicine: the treatment of diseases with acupuncture and Chinese herbs. London: Churchill Livingstone; 1994.
37. Sudhakaran P. How do you treat benign paroxysmal positional vertigo in your practice? Medical Acupuncture 2012;24(2):129–30.
38. Bensky D, Barolet R. Chinese herbal medicine: formulas & strategies. Seattle (WA): Eastland Press; 1990.
39. Plum flower–Tian ma gou teng yin wan. 2007. Available at: http://www.morningstarhealth.com/3993483337.html. Accessed July 25, 2012.
40. Ramachandran U, Manavalan A, Sundaramurthi H, et al. Tianma modulates proteins with various neuro-regenerative modalities in differentiated human neuronal SH-SY5Y cells. Neurochem Int 2012;60(8):827–36.
41. Kane E. Vertigo: natural treatments. 2004. Available at: http://dremilykane.com/2004/08/31/vertigo-natural-treatments/. Accessed July 18, 2012.
42. Steinberger A, Pansini M. The treatment of Meniere's disease by acupuncture. Am J Chin Med 1983;11(1–4):102–5.
43. Bergamaschi M, Ferrari G, Gallamini M, et al. Laser acupuncture and auriculotherapy in postural instability–a preliminary report. J Acupunct Meridian Stud 2011;4(1):69–74.
44. Liu SY, Hsieh CL, Wei TS, et al. Acupuncture stimulation improves balance function in stroke patients: a single-blinded controlled, randomized study. Am J Chin Med 2009;37(3):483–94.
45. Liao W. T'ai chi classics. Boston: Shambhala; 1990.
46. Nguyen MH, Kruse A. A randomized controlled trial of Tai chi for balance, sleep quality and cognitive performance in elderly Vietnamese. Clin Interv Aging 2012; 7:185–90.
47. Low S, Ang LW, Goh KS, et al. A systematic review of the effectiveness of Tai Chi on fall reduction among the elderly. Arch Gerontol Geriatr 2009;48(3):325–31.
48. Leung DP, Chan CK, Tsang HW, et al. Tai chi as an intervention to improve balance and reduce falls in older adults: a systematic and meta-analytical review. Altern Ther Health Med 2011;17(1):40–8.
49. Manual medicine–osteopathy: history and philosophy. Available at: http://integrativemedicine.arizona.edu/program/2011w/manual_medicine/osteopathy/2.html. Accessed July 25, 2012.
50. Lopez D, King HH, Knebl JA, et al. Effects of comprehensive osteopathic manipulative treatment on balance in elderly patients: a pilot study. J Am Osteopath Assoc 2011;111(6):382–8.
51. Fraix M. Osteopathic manipulative treatment and vertigo: a pilot study. PM R 2010;2(7):612–8.
52. Channell MK. Modified Muncie technique: osteopathic manipulation. J Am Osteopath Assoc 2008;108:260–3.

53. Naber CM, Water-Schmeder O, Bohrer PS, et al. Interdisciplinary treatment for vestibular dysfunction: the effectiveness of mindfulness, cognitive-behavioral techniques, and vestibular rehabilitation. Otolaryngol Head Neck Surg 2011; 145(1):117–24.
54. Kabat-Zinn J. Full catastrophe living: using the wisdom of your body and mind to face stress, pain, and illness. New York: Delta Trade Paperbacks; 1990.
55. Lin HW, Bhattacharyya N. Balance disorders in the elderly: epidemiology and functional impact. Laryngoscope 2012;122(8):1858–61.

Complementary and Integrative Treatments Thyroid Disease

Jennifer E. Rosen, MD[a],*, Paula Gardiner, MD, MPH[b],
Stephanie L. Lee, MD, PhD[c]

KEYWORDS

- Complementary and integrative medicine • Thyroid disease • Hyperthyroidism
- Otolaryngology

KEY POINTS

- Complementary and integrative medicine (CIM) use is common; many patients use it to compliment their allopathic treatment.
- Hyperthyroidism and, in particular, thyrotoxicosis may be induced by the use of natural products, in particular, the use of kelp as seaweed or in tea.
- Diet modulation to avoid iodine-containing products, such as kelp and seaweed, is recommended to patients undergoing radioactive iodine treatment of papillary thyroid cancer.

COMPLEMENTARY AND INTEGRATIVE MEDICINE OVERVIEW

Complementary and Integrative Medicine (CIM) is defined by the National Institutes of Health as a group of diverse medical and health care systems, practices, and products that are not generally considered part of conventional medicine. In the 2007 National Health Interview Survey, approximately one-third of US adults were estimated to have used some form of CIM, with annual costs estimated as exceeding $4 billion.[1,2] CIM use in patients is common and a working knowledge is relevant to practicing physicians. The purpose of this article is to review the common forms of CIM, review the data regarding use of CIM in disease states relevant to otolaryngologists, and provide an overview to facilitate communication with patients regarding CIM for physicians. CIM practices are usually grouped into 4 broad categories:

1. Natural products
2. Mind and body medicine practices

No Disclosures.
[a] Section of Surgical Oncology, Department of Surgery, Boston University, 820 Harrison Avenue, Suite 5007, Boston, MA 02118, USA; [b] Department of Family Medicine, Boston University Medical Center, Boston University, 1 Boston Medical Center Place, Dowling 5 South, Boston, MA 02118, USA; [c] Section of Endocrinology, Diabetes, and Nutrition, Department of Medicine, Boston Medical Center, Boston University School of Medicine, Endocrinology Evans-201, 88 East Newton Street, Boston, MA 02111, USA
* Corresponding author.
E-mail address: Jennifer.Rosen@bmc.org

Otolaryngol Clin N Am 46 (2013) 423–435
http://dx.doi.org/10.1016/j.otc.2013.02.004
0030-6665/13/$ – see front matter © 2013 Elsevier Inc. All rights reserved.

3. Manipulative practices
4. Body-based practices

A comprehensive discussion of all forms of CIM is outside of the scope of this article; however, helpful Web sites for this information include the following: www. cancer.gov, www.nccam.nih.gov, and www.fda.gov.

Practices considered CIM may become more widely accepted over time and become part of conventional medicine (eg, biofeedback and nasal clearing techniques). Most CIM practices have the following elements in common:

1. A philosophic or theoretic framework that arises from their indigenous culture
2. A model of the body and its functions
3. A concept of disease types and causes
4. A method of diagnosis of disease
5. Unique disease treatments
6. A method of evaluation of efficacy

An overview of the most common forms of CIM, their theoretic framework, and the evidence for or against their use is presented.

CIM IN OTOLARYNGOLOGY

CIM use in the United States is common, as evidenced by the 2007 National Health Interview Survey findings that 34% of Americans use some form of CIM, with an annual estimated cost of approximately $4 billion.[1,2] Insurance coverage for some forms of CIM has become more common, from therapeutic massage during physical therapy to acupuncture or reimbursement for health club membership, where classes can include Pilates or yoga. Similar studies demonstrate a high use of CIM in patients in otolaryngology clinics.[3–23] Practitioners should be aware that use of these CIM is likely to be greatest in those treatment areas where allopathic medicine may be less than effective, patients are refractory to treatment, or patients find that the side effects of conventional therapies are less than ideal.

Symptoms

Patients use CIM for many reasons: as an adjunct to conventional therapy, as a way to support their overall health and well-being, in place of conventional therapy, and as a means to improve the symptoms that come from their disease and the symptoms that can come from conventional medical treatment.[11,24–27] These symptoms can include fatigue, nausea, headache, pain, nasal congestion, dry mouth, and hoarseness.

Patient Self-treatments

Most forms of CIM that are non–practitioner based are based on patient self-treatment. Despite the high prevalence of patient use, fewer than half of the patients who use CIM typically discuss it with their clinician, and health care professionals do not consistently inquire about or record patients' use of CIM.[28–31] This is concerning because the potential for interactions between CIM modalities and patients' thyroid cancer treatment is unknown, for example, the potential drug-herb interactions or the interaction with anesthetics. Despite the evidence that patients are using CIM modalities at a significant rate and the significant data on CIM use available to clinicians, there is room for improvement in communication between providers and patients.

Physicians and patients may have a lack of confidence in communication and a lack of knowledge of CIM and its effect on health care outcomes. Physicians and trainees in all health professions represent a prime target for curricula about CIM. Physicians may be aware that patients are using CIM, but many respondents report that being asked meant only filling in a box on forms without a physician asking any further questions. This indicates that CIM use is not treated in the same manner as other types of medications. Because the data are poor, knowledge of side effects and medication interactions is limited. Additionally, because most CIM modalities are accessible without prescription, patients may not turn to a physician for information on CIM use, which potentially harms patient-provider communication further. Physicians should ask their patients about any CIM, including both patient-based and practitioner-based therapies, and be prepared to discuss them to the best of their ability.

INTEGRATIVE TREATMENT APPROACHES AND OUTCOMES
Natural Products

Natural products cover a wide span. They may include the use of

- Herbal medicines
- Vitamins
- Minerals
- Dietary supplements
- Specific foods (eg, kelp), diets, aka "nutritional" food supplements, including probiotics

The term "natural products" can be confusing, because use of a daily multivitamin or regular use of calcium or other mineral supplements is not universally considered to constitute CIM, and many patients may follow a specific diet for reasons other than their current medical issue. The most popular products include fish oil/omega-3 fatty acids and Echinacea among children.[1] Not all natural products must be taken orally; for example, eucalyptus oil is often used for patients with upper respiratory symptoms[32–73] and has transitioned from practitioner-applied therapy to self-medication because it is widely available as a rub or application oil over the counter.

The Food and Drug Administration (FDA) evaluates dietary supplement products and ingredients under a different set of regulations from those covering conventional foods and drug products. Under the Dietary Supplement Health and Education Act of 1994, the dietary supplement or dietary ingredient manufacturer is responsible for ensuring that a dietary supplement or ingredient is safe before it is marketed and the FDA is responsible for taking action against any unsafe dietary supplement product after it reaches the market. Most importantly, manufacturers only need to register their products with the FDA if it is a new ingredient to get FDA approval before producing or selling dietary supplements, but manufacturers must comply with the dietary supplement Current Good Manufacturing Practices for quality control. In addition, the manufacturer, packer, or distributor whose name appears on the label of a dietary supplement marketed in the United States is required to submit to the FDA all serious adverse event reports associated with use of the dietary supplement in the United States. Enforcement of these regulations is difficult and onerous given the widespread nature of these products.

On a historical note, natural products have been used since the earliest times known to improve health. The personal effects of the mummified prehistoric iceman found in the Italian Alps in 1991 included medicinal herbs. The Ebers Papyrus and the writings of Galen and Hippocrates evaluated and recommended specific herbs for specific disease states and contained numerous herbal prescriptions and remedies. By the Middle Ages, thousands of botanic products had been grown specifically for their medicinal effects and cataloged extensively.

Any discussion of natural products also needs to refer to the area of whole medical systems, because many of these, including ayurveda, Chinese medicine, and homeopathy, incorporate natural products in their approach.

Mind and Body Medicine

CIM mind and body practices focus on the potential (and potent) interactions between the brain, mind, and body through the use of behaviors to promote health. The most common forms of mind and body medicine are

- Deep breathing
- Meditation
- Yoga

This idea that the mind is important in the treatment of illness is an ancient one. Humanity has used behaviors to try to alter the world around them from the Neanderthals' use of cave drawings to Anasazi rain dances and Haitian voodoo. Hippocrates and Galen reference the use of massage for healing, and the Vedas documented Indian yoga sutras for the treatment of body ailments from seals thousands of years old. This concept is used today in using placebos as controls (and the unfortunately common nocebo effect).

Meditation techniques may include specific postures, focused attention, or a recommended inward focus to reduce distractions. The concept is to relax the body and mind by suspending or removing constant thoughts and attitudes. The intended goal is to improve calmness and balance and thereby improve patients' ability to cope with illness and possibly to enhance overall health and well-being.

Yoga (to use or to unite) as a discipline incorporates not only the physical practice but also mental and spiritual practice. Yoga used for health purposes typically combines physical postures, breathing techniques, meditation, and mental focus. As with many of these practices, yoga can be used not just for specific health conditions but also for overall well-being.

There are innumerable mind-body practices, including deep breathing, guided imagery, hypnotherapy, guided relaxation, qigong, and tai chi, all of which have as their goals focus and attention for health.

Manipulative and Body-based Practices

Manipulative and body-based practices mostly focus on bodily structures and systems, primarily the spine, bones and joints, soft tissue, and circulatory and lymphatic systems. The 2 most common of these are

- Chiropractic/osteopathic manipulation
- Massage

In chiropraxy/osteopathic manipulation, practitioners use their hands (*chiro*, in Greek, means hand) or, on occasion, a device to perform manipulation, most commonly around a joint with a degree of force. A wide variety of practitioners incorporate this form of manipulation, including chiropractors, osteopathic physicians, naturopathic physicians, physical therapists, and some allopathic physicians. The goal of the treatment is to relieve pain and improve physical functioning.

Massage is a hands-on technique that involves manipulating muscle and soft tissue with the aim of increasing the flow of blood and oxygen to that area. Massage not only can be used for relief of pain but can also incorporate other approaches, including acupressure points to alleviate stress, improve relaxation, and aid with anxiety and depression.

Acupuncture is an alternative approach originating in ancient China that uses the manipulation of acupuncture points by the use of insertion of thin, solid needles to achieve health through the correction of perceived imbalances in the flow of qi through channels known as meridians. Acupressure is the manipulation of these points by the use of pressure rather than through the needles.

Additional practitioner-based approaches include

- Chelation, where products are taken orally to detoxify heavy metals believed to be causing deleterious effects
- Cupping, where local suction is created on the skin with heat or mechanical devices with the intent of improving blood flow and thereby overall health
- Thermal-auricular therapy (also known as ear candling)
- Moxibustion using the burning of the mugwort herb, often in conjunction with acupuncture

There are several folk remedies still in common use, including talismans that can be worn, copper bracelets, and poultices applied to the skin. Alternative approaches to wound healing include the use of maggots for infected wounds, leaches for skin grafts, sugar/honey for chronic ulceration, and various forms of urea/papaya enzyme (papain) for decubitus ulcers.

Many practitioner-based therapies have licensing requirements that may vary from state to state; these serve to ensure a basis for training, practice, and patient information that practitioners meet the basic standards as set by national guidelines (eg, massage therapy and chiropraxy).

Whole Medical Systems

Just as patients come from different cultures that have evolved over time, so have whole medical systems developed apart from conventional or Western medicine. Most of these incorporate a worldview with a combination of botanic products and physical and spiritual practices with a unique view toward the meaning or cause of disease. For example, traditional Chinese medicine incorporates the theory of balance (yin/yang) with the 5 phases of process and change. Most commonly, traditional Chinese medicine incurs the use of botanic products, yoga, and so forth to restore harmony in the body because disease is viewed as disharmony.

Ayurvedic medicine arose in India and is based on the 3 energies, or dosas, and 5 elements that must be in balance; treatments include hygiene, plant-based medicines, elimination of toxins, and restoration of proper fluid movement.

Homeopathy arose in Europe as a way to stimulate the body's ability to heal itself through the like-cures-like approach of giving very small doses of substances that can be toxic in larger amounts. Naturopathy also supports the body's presumed ability to heal itself through dietary and lifestyle manipulations along with other CIM therapies.

Other CIM Practices

Movement therapies are additional forms of CIM, also intended to improve stress and encourage overall health and well-being. These can include

- The Feldenkrais method
- The Alexander technique
- Pilates
- Rolfing
- Structural integration

Traditional healers can be considered a form of CIM, because they use methods often based on cultural theories, beliefs, and worldviews. Examples include

- Shamans
- Native American healers
- Medicine men

Energy field manipulation is an ancient concept, based on either theoretic energy fields or known measurable energy forms (eg, magnet therapy and light therapy). The theoretic fields are also called putative or biofields and center around the concept that humans have subtle, often unmeasurable, energy. These practices include the transfer of energy to a patient either from a practitioner or from a universal energy and include qigong and Reiki, among others.

There are several practices not commonly considered CIM but that do not fit into the status of allopathic medicine. These include

- Biofeedback
- Spiritual practices or prayer
- The use of marijuana or other mind-altering substances for medicinal purposes

Espiritism and vodun are more commonly practiced among patients with African heritage, and are more centered on religious aspects of the spiritual health of patients.

THYROID DISEASE
Hyperthyroidism

Hyperthyroidism, in particular, thyrotoxicosis, may be induced by the use of natural products (for example, the use of kelp as seaweed or in tea).[74,75] Over-the-counter supplements may contain traces of iodine. There are approximately 4 million hits through online search engines for "thyroid" and "health," the vast majority of which are for weight reduction and are associated with products for sale. Factitious thyrotoxicosis has been reported worldwide in patients taking either animal thyroid hormone or products intended for weight loss.[76–80] There are few clinical trials supporting CIM approaches to the treatment of hyperthyroidism. Acupuncture was considered useful in a selective group of Chinese patients both for symptoms of thyroid hormone excess and for associated orbitopathy, but these results have not been validated.[81–83] There is a similar lack of evidence for the efficacy of kinesiology or homeopathy for treatment of Graves orbitopathy. It is difficult to support use of CIM for the treatment of hyperthyroidism given this lack of substantial, well-designed trials.

Hypothyroidism

Use of alternative approaches in patients with hypothyroidism is difficult to evaluate, because many patients may have been self-treating at the time of their laboratory evaluation, which may cause false-negative results. In female patients with infertility related to hypothyroidism, the medical literature has little comment, but the Internet yields approximately 5 million hits. Some of the most common types of CIM for fertility believed related to thyroid hormone dysfunction are

- Acupuncture
- Acupressure
- Yoga
- Massage

Most of these treatments are extrapolated from clinical trials designed to test CIM for women with infertility[84] but not specifically women with hypothyroidism. Common approaches for CIM in patients with hypothyroidism include

- The use of natural products, especially kelp and iodine or animal preparations of thyroid hormone
- Whole medical system approaches to bring the body into a sense of well-being, in particular, through the use of homeopathy
- Naturopathy or Chinese herbal medicine
- Mind-body practices, including yoga and massage

Patients with hypothyroidism often use CIM to treat side effects, such as weight gain, constipation, and fatigue. The literature for use of CIM in treatment of weight gain, constipation or fatigue is vast. However, there are no published data in the conventional literature to support or disprove use of any specific CIM for treatment of these symptoms in patients known to have hypothyroidism.

Thyroid Nodules and Symptomatic Multinodular Goiter

Treatment of goiter with CIM in the lay literature includes the use of acupuncture and seaweed. None of these has been studied in a clinical trial or under well-controlled circumstances. Few people recommend use of CIM alone for the treatment of thyroid nodules although there are reports of use of acupuncture or electrical stimulation for this purpose. Several of the side effects or symptoms for patients with large goiters, such as neck pain, can be treated with massage, but this is only of short-term benefit. CIM after surgery for these indications is discussed along with the surgical management of thyroid cancer.

Thyroid Cancer

Thyroid cancer is the most common endocrine malignancy and its incidence is rising.[85–87] The vast majority of patients with thyroid cancer have papillary thyroid cancer, which generally has an excellent prognosis. There are no reports of the induction of thyroid cancer caused by the use of CIM that can be well substantiated. Use of CIM alone for the treatment of papillary thyroid cancer is not supported by the literature.

There are several natural products currently being investigated for their efficacy in medullary thyroid cancer, a specific form of thyroid cancer that can be difficult to treat. In particular, natural withanolides hold some promise in preclinical trials for the treatment of medullary thyroid cancer.[88,89] Theoretically, because patients with medullary thyroid cancer have a high likelihood of recurrence and the cancer itself is not believed to be radioactive iodine sensitive, use of kelp and seaweed products is not clearly contraindicated, although they may interfere with the ability to regulate postoperative thyroid hormone levels. Anaplastic thyroid cancer is a particularly aggressive form of thyroid cancer that carries a poor prognosis; there are no known alternative approaches to treatment. Likewise, Hürthle cell carcinoma and follicular carcinoma do not have specific CIM recommended for their treatment. Diet modulation to avoid iodine-containing foods is recommended most commonly to patients undergoing treatment of papillary thyroid cancer.[86] Iodine could cross-react with conventional thyroid hormone supplementation or make it difficult to induce thyroid hormone suppression for therapy. Interference with PET or CT scans may also occur. Side effects from radioactive iodine ablation can include dry mouth, which the use of sialogogues, such as lemon drops or parotid massage, may alleviate.

Patients with thyroid cancer may use CIM for a variety of reasons, such as

- To help them cope with the side effects of cancer treatments
- To help their overall sense of well-being
- To cope with the stress and worry
- To try and treat or cure their cancer

There is a wide range of CIM with proved efficacy in other cancer types that coincide with the symptoms that patients with thyroid cancer may have, including fatigue,[90,91] nausea,[92] anxiety and depression,[93] and pain.[94] Patients who undergo surgical intervention for thyroid cancer may develop postoperative symptomatology similar to other patients with head and neck cancer, including neck pain, stiffness, and dysphagia. Acupuncture and massage have shown benefit for the treatment of neck pain after neck dissection.[95,96] Biofeedback and acupuncture have yielded less confident results for the treatment of dysphagia.[97–100]

Additional symptoms in thyroid cancer patients include hoarseness or other voice changes and hypocalcemia referable to hypoparathyroidism. Voice therapy is well supported for patients with postoperative surgery-induced dysphonia but use of biofeedback and acupuncture has not been tested in clinical trials of patients with recurrent laryngeal nerve injury. Postoperative hypocalcemia is usually well treated with oral calcium supplementation; vitamin D supplementation may be considered an adjunct to treatment but is not alternative because its mechanism in hypocalcemia is well described. Use of the different forms of calcium (oyster calcium, liquid calcium, and chewable tablets) is hotly debated. The different forms of calcium probably vary slightly in bioavailability and are not worth substantial out-of-pocket investment for any specific natural or purported organic formulation.

In general, CIM that supports the general sense of well-being for patients with thyroid cancer could be beneficial for patients as a whole and not specifically for the treatment of their cancer. These could include

- Spiritualism or prayer
- Yoga or massage
- Meditation
- Daily exercise

SUMMARY

In summary, patients often use CIM; physicians often do not deeply inquire about the use of CIM, and this miscommunication can be a contributing factor to the lack of adequate data that could support or disprove the use of CIM. The most appropriate strategy for physicians for incorporating CIM remains controversial but should be centered on alleviation of patient symptoms. There is insufficient evidence to recommend one management strategy over another for many common problems because the current literature is limited by inadequately powered studies. Large, multi-institutional clinical trials with well-defined outcomes are needed to properly define the role of CIM in thyroid disease.

REFERENCES

1. Barnes PM, Bloom B, Nahin RL. 2008 Complementary and alternative medicine use among adults and children: United States. Natl Health Stat Report 2007;(12):1–23.

2. Nahin RL, Barnes PM, Stussman BJ, et al. 2009 Costs of complementary and alternative medicine (CAM) and frequency of visits to CAM practitioners: United States. Natl Health Stat Report 2007;(18):1–14.

3. Krouse JH, Krouse HJ. Patient use of traditional and complementary therapies in treating rhinosinusitis before consulting an otolaryngologist. Laryngoscope 1999;109:1223–7.

4. Roehm CE, Tessema B, Brown SM. The role of alternative medicine in rhinology. Facial Plast Surg Clin North Am 2012;20:73–81.

5. Brake MK, Bartlett C, Hart RD, et al. Complementary and alternative medicine use in the thyroid patients of a head and neck practice. Otolaryngol Head Neck Surg 2011;145:208–12.

6. Trinidade A, Shakeel M, Hurman D, et al. Traditional and complementary and alternative medicines make for unwilling bedfellows in the management of cancer: a case report with a tragic outcome. J Laryngol Otol 2011;125:1193–5.

7. Amin M, Glynn F, Rowley S, et al. Complementary medicine use in patients with head and neck cancer in Ireland. Eur Arch Otorhinolaryngol 2010;267:1291–7.

8. Miller MC, Pribitkin EA, Difabio T, et al. Prevalence of complementary and alternative medicine use among a population of head and neck cancer patients: a survey-based study. Ear Nose Throat J 2010;89:E23–7.

9. Lim CM, Ng A, Loh KS. Use of complementary and alternative medicine in head and neck cancer patients. J Laryngol Otol 2010;124:529–32.

10. Vyas T, Hart RD, Trites JR, et al. Complementary and alternative medicine use in patients presenting to a head and neck oncology clinic. Head Neck 2010;32:793–9.

11. Shakeel M, Trinidade A, Ah-See KW. Complementary and alternative medicine use by otolaryngology patients: a paradigm for practitioners in all surgical specialties. Eur Arch Otorhinolaryngol 2010;267:961–71.

12. Yap L, Pothula VB, Warner J, et al. The root and development of otorhinolaryngology in traditional Chinese medicine. Eur Arch Otorhinolaryngol 2009;266:1353–9.

13. Shakeel M, Newton JR, Ah-See KW. Complementary and alternative medicine use among patients undergoing otolaryngologic surgery. J Otolaryngol Head Neck Surg 2009;38:355–61.

14. Newton JR, Santangeli L, Shakeel M, et al. Use of complementary and alternative medicine by patients attending a rhinology outpatient clinic. Am J Rhinol Allergy 2009;23:59–63.

15. Man LX. Complementary and alternative medicine for allergic rhinitis. Curr Opin Otolaryngol Head Neck Surg 2009;17:226–31.

16. Amin M, Hughes J, Timon C, et al. Quackery in head and neck cancer. Ir Med J 2008;101:82–4.

17. Shakeel M, Little SA, Bruce J, et al. Use of complementary and alternative medicine in pediatric otolaryngology patients attending a tertiary hospital in the UK. Int J Pediatr Otorhinolaryngol 2007;71:1725–30.

18. Karkos PD, Leong SC, Arya AK, et al. 'Complementary ENT': a systematic review of commonly used supplements. J Laryngol Otol 2007;121:779–82.

19. Pletcher SD, Goldberg AN, Lee J, et al. Use of acupuncture in the treatment of sinus and nasal symptoms: results of a practitioner survey. Am J Rhinol 2006;20:235–7.

20. Karmody CS. Alternative therapies in the management of headache and facial pain. Otolaryngol Clin North Am 2003;36:1221–30.

21. Ferguson BJ. New horizons in the management of allergy. Otolaryngol Clin North Am 2003;36:771–9, v.
22. Sarrell EM, Cohen HA, Kahan E. Naturopathic treatment for ear pain in children. Pediatrics 2003;111:e574–9.
23. Asher BF, Seidman M, Snyderman C. Complementary and alternative medicine in otolaryngology. Laryngoscope 2001;111:1383–9.
24. Verhoef MJ, Balneaves LG, Boon HS, et al. Reasons for and characteristics associated with complementary and alternative medicine use among adult cancer patients: a systematic review. Integr Cancer Ther 2005;4:274–86.
25. Richardson MA, Masse LC, Nanny K, et al. Discrepant views of oncologists and cancer patients on complementary/alternative medicine. Support Care Cancer 2004;12:797–804.
26. Hyodo I, Eguchi K, Nishina T, et al. Perceptions and attitudes of clinical oncologists on complementary and alternative medicine: a nationwide survey in Japan. Cancer 2003;97:2861–8.
27. Weiger WA, Smith M, Boon H, et al. Advising patients who seek complementary and alternative medical therapies for cancer. Ann Intern Med 2002;137: 889–903.
28. Tasaki K, Maskarinec G, Shumay DM, et al. Communication between physicians and cancer patients about complementary and alternative medicine: exploring patients' perspectives. Psychooncology 2002;11:212–20.
29. Eisenberg DM, Kessler RC, Foster C, et al. Unconventional medicine in the United States. Prevalence, costs, and patterns of use. N Engl J Med 1993; 328:246–52.
30. Cohen MH, Eisenberg DM. Potential physician malpractice liability associated with complementary and integrative medical therapies. Ann Intern Med 2002; 136:596–603.
31. Kemper KJ, Amata-Kynvi A, Dvorkin L, et al. Herbs and other dietary supplements: healthcare professionals' knowledge, attitudes, and practices. Altern Ther Health Med 2003;9:42–9.
32. Cohen HA, Rozen J, Kristal H, et al. Effect of honey on nocturnal cough and sleep quality: a double-blind, randomized, placebo-controlled study. Pediatrics 2012;130:465–71.
33. Ben-Arye E, Dudai N, Eini A, et al. 2011 Treatment of upper respiratory tract infections in primary care: a randomized study using aromatic herbs. Evid Based Complement Alternat Med 2011;2011:690346.
34. Kutz JW Jr, Fayad JN. Ear candling. Ear Nose Throat J 2008;87:499.
35. Pulec JL. Cerumen and coning candle chicanery. Ear Nose Throat J 1996;75: 574.
36. Rafferty J, Tsikoudas A, Davis BC. Ear candling: should general practitioners recommend it? Can Fam Physician 2007;53:2121–2.
37. Seely DR, Langman AW. Coning candles—an alert for otolaryngologists? Ear Nose Throat J 1997;76:47.
38. Seely DR, Quigley SM, Langman AW. Ear candles—efficacy and safety. Laryngoscope 1996;106:1226–9.
39. Zackaria M, Aymat A. Ear candling: a case report. Eur J Gen Pract 2009;15: 168–9.
40. Park JE, Lee SS, Lee MS, et al. Adverse events of moxibustion: a systematic review. Complement Ther Med 2010;18:215–23.
41. Cao H, Li X, Liu J. An updated review of the efficacy of cupping therapy. PLoS One 2012;7:e31793.

42. Ciocon JO, Ciocon DG, Galindo DJ. Dietary supplements in primary care. Botanicals can affect surgical outcomes and follow-up. Geriatrics 2004;59:20–4.
43. Ciordia R. Beware "St. John's Wort," potential herbal danger. J Clin Monit Comput 1998;14:215.
44. Crowe S, Lyons B. Herbal medicine use by children presenting for ambulatory anesthesia and surgery. Paediatr Anaesth 2004;14:916–9.
45. Crowe S, McKeating K. Delayed emergence and St. John's wort. Anesthesiology 2002;96:1025–7.
46. Grauer RP, Thomas RD, Tronson MD, et al. Preoperative use of herbal medicines and vitamin supplements. Anaesth Intensive Care 2004;32:173–7.
47. Irefin S, Sprung J. A possible cause of cardiovascular collapse during anesthesia: long-term use of St. John's Wort. J Clin Anesth 2000;12:498–9.
48. Meijerman I, Beijnen JH, Schellens JH. Herb-drug interactions in oncology: focus on mechanisms of induction. Oncologist 2006;11:742–52.
49. Ang-Lee MK, Moss J, Yuan CS. Herbal medicines and perioperative care. JAMA 2001;286:208–16.
50. Raduege KM, Kleshinski JF, Ryckman JV, et al. Anesthetic considerations of the herbal, kava. J Clin Anesth 2004;16:305–11.
51. Figueredo VM. Chemical cardiomyopathies: the negative effects of medications and nonprescribed drugs on the heart. Am J Med 2011;124:480–8.
52. O'Neil J, Hughes S, Lourie A, et al. Effects of echinacea on the frequency of upper respiratory tract symptoms: a randomized, double-blind, placebo-controlled trial. Ann Allergy Asthma Immunol 2008;100:384–8.
53. Quimby EL. The use of herbal therapies in pediatric oncology patients: treating symptoms of cancer and side effects of standard therapies. J Pediatr Oncol Nurs 2007;24:35–40.
54. Carr RR, Nahata MC. Complementary and alternative medicine for upper-respiratory-tract infection in children. Am J Health Syst Pharm 2006;63:33–9.
55. Bielory L. Complementary and alternative interventions in asthma, allergy, and immunology. Ann Allergy Asthma Immunol 2004;93:S45–54.
56. Eriksen K, Rochester RP, Hurwitz EL. Symptomatic reactions, clinical outcomes and patient satisfaction associated with upper cervical chiropractic care: a prospective, multicenter, cohort study. BMC Musculoskelet Disord 2011;12:219.
57. Saper RB, Sherman KJ, Cullum-Dugan D, et al. Yoga for chronic low back pain in a predominantly minority population: a pilot randomized controlled trial. Altern Ther Health Med 2009;15:18–27.
58. Cohen AJ, Menter A, Hale L. Acupuncture: role in comprehensive cancer care— a primer for the oncologist and review of the literature. Integr Cancer Ther 2005; 4:131–43.
59. Herbert V. Unproven (questionable) dietary and nutritional methods in cancer prevention and treatment. Cancer 1986;58:1930–41.
60. Saper RB, Kales SN, Paquin J, et al. Heavy metal content of ayurvedic herbal medicine products. JAMA 2004;292:2868–73.
61. Over-the-counter medications: Zicam nasal products may cause loss of sense of smell. Child Health Alert 2009;27:3.
62. Prasad HR, Malhotra AK, Hanna N, et al. Arsenicosis from homeopathic medicines: a growing concern. Clin Exp Dermatol 2006;31:497–8.
63. Chakraborti D, Mukherjee SC, Saha KC, et al. Arsenic toxicity from homeopathic treatment. J Toxicol Clin Toxicol 2003;41:963–7.
64. Demeester K, van Wieringen A, Hendrickx JJ, et al. Prevalence of tinnitus and audiometric shape. B-ENT 2007;3(Suppl 7):37–49.

65. Salvi R, Lobarinas E, Sun W. Pharmacological treatments for tinnitus: new and old. Drugs Future 2009;34:381–400.
66. Coelho CB, Tyler R, Hansen M. Zinc as a possible treatment for tinnitus. Prog Brain Res 2007;166:279–85.
67. Paaske PB, Pedersen CB, Kjems G, et al. Zinc in the management of tinnitus. Placebo-controlled trial. Ann Otol Rhinol Laryngol 1991;100:647–9.
68. Heinecke K, Weise C, Rief W. Psychophysiological effects of biofeedback treatment in tinnitus sufferers. Br J Clin Psychol 2009;48:223–39.
69. Weise C, Heinecke K, Rief W. Biofeedback-based behavioral treatment for chronic tinnitus: results of a randomized controlled trial. J Consult Clin Psychol 2008;76:1046–57.
70. Simcock R, Fallowfield L, Monson K, et al. ARIX: a randomised trial of acupuncture v oral care sessions in patients with chronic xerostomia following treatment of head and neck cancer. Ann Oncol 2013;24(3):776–83.
71. Zhuang L, Yang Z, Zeng X, et al. The preventive and therapeutic effect of acupuncture for radiation-induced xerostomia in patients with head and neck cancer: a systematic review. Integr Cancer Ther 2012. [Epub ahead of print].
72. Meng Z, Kay Garcia M, Hu C, et al. Sham-controlled, randomised, feasibility trial of acupuncture for prevention of radiation-induced xerostomia among patients with nasopharyngeal carcinoma. Eur J Cancer 2012;48:1692–9.
73. Wong RK, James JL, Sagar S, et al. Phase 2 results from Radiation Therapy Oncology Group Study 0537: a phase 2/3 study comparing acupuncture-like transcutaneous electrical nerve stimulation versus pilocarpine in treating early radiation-induced xerostomia. Cancer 2012;118:4244–52.
74. Arum SM, He X, Braverman LE. Excess iodine from an unexpected source. N Engl J Med 2009;360:424–6.
75. Mussig K, Thamer C, Bares R, et al. Iodine-induced thyrotoxicosis after ingestion of kelp-containing tea. J Gen Intern Med 2006;21:C11–4.
76. Ohye H, Fukata S, Kanoh M, et al. Thyrotoxicosis caused by weight-reducing herbal medicines. Arch Intern Med 2005;165:831–4.
77. Diez JJ. Hyperthyroidism in patients older than 55 years: an analysis of the etiology and management. Gerontology 2003;49:316–23.
78. Bogazzi F, Bartalena L, Scarcello G, et al. The age of patients with thyrotoxicosis factitia in Italy from 1973 to 1996. J Endocrinol Invest 1999;22:128–33.
79. Locker GJ, Kotzmann H, Frey B, et al. Factitious hyperthyroidism causing acute myocardial infarction. Thyroid 1995;5:465–7.
80. Bricaire H, Moreau L, Joly J, et al. Factitious thyrotoxicosis. Rev Fr Endocrinol Clin 1967;8:99–112.
81. Zhang Y, Wang X. Treatment of 51 cases of hyperthyroidism by puncturing effective points. J Tradit Chin Med 1994;14:167–70.
82. Ge TY, Du J, Shi XQ. An approach to the mechanisms of laser acupuncture in treatment of exophthalmic hyperthyroidism. J Tradit Chin Med 1988;8:85–8.
83. He JS, Jin SB, Heng JS, et al. Comparative analysis of therapeutic effects of acupuncture in the treatment of hyperthyroidism. J Tradit Chin Med 1988;8:79–82.
84. Moy I, Milad MP, Barnes R, et al. Randomized controlled trial: effects of acupuncture on pregnancy rates in women undergoing in vitro fertilization. Fertil Steril 2011;95:583–7.
85. Davies L, Welch HG. Increasing incidence of thyroid cancer in the United States, 1973-2002. JAMA 2006;295:2164–7.

86. Cooper DS, Doherty GM, Haugen BR, et al. Revised American Thyroid Association management guidelines for patients with thyroid nodules and differentiated thyroid cancer. Thyroid 2009;19:1167–214.

87. Siegel R, Desantis C, Virgo K, et al. 2012 Cancer treatment and survivorship statistics. CA Cancer J Clin 2012;62(4):220–41.

88. Samadi AK, Bazzill J, Zhang X, et al. Novel withanolides target medullary thyroid cancer through inhibition of both RET phosphorylation and the mammalian target of rapamycin pathway. Surgery 2012;152:1238–47.

89. Samadi AK, Mukerji R, Shah A, et al. A novel RET inhibitor with potent efficacy against medullary thyroid cancer in vivo. Surgery 2010;148:1228–36 [discussion: 1236].

90. Cruciani RA, Zhang JJ, Manola J, et al. L-Carnitine supplementation for the management of fatigue in patients with cancer: an Eastern Cooperative Oncology Group phase III, randomized, double-blind, placebo-controlled trial. J Clin Oncol 2012;30:3864–9.

91. Ernst E. Massage therapy for cancer palliation and supportive care: a systematic review of randomised clinical trials. Support Care Cancer 2009;17:333–7.

92. Rangwala F, Zafar SY, Abernethy AP. Gastrointestinal symptoms in cancer patients with advanced disease: new methodologies, insights, and a proposed approach. Curr Opin Support Palliat Care 2012;6:69–76.

93. Yun YH, Lee MK, Park SM, et al. Effect of complementary and alternative medicine on the survival and health-related quality of life among terminally ill cancer patients: a prospective cohort study. Ann Oncol 2013;24(2):489–94.

94. McNeely ML, Parliament MB, Seikaly H, et al. Effect of exercise on upper extremity pain and dysfunction in head and neck cancer survivors: a randomized controlled trial. Cancer 2008;113:214–22.

95. Lu W, Rosenthal DS. Recent advances in oncology acupuncture and safety considerations in practice. Curr Treat Options Oncol 2010;11:141–6.

96. Pfister DG, Cassileth BR, Deng GE, et al. Acupuncture for pain and dysfunction after neck dissection: results of a randomized controlled trial. J Clin Oncol 2010;28:2565–70.

97. Crary MA, Carnaby Mann GD, Groher ME, et al. Functional benefits of dysphagia therapy using adjunctive sEMG biofeedback. Dysphagia 2004;19:160–4.

98. Gaziano JE. Evaluation and management of oropharyngeal Dysphagia in head and neck cancer. Cancer Control 2002;9:400–9.

99. Lu W, Wayne PM, Davis RB, et al. Acupuncture for dysphagia after chemoradiation in head and neck cancer: rationale and design of a randomized, sham-controlled trial. Contemp Clin Trials 2012;33:700–11.

100. Lu W, Posner MR, Wayne P, et al. Acupuncture for dysphagia after chemoradiation therapy in head and neck cancer: a case series report. Integr Cancer Ther 2010;9:284–90.

Complementary and Integrative Treatments
The Voice

Benjamin F. Asher, MD

KEYWORDS

- Complementary treatments • Integrative treatments • Voice • Integrative approach

KEY POINTS

- Voice professionals seek integrative care to minimize potential side effects on the voice.
- The antioxidant glutathione seems to reduce vocal fatigue and the effects of phonotrauma.
- Myofascial release and laryngeal massage are effective in improving vocal function and helping minimize throat pain.
- There are supplements that effectively modulate the immune system and prevent or treat allergies and upper respiratory infections.

OVERVIEW

Most benign voice disorders are the result of phonotrauma, infection, or inflammation. Voice professionals often seek integrative physicians because of concerns about the limitations and potential side effects of most conventional treatments for their voice disorders. The armamentarium of the conventional voice physician, for the most part, includes antibiotics for infections, steroids for inflammation, and stomach acid–reducing medications for reflux-related voice issues. I have more than 25 years of experience using an integrative approach in the evaluation and management of the voice. This approach includes both conventional and integrative modalities, with an attempt at restoring health and balance to the individual and managing any problems with the fewest possible side effects. I particularly focus on reducing oxidative stress to the larynx, eliminating all muscle tension issues, and using nutritional supplements and herbal therapies when possible to treat infections, allergies, and reflux. This article is a distillation of my experience based on the best possible evidence and empirical data.

INTEGRATIVE TREATMENT APPROACHES AND OUTCOMES
Antioxidant Therapy

The larynx, being continually exposed to oxygen and irritants that promote inflammation, is a prime candidate for oxidative stress. Hydrochloric acid, pepsin, air pollution,

Private Practice, Asher Integrative Ear, Nose, and Throat, 127 East 61st Street, New York, NY 10065, USA
E-mail address: drasher@asherentd.com

Otolaryngol Clin N Am 46 (2013) 437–445
http://dx.doi.org/10.1016/j.otc.2013.02.008
0030-6665/13/$ – see front matter © 2013 Elsevier Inc. All rights reserved.
oto.theclinics.com

toxic fumes, and allergens are all agents that promote laryngeal inflammation. Reactive oxygen species (ROS) are a wide variety of unstable molecules that cause tissue damage, which is known as oxidative stress.[1–3] Glutathione (GSH), a tripeptide synthesized intracellularly from L-cysteine, L-glutamic acid, and glycine, has multiple functions, including protecting cells from ROS. It has a high electron-donating capacity and is found in high concentrations within cells, which allows it to be a potent antioxidant. The larynx naturally contains high levels of GSH and other antioxidants (superoxide dismutase) as protection against ROS.[4,5] GSH depletion has been found in numerous disease states including:

- asthma
- neurodegenerative diseases[6]
- diabetes[7]

GSH levels are also found to decrease with:

- aging[8]
- ultraviolet light and other radiation exposure[9]
- viral infections[10,11]
- exposure to environmental toxins[12]
- after surgery[13]
- among burn patients[14]

Generalized inflammation also decreases GSH levels.[15] When the cellular antioxidant defenses are insufficient to keep levels of ROS lower than a toxic level, then oxidative stress occurs. Oxidative stress is a product of either insufficient antioxidants or increased levels of ROS or both.

I have now used GSH in more than 150 patients with acute and chronic vocal fold inflammation. GSH is poorly absorbed orally, and intravenous administration is required to achieve an adequate dose. However, N-acetyl cysteine, undenatured whey protein, and α-lipoic acid seem to increase GSH levels in the body.[16,17] GSH is available as a compounded intravenous nutritional supplement, which has been safely used in patients with Parkinson disease to their benefit.[18] It has also been safely used for many years by integrative physicians for many chronic health problems. Voice patients receiving GSH report:

- increased vocal range and stamina
- less laryngeal mucus
- reduced burning sensations

GSH was also found to benefit some of my patients with refractory laryngopharyngeal reflux and laryngeal allergies. Some performers with phonotraumatic vocal fold lesions such as nodules, pseudocysts, and polyps have been able to maintain the high level of functioning required to continue performing even with these lesions. I have also seen phonotraumatic lesions disappear. The following case shows the benefit of GSH for acute phonotrauma.

Case 1

A 60-year-old male voice teacher presented with acute onset of hoarseness after holding back a sneeze. Initial strobovidolaryngoscopy revealed a small hemorrhagic polyp of the right posterior true vocal cord along the free margin of the fold (**Fig. 1**).

The patient was given 2 g of intravenous GSH weekly for 8 consecutive weeks and his voice completely returned to normal, with a vocal range that was better than before the injury. A proton pump inhibitor was recommended, but the patient did not take it.

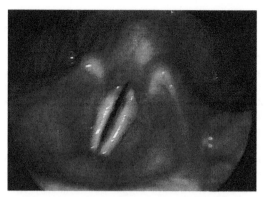

Fig. 1. Hemorrhagic polyp along margin of right posterior true cord.

Examination of the larynx at the end of 8 weeks showed complete resolution of the polyp (**Fig. 2**).

Myofascial Pain

Muscle tension dysponia

Muscle tension often plagues vocalists, and circumlaryngeal massage has been shown to be effective for muscle tension dysphonia (MTD).[19] MTD can often mimic spasmodic dysphonia. MTD is considered to be a functional voice disorder. Symptoms include nondystonic laryngeal or paralaryngeal muscle tension, with impaired, strained vocal quality. Other symptoms of MTD may include pain, hoarseness, and burning in the throat. The pathophysiology of MTD has yet to be characterized. Roy[20] has suggested that MTD is the result of a central conditioning of the laryngeal and paralaryngeal muscle groups, which function in an inhibitory fashion to restrain voice production. Roy and others have described the use of circumlaryngeal massage in the successful management of this disorder. The mechanisms for the beneficial results of this therapy have yet to be completely understood. Most theories have postulated that the manual reduction of extralaryngeal musculoskeletal tension results in reduced laryngeal hyperfunction.[19,20] In my personal experience, patients with MTD and other function laryngeal complaints such as diminished vocal range, vocal fatigue, and throat pain are often suffering from a subset of myofascial pain.

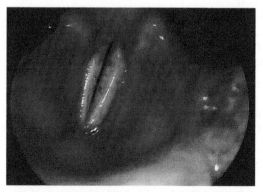

Fig. 2. Hemorrhagic polyp has disappeared after 8 consecutive weeks of 2 g of intravenous GSH.

Myofascial trigger points

The concept of myofascial pain and myofascial trigger points was developed by Dr Janet Travell in the middle of the twentieth century. She recognized that patients who had been bedridden with tuberculosis often suffered from severe pain in the shoulders and arms. She noted that the origin of this pain appeared to be coming from trigger areas in the chest muscles and scapula. She went on to postulate and then to identify focal points in muscles that referred pain to distant locations. These points were termed trigger points.[21] Myofascial pain and trigger points have been understood and researched by physiatrists, pain specialists, physical therapists, and massage therapists, but the concept is not taught to otolaryngologists and speech pathologists.

Trigger points are hyperirritable spots in skeletal muscles that give rise to referred pain, referred tenderness, motor dysfunction, and autonomic phenomenon. Trigger points may be active or latent. Active trigger points usually cause pain locally on compression but also refer pain in a characteristic pattern. Latent trigger points, on the other hand, cause symptoms other than pain, such as increased muscular tension, restriction of motion, and autonomic phenomenon. Trigger point pain distributions and the effects of latent trigger points have been well delineated by Travell and Simmons.[21] Each trigger point has a characteristic pattern of pain, specific to individual muscles. An active trigger point in the sternal division of the sternocleidomastoid muscle, for example, refers pain to the occiput, the parietal region, the supraorbital rim, the submandibular area, and the mentum.[21]

Trigger points arise from multiple causes; they may be activated indirectly by:

- other trigger points
- acute or chronic overload stress
- exposure to cold
- visceral disease
- arthritic joints
- emotional distress

Once a trigger point is created, if it is not treated, it has a tendency to propagate further trigger points, further aggravating symptoms. Activation of trigger points in the neck often gives rise to neck pain, facial pain, throat pain, and shoulder pain. Activation of trigger points in the muscles supporting laryngeal function gives rise not only to pain, but also to several other symptoms, including burning, hoarseness, and autonomic dysfunction. Active myofascial trigger points vary in irritability from hour to hour and day to day. Signs and symptoms of trigger point activity long outlast the precipitating event.

In general, myofascial pain and trigger points should be suspected when the symptoms arise shortly after acute overload stress or there is a history of gradual onset of symptoms with chronic overload of the affected muscle. Other characteristics of myofascial pain include:

- characteristic patterns of pain, specific to individual muscles
- weakness and restriction in the stretch range of motion of the affected muscle
- a taut palpable band in the affected muscle
- exquisite and focal tenderness to digital pressure in the taut band

Trigger points are diagnosed by direct palpation. Palpation of a trigger point may cause a characteristic twitch response. With palpation, pain may also be experienced at the trigger point or in its distribution pattern. The distribution pattern of myofascial pain does not follow neural pathways. The pathophysiology of myofascial pain is not completely known.

Treatment is directed to the trigger point. Treatment techniques vary, including:

- injection of the trigger point with lidocaine or saline
- dry needling the trigger point
- spraying the trigger point with a cooling agent, such as ethylene chloride
- ischemic massage.

The affected muscle must always be stretched after the trigger point is treated. Treating a trigger point without stretching the muscle does not eliminate the symptom.

I find that massage and stretching are my most effective tools in the treatment of vocal fatigue and throat pain. The following 2 cases are examples of patients with throat and voice symptoms, who were treated successfully with myofascial release.

Case 2

N.H. is a 47-year-old woman, who presented with the sudden onset of pain in the base of her tongue. Although on initial examination, there were no physical findings, she was treated by another otolaryngologist for an infection with a course of antibiotics, which were ineffective. She also did not benefit from proton pump inhibitors. Head and neck examination was normal, except for finding exquisite tenderness in the left scalenes, trapezius muscle, and her supralaryngeal musculature. She was treated with myofascial release of the affected muscles on 3 separate visits and her symptoms were eliminated.

Case 3

I.R. is a 48-year-old woman, who developed persistent throat pain and vocal fatigue after a bout of shouting. She also complained of a right hemicranial headache and pain in the right posterior neck. She had a normal laryngeal examination. She had exquisite tension in the right posterior neck along the nuchal line and suboccipital muscles. She was also tender along her right scalenes. Myofascial release of the affected areas eliminated her pain and improved her vocal fatigue.

Herbs and Supplements

Herbs and supplements for the vocalist may be used to replace conventional medications in allergies and reflux, often with fewer side effects. Immune-modulating herbs and supplements are available to prevent and treat upper respiratory infections (URIs) and have no conventional counterpart.

Butterbur

In the management of seasonal and perennial allergic symptoms, natural and nutritional products have been researched. Perhaps the most well-researched herb is butterbur. This herb has been found in head-to-head trials to be as effective as cetirizine in the relief of allergic symptoms and has less of a drying effect on the voice. It seems to work as a leukotriene inhibitor.[22,23]

Stinging nettle and quercetin

Less rigorous studies have shown that plant sterols balance the T helper type 1 (Th1) and Th2 lymphocytes and thereby reduce the allergic response, and daily use of probiotics reduces allergy symptoms.[24–26] In vitro studies of the herb stinging nettle and the antioxidant quercetin provide a theoretic basis for allergy relief.[27,28] Stinging nettle has antagonistic and negative agonist activity against the histamine 1 (H_1) receptors and causes inhibition of mast cell tryptase, preventing mast cell degranulation. It also inhibits prostaglandin formation through inhibition of cyclooxygenase 1 (COX-1), COX-2, and hematopoietic prostaglandin D_2 synthase.

Quercetin is a natural antioxidant that blocks substances involved in allergies and acts as an inhibitor of mast cell secretion, causing a decrease in the release of tryptase, monocyte chemotactic protein 1, and interleukin 6 and the downregulation of histidine decarboxylase mRNA from a few mast cell lines.[27,28] Quercetin and stinging nettle are often together in many herbal allergy products.

Chinese herbs
A combination of Chinese herbs for asthma has been compared with prednisone in a double-blind placebo-controlled trial, and it was shown that the herbs were as effective as prednisone in improving pulmonary function; they increased serum cortisol levels rather than suppressing the adrenal glands.[29]

Other natural treatments
Natural treatments for reflux abound, but there are no studies validating their efficacy. In my own practice, I find that they help some people and do recommend them in cases that are not severe. Digestive enzymes and calcium citrate powder are used with each meal to theoretically increase gastric emptying time and slightly buffer the stomach acid. Other products used include:

- D-Limonene
- Betaine hydrochloride (HCL)
- Magnolia extract
- Black raspberry

The mechanism of action of D-limonene is unknown, but it does relieve symptoms in some patients. Betaine HCL purportedly increases stomach acid, and those who use it once again believe that it increases gastric emptying time by speeding up digestion. Magnolia extract purportedly increases the sphincter tone to the lower esophageal sphincter, thereby reducing reflux. Black raspberry has been shown to protect the esophagus against stomach acid and convert Barrett esophagus to normal mucosa.

URIs
Supplements Supplements for immune modulation for the prevention and treatment of URIs, which are the bane of most vocalists, have been well researched and have been shown to be effective. CVT-002, a proprietary North American ginseng extract, has been shown in several double-blind placebo-controlled trials to both prevent and enhance recovery from viral URIs.[30,31] Ginseng has multiple known effects in vitro on immune function. The Cochrane database has reported that evidence supports the use of zinc supplements in the treatment of URIs, even although the exact dose has not yet been established.[32] Zinc can cause nausea as a side effect and caution is advised. The African herb *Pelargonium sidoides* has also been shown in double-blind placebo-controlled studies to be an effective nonantibiotic treatment of acute

Table 1 Brand names for herbal supplements	
Herb	**Brand Name**
Butterbur	Petadolex
Pelargonium Sidoides	Umcka Viraclear EPS 7640 Umckaloabo Kaloba
CVT-E002 (Proprietary North American ginseng)	Cold FX

bronchitis and sinusitis.[33] The active ingredient is EPs-7630. It seems to modulate salivary secretory immunoglobulin A and serum and nasal inflammatory cytokines.[34] This herbal treatment is also supported in the Cochrane database (**Table 1** gives the product names of these supplements).[35]

SUMMARY

An integrative and holistic medical approach is often greatly appreciated by the voice patient. Many vocalists seek complementary and integrative treatments because of their appreciation that their body is their instrument. They understand that most practitioners of complementary and integrative medicine operate from a belief (whether correct or not) that there is a place of balance in the body that reflects a state of optimal health. When the body is functioning optimally, the voice reflects that state. These vocalists attempt to minimize therapeutic modalities that have significant side effects that tip the scale away from well-being. The approaches delineated in this article have been used successfully to treat patients with a wide array of benign voice disorders.

REFERENCES

1. Inci E, Civelek S, Seven A, et al. Laryngeal cancer: in relation to oxidative stress. Tohoku J Exp Med 2003;200(1):17–23.
2. Diamond J, Skaggs J, Manaligod JM. Free-radical damage: a possible mechanism of laryngeal aging. Ear Nose Throat J 2002;81(8):531–3.
3. Fitzpatrick AM, Teague WG, Burwell L, et al. Glutathione oxidation is associated with airway macrophage functional impairment in children with severe asthma. Pediatr Res 2011;69:154–9.
4. Seven A, Civelek S, Inci E, et al. Evaluation of oxidative stress parameters in blood of patients with laryngeal carcinoma. Clin Biochem 1999;32(5):369–73.
5. Kalayci A, Ozturk A, Ozturk K, et al. Superoxide dismutase and glutathione peroxidase enzyme activities in larynx carcinoma. Acta Otolaryngol 2005; 125(3):312–5.
6. Schulz JB, Lindenau J, Seyfried J, et al. Glutathione, oxidative stress and neurodegeneration. Eur J Biochem 2000;267:4904–11.
7. Parthiban A, Vijayalingam S, Shanmugasundaram KR, et al. Oxidative stress and the development of diabetic complications–antioxidants and lipid peroxidation in erythrocytes and cell membrane. Cell Biol Int 1995;19(12):987–93.
8. Gautam N, Das S, Mahapatra SK, et al. Age associated oxidative damage in lymphocytes. Oxid Med Cell Longev 2010;3(4):275–82.
9. Schafer M, Dutsch S, auf dem Keller U, et al. Nrf2 establishes a glutathione-mediated gradient of UVB cytoprotection in the epidermis. Genes Dev 2010; 24(10):1045–58.
10. Witschi A, Junker E, Schranz C, et al. Supplementation of N-acetylcysteine fails to increase glutathione in lymphocytes and plasma of patients with AIDS. AIDS Res Hum Retroviruses 1995;11(1):141–3.
11. Bounous G, Molson J. Competition for glutathione precursors between the immune system and the skeletal muscle: pathogenesis of chronic fatigue syndrome. Med Hypotheses 1999;53(4):347–9.
12. Gul M, Kutay FZ, Temocin S, et al. Cellular and clinical implications of glutathione. Indian J Exp Biol 2000;38(7):625–34.
13. Luo JL, Hammarqvist F, Andersson K, et al. Surgical trauma decreases glutathione synthetic capacity in human skeletal muscle tissue. Am J Physiol 1998; 275(2 Pt 1):E359–65.

14. Wernerman J, Luo JL, Hammarqvist F. Glutathione status in critically-ill patients: possibility of modulation by antioxidants. Proc Nutr Soc 1999;58(3):677–80.
15. Beloqui O, Prieto J, Suarez M, et al. N-acetyl cysteine enhances the response to interferon-alpha in chronic hepatitis C: a pilot study. J Interferon Res 1993;13(4): 279–82.
16. Witschi A, Reddy S, Stofer B, et al. The systemic availability of oral glutathione. Eur J Pharmacol 1992;43(6):667–9.
17. Bounous G. Whey protein concentrate (WPC) and glutathione modulation in cancer treatment. Anticancer Res 2000;20(6C):4785–92.
18. Hauser RA, Lyons KE, McClain T, et al. Randomized, double-blind, pilot evaluation of intravenous glutathione in Parkinson's disease. Mov Disord 2009;24(7):979–83.
19. Van Lierde KM, DeLey S, Clement G, et al. Outcome of laryngeal manual therapy in four Dutch adults with persistent moderate to severe vocal hyperfunction: a pilot study. J Voice 2004;18(4):467–74.
20. Roy N. Functional dysphonia. Curr Opin Otolaryngol Head Neck Surg 2003;11(3): 144–8.
21. Simons D, Travell J, Simons L. Myofascial pain and dysfunction: the trigger point manual, vol. 1. Williams and Wilkins; 1999.
22. Schapowal A, Petasites Study Group. Butterbur Ze 339 for the treatment of intermittent allergic rhinitis: dose-dependent efficacy in a prospective, randomized, double blind placebo controlled study. Arch Otolaryngol Head Neck Surg 2004;130:1381–6.
23. Schapowal A, Petasites Study Group. Randomised controlled trial of butterbur and cetirizine for treating seasonal allergic rhinitis. BMJ 2002;324(7330):144–6.
24. Bouci PJ, Lamprecht JH. Plant sterols and sterolins: a review of their immune-modulating properties. Altern Med Rev 1999;4(3):170–7.
25. Bjorksten B. Evidence of probiotics in prevention of allergy and asthma. Curr Drug Targets Inflamm Allergy 2005;4(5):599–604.
26. de Vresem M, Winkler P, Rautenberg P, et al. Effect of Lactobacillus gasseri PA 16/8, Bifidobacterium longum SP 07/3, B. bifidum MF 20/5 on common cold episodes: a double blind, randomized controlled trial. Clin Nutr 2005;24(4):481–91.
27. Shaik YB, Castellani ML, Parrella A, et al. Role of quercetin (a natural herbal compound) in allergy and inflammation. J Biol Regul Homeost Agents 2006;20(3–4): 47–52.
28. Roscheek B Jr, Fink RC, McMichael M, et al. Nettle extract (Urtica dioica) affects key receptors and enzymes associated with allergic rhinitis. Phytother Res 2009; 23(7):920–6.
29. Wen MC, Wei CH, Hu J, et al. Efficacy and tolerability of anti-asthma herbal medicine intervention in adult patients with moderate-severe allergic asthma. J Allergy Clin Immunol 2005;116:517–24.
30. McElhaney JE, Goel V, Toane B, et al. Efficacy of Cold-fX in the prevention of respiratory symptoms in community-dwelling adults: a randomized double-blinded, placebo controlled trial. J Altern Complement Med 2006;12(2):153–7.
31. Predy GN, Goel V, Lovlin R, et al. Efficacy of an extract of North American ginseng containing poly-furanosyl-pyranosyl-saccharides for preventing upper respiratory tract infections: a randomized controlled trial. CMAJ 2005;173(9):1043–8.
32. Singh M, Das RR. Zinc for the common cold. Cochrane Database Syst Rev 2011;(2):CD001364.
33. Bachert C, Schapowal A, Funk P, et al. Treatment of acute rhinosinusitis with the preparation from Pelargonium sidoides EPs 7630: a randomized, double-blind, placebo-controlled trial. Rhinology 2009;47(1):51–8.

34. Luna LA Jr, Bachi AL, Novaes e Brito RR, et al. Immune responses induced by *Pelargonium sidoides* extract in serum and nasal mucosa after exhaustive exercise: modulation of secretory IgA, IL-6 and IL-15. Phytomedicine 2011; 18(4):303–8.
35. Timmer A, Gunther J, Rucjker G, et al. *Pelargonium sidoides* extract for acute respiratory tract infections. Cochrane Database Syst Rev 2008;(3):CD006023.

Complementary and Integrative Treatments Swallowing Disorders

Jennifer M. Lavin, MD[a],*, David Tieu, MD[b],
John Maddalozzo, MD[a,c]

KEYWORDS

- Integrative medicine • Dysphagia • Alternative medicine

KEY POINTS

- Swallowing disorders can be grouped by etiology into oropharyngeal and esophageal as well as neuromuscular and structural causes.
- Whenever possible, attempts should be made at medical or surgical treatment of the underlying cause of a swallowing disorder.
- When no treatment of the underlying cause is available, medical supportive management includes speech therapy and diet modification.
- Surgical supportive management options include gastrostomy tube placement or laryngeal separation procedures.
- Integrative treatment modalities such as acupuncture and Banxia Houpo Tang have been described in conjunction with other medical and surgical treatments.

OVERVIEW

Swallowing disorders are of many different causes and may lead to significant morbidity and mortality if not addressed. These disorders affect patients of all ages; however, their prevalence increases in the elderly population, not because of the normal aging process but rather the fact that, as patients age, they are more likely to be affected by disorders that lead to dysphagia such as stroke and neurodegenerative disorders.[1] Dysphagia has been associated with increased incidence of malnutrition, aspiration pneumonia, and death, especially in the elderly population.[2] Due to

Disclosures: None.
[a] Department of Otolaryngology-Head and Neck Surgery, Northwestern, University Feinberg School of Medicine, 676 North Saint Clair Street, #1325, Chicago, IL 60611, USA; [b] Department of Otolaryngology-Head and Neck Surgery, Kaiser Foundation Hospital, 4900 Sunset Boulevard, 6th floor, Los Angeles, CA 90027, USA; [c] Department of Surgery, Division of Otolaryngology, Anne & Robert H. Lurie Children's Hospital of Chicago, 225 East Chicago Avenue, Box #25, Chicago, IL 60611, USA
* Corresponding author. Department of Otolaryngology-Head and Neck Surgery, Northwestern University Feinberg School of Medicine, 676 North Saint Clair Street, #1325, Chicago, IL 60611.
E-mail address: j-lavin@fsm.northwestern.edu

this, aggressive management of swallowing disorders is essential to limit their associated morbidity and mortality. Treatments of swallowing disorders either address the underlying cause of the patient's dysphagia or aim to decrease the incidence of dysphagia-associated complications. Although medical and surgical therapies have been the mainstays of managing these patients, complementary and integrative medicine approaches have also been described and may play a role in treatment of swallowing disorders.

PHYSIOLOGY AND ANATOMY

The upper aerodigestive tract participates in swallowing, and normal swallowing has phases under volitional and reflexive control. Structures involved in swallowing are located in the oral cavity, oropharynx, larynx, and esophagus (**Fig. 1**). The upper aerodigestive tract has been described as a series of 6 valves.[3] These valves include

- Lips
- Tongue
- Glossopalatal valve
- Velopharyngeal valve
- Larynx
- Cricopharyngeal sphincter

At the initiation of feeding, the lips, via the orbicularis oris muscle, form the first valve by forming a seal around the eating utensil. This valve also contributes to oral competence during mastication.

Next, the tongue acts as the second valve, moving food around the mouth permitting mastication, intermixing of saliva produced by the salivary glands, and finally, forming a bolus of food to begin the oral phase of deglutition. At the same time, the buccinator muscles act to hold the cheeks to the alveolar ridges to prevent food from being displaced into the lateral sulci during mastication. The soft palate, which acts as the third (glossopalatal) valve, makes contact with the back of the tongue to prevent the bolus from prematurely entering the oropharynx. The oral phase of the swallow is then initiated when the tongue makes contact with the hard palate in an anterior to posterior direction, allowing the bolus to be transported to the oropharynx.[4]

When the bolus reaches the faucial arches, the pharyngeal swallow is triggered. From this point forward, the swallow is no longer under voluntary control. During the

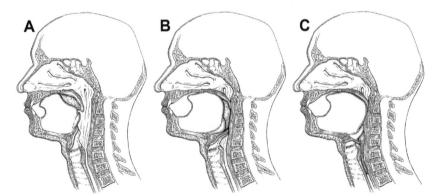

Fig. 1. Normal anatomy and physiology of swallowing. (*A*) Oral phase, (*B*) pharyngeal phase, and (*C*) esophageal phase. (*Courtesy of* M. Gallagher, MS, Chicago, Illinois.)

pharyngeal phase, the base of tongue moves posteriorly to contact the posterior pharyngeal wall, thus pushing the bolus inferiorly. At the same time, the fourth (velopharyngeal) valve closes to prevent reflux of material into the nasopharynx. Next, the larynx acts as the fifth valve protecting the airway with the approximation of the true and false vocal cords. In addition, the larynx and hyoid bone elevate, which causes the epiglottis to fold down over the airway providing additional protection. Finally, the bolus reaches the cricopharyngeal valve (upper esophageal sphincter). This valve relaxes, and food can pass into the esophagus and then into the stomach via peristalsis.

SYMPTOMS

Swallowing disorders have many different causes, and symptoms vary with each underlying cause. These disorders are grouped into 2 categories based on the location of the dysfunction:

- Oropharyngeal
- Esophageal

Oropharyngeal dysphagia is further categorized into neuromuscular and structural causes. Similarly, esophageal dysphagia is categorized as either esophageal dysmotility or structural esophageal dysphagia. Understanding the different symptoms associated with each underlying cause of dysphagia can help the physician pinpoint the cause of the swallowing disorder and can direct further management.

Dysphagia of all causes may present with malnutrition and weight loss. One study found a statistically significant increase in malnutrition in patients with oropharyngeal dysphagia compared with patients without, as determined by the mini nutritional assessment.[5] Similarly, in a study by Caporali, 160 patients with systemic sclerosis were studied for malnutrition, as defined by body mass index less than 20 or a 6-month weight loss greater than 10% and determined that 15% of these patients had evidence of malnutrition according to this criterion.[6] Malnutrition, however, is very nonspecific and does not suggest the etiology of the underlying cause.

Oropharyngeal dysphagia is distinguished from esophageal dysphagia by symptoms involving structures above the esophageal inlet. The patient with oropharyngeal dysphagia may present with recurrent aspiration pneumonia or frequent cough after swallowing.[1] If residual food is present in the vallecula after swallowing, the patient may note the need to swallow multiple times to clear the bolus. Further determination of timing of symptom onset and associated symptoms helps further delineate the underlying cause of oropharyngeal dysphagia.

Oropharyngeal dysphagia can further be categorized according to whether it has

- Neuromuscular cause
- Structural cause

The most common neuromuscular cause of dysphagia is stroke,[1] with 25% to 40% of stroke patients experiencing dysphagia.[7,8] About 45% to 68% of patients with dysphagia after stroke die within 6 months, and this death rate is largely attributed to malnutrition and aspiration pneumonia.[7,9] In patients with oropharyngeal dysphagia due to stroke, symptoms of dysphagia are acute in onset and are associated with other stigmata of stroke such as hemiparesis or bulbar symptoms.

As patients age, neurodegenerative diseases such as dementia and Parkinson disease become more prevalent. In one study, pneumonia was found to be the cause of death in 55% and 33% of patients with Alzheimer and vascular dementia, respectively.[10] Similarly, in patients with Parkinson disease, the median duration between dysphagia onset and death is 15 to 24 months.[11] Dysphagia in both dementia and Parkinson disease is often slow and progressive in nature. On esophageal manometry, patients with Parkinson frequently have diminished cricopharyngeal relaxation.[12]

Patients with other, less common, neuromuscular diseases may also present with symptoms of dysphagia. Dysarthria and dysphagia are the presenting complaints in 25% to 30% of patients with amyotrophic lateral sclerosis.[13] These patients note symptoms that are gradual in onset and are associated with focal areas of weakness. Physical examination of these patients frequently reveals fasciculations of the tongue. Dysphagia affects 30% to 60% of patients with polymyositis and dermatomyositis.[14] Patients with these inflammatory myopathies present gradual onset dysphagia with proximal limb weakness. Patients with dermatomyositis also have skin manifestations such as the heliotrope rash. Patients with myasthenia gravis may also present with dysphagia, which may wax and wane and increase in magnitude with fatigue.

In contrast to neuromuscular causes, structural anomalies are also associated with oropharyngeal dysphagia. Patients with Zenker diverticulum complain of dysphagia that is gradual in onset. If food falls into the diverticulum, the patient may complain of regurgitation of undigested food or may even present with symptoms of aspiration. As the pouch enlarges over time, it may lead to extrinsic compression of the esophagus and further dysphagia, especially to solid foods.

Another structural cause of oropharyngeal dysphagia is secondary to head and neck neoplasm. Dysphagia may be due to tethering of the tongue, abnormal pharyngeal wall motion, or obstruction of the esophageal inlet. Although less common, it is also possible for masses outside the aerodigestive tract, such as large thyroid neoplasms, to cause extrinsic compression leading to dysphagia.[15] Patients can often develop dysphagia following medical and surgical treatment of head and neck cancer. For instance, surgical resection of oral and oropharyngeal tumors historically resulted in poor swallowing outcomes, but swallowing function after these surgeries has improved with the advent of free flap reconstruction.[16–19] Combined chemotherapy and radiation has been associated with swallowing impairment with 50% of patients having long-term dysphagia and 70% having xerostomia.[20–23] In a study by El-Deiry, surgical resection with postoperative radiation had a similar degree of swallowing dysfunction as combined chemotherapy and radiation.[24]

The symptomatic presentation of esophageal dysphagia can differ from that of oropharyngeal dysphagia. Patients with esophageal dysphagia often note a sensation of food getting "stuck" several seconds after swallowing and frequently localize the sensation to an area deep to the sternum. Because patients with esophageal dysphagia occasionally have referred sensation in the neck, care must be taken when relying on these symptoms for localization.[1]

Similar to oropharyngeal dysphagia, esophageal dysphagia is divided into 2 main underlying causes:

- Structural causes
- Esophageal dysmotility

Structural causes present with gradual onset of dysphagia to solids before liquids. Some examples include esophageal strictures, rings, webs, or malignancy. In contrast, patients with esophageal dysmotility present with dysphagia to both solids and liquids. Symptoms that are intermittent in nature suggest diffuse esophageal spasm as the underlying cause of dysmotility whereas constant, progressive symptoms point to achalasia or scleroderma.

Furthermore, swallowing disorders in the pediatric population can have different presentations and causes as compared with adults. Common symptoms in this population include poor coordination of the suck-swallow-breathe reflex, coughing while feeding, drooling, failure to thrive, and prolonged feeding times.[25] Dysphagia and feeding difficulties are also prevalent in prematurity.[26] In one study, patients with prematurity-associated bronchopulmonary dysplasia were found to have poor suck-swallow-breathe coordination, weak sucking pressures, less frequent swallowing, and prolonged deglutition apnea.[27] Other common disorders associated with pediatric dysphagia are neuromuscular diseases such as cerebral palsy and spinal muscular atrophy type II, laryngomalacia, vocal cord paralysis, and vascular rings/slings.[26,28,29]

Although eosinophilic esophagitis, an entity associated with swallowing dysfunction, is typically diagnosed in childhood, it can present in patients of any age. Symptoms can vary depending upon age.[30] Presentation during infancy includes vomiting, food refusal, and choking with meals.[31] On the other hand, dysphagia, food impaction, gagging with meals, and occasionally chest pain are symptoms commonly encountered in older children and adolescents. Adults typically present with dysphagia, heartburn, and food impaction secondary to esophageal rings and webs. In patients of all ages, there is a lack of response to acid-reducing medications and an association with food and environmental allergy.[30]

MEDICAL TREATMENT APPROACHES AND OUTCOMES

Whenever possible, the primary goal of management of swallowing disorders should be to treat the underlying cause. In most types of oropharyngeal dysphagia of neuromuscular cause, treating the underlying cause does not improve dysphagia. In a meta-analysis of patients with Parkinson disease, treatment with levodopa did not improve swallowing dysfunction despite improvement in other symptoms.[32] In contrast to other neuromuscular causes of oropharyngeal dysphagia, treatment of inflammatory myopathies has led to decreased symptoms of dysphagia. In 2 randomized controlled trials, patients with severe inflammatory myopathies demonstrated improvement in dysphagia when intravenous immunoglobulin was administered over several sessions.[33,34] In a case series by Kiely, all 4 patients with severe dysphagia and a diagnosis of inflammatory myopathy who underwent intravenous immunoglobulin treatment became gastrostomy-tube independent after therapy.[35]

In addition to medical therapies, nonsurgical, procedural treatments are available to address specific causes of dysphagia. In cases of dysphagia induced by late-stage, unresectable esophageal neoplasm, a statistically significant improvement in swallowing was found in patients undergoing esophageal stent placement.[36] Botulinum toxin (Botox) injection has also been used to treat several types of dysphagia. In a study by Storr, endoscopic injection of Botox into the esophageal wall was performed on patients with diffuse esophageal spasm, resulting in an elimination of symptoms in 8 of 9 patients;[37] this is in contrast to the traditional medical management with anticholinergics, nitrates, calcium channel antagonists, and antidepressants, in which clinical trials have shown mixed results regarding efficacy.[38–41] Injection of Botox into the lower esophageal sphincter (LES) in patients with achalasia has demonstrated short-term resolution of symptoms in 78% to 90% of patients, but recurrence of symptoms is relatively common.[42,43] Cricopharyngeus injection of Botox has been described, but outcomes remain better in patients undergoing surgical myotomy for cricopharyngeal dysfunction.[44]

In cases where treatment of the underlying condition is not possible, management goals should be supportive, including decreasing symptoms of dysphagia and preventing aspiration. The most noninvasive means of doing so involves dietary modification (eg, thickening of liquids) and speech and swallow therapy. Speech and swallow therapy aims to strengthen weakened oropharyngeal muscle groups or to modify dysfunctional portions of the swallow apparatus to prevent aspiration. In a randomized controlled trial, there appeared to be no significant difference when comparing the chin-down technique during swallowing versus thickening of liquids.[45] Because no randomized trials to date have included a nontreatment group, the true benefit of these interventions remains unknown. In the infant and young child, swallow therapy and transition to oral feedings differ slightly from that of the adult, with increased emphasis on oral stimulation and nonnutritive stimulation. These interventions have been associated with faster transition to oral feeding and shorter hospital stays in preterm infants.[46]

When dietary modifications and swallow therapy alone are insufficient in preventing pneumonia, alternative means of feeding may be required. Nasogastric tube (NGT) feeding is a nonsurgical alternative to feeding via a percutaneous endoscopic gastrostomy (PEG) tube. Studies have compared feeding via NGT to that of PEG tube in stroke patients and have shown no difference in aspiration rates between either method.[47,48] One benefit to PEG over NGT is that PEG was found to be superior to NGT with regards to delivering the prescribed number of calories and maintaining adequate long-term nutrition.[49,50] On the other hand, PEG was associated with higher risk of death at 6 months when compared with NGT.[51]

SURGICAL TREATMENT APPROACHES AND OUTCOMES

Similar to medical management, the initial goals of surgical management should be directed toward treatment of the underlying condition. In patients with Zenker diverticulum, treatment is surgical and may be approached with either an endoscopic or an open, transcervical approach. When endoscopic stapler-assisted esophago diverticulostomy was compared with open cricopharyngeal myotomy, endoscopic approaches have resulted in shorter operating duration, faster recovery, shorter time to oral intake, and shorter hospital stays.[52–55] Both surgeries have similar success rates ranging from 90% to 100%.[56–58] The major disadvantage of endoscopic stapler-assisted repair is the limited benefit in very small (<2 cm) diverticula where the anvil of the stapler is too long to fit in the pouch.[59] Endoscopic carbon dioxide laser-assisted diverticulectomy has been studied; however, results are mixed when compared with stapler-assisted procedures.[60,61]

In addition to patients with Zenker diverticulum, select patients with neuromuscular causes of oropharyngeal dysphagia may be candidates for cricopharyngeal myotomy. Parkinson disease and the inflammatory myopathies have been associated with dysfunction of the upper esophageal sphincter. Outcomes after cricopharyngeal myotomy in these patients are worse with published success rates of 60%.[62,63]

There are various surgical interventions for the many causes of esophageal dysphagia. The surgical treatment of achalasia is laparoscopic Heller myotomy (LHM) with fundoplication. In one study, 90% of patients with achalasia who underwent LHM reported resolution of symptoms.[64] Pneumatic dilation of the LES is also an alternative to surgery in these patients. In a multicenter, randomized controlled trial, there was no difference between the 2 procedures with respect to symptoms, LES pressure, esophageal emptying, and quality of life.[65] The authors argue that balloon dilation carries a high risk of perforation even in experienced hands, and multiple dilation procedures must be performed to achieve the same result as LHM.[66] In patients with esophageal cancer who have resectable disease, removal of the mass is the treatment of choice to improve the patient's dysphagia. One common complication of Ivor-Lewis esophagectomy, however, is anastomotic stricture, with postoperative rates of dysphagia to solid foods quoted at 25% to 35%.[67,68]

When PEG or NGT feeding fails to prevent aspiration events, more radical measures may be required to prevent aspiration, such as

- Glottis closure
- Laryngotracheal separation
- Total laryngectomy

Most studies published in the literature have been small in scale and no prospective trails have been performed. Laryngotracheal separation is most commonly performed on the neurologically impaired pediatric patient; however, it also has been described as a treatment of the elderly patient with intractable aspiration.[69] In a retrospective review of 56 neurologically impaired pediatric patients with intractable aspiration, laryngotracheal separation resulted in control of aspiration in 100% of patients.[70]

PATIENT SELF-TREATMENTS

In certain circumstances, patients can use self-directed measures to improve symptoms of dysphagia. There are currently 2 studies in the literature that have investigated the benefit of pretreatment swallowing exercises in patients with head and neck cancer who undergo chemoradiation. The first study prospectively compared patients who performed pretreatment swallowing exercises to those who performed the same exercises post-treatment. Exercises included Mendelsohn maneuver, Shaker exercises, tongue hold, and tongue resistance exercises. Patients who participated in pretreatment swallow exercises scored higher on the M.D. Anderson Dysphagia Inventory and quality-of-life questionnaires than patients who performed the same exercises post-treatment.[71] A second retrospective study demonstrated that performance of these exercises pretreatment was associated with better epiglottis inversion and tongue retropulsion on videofluoroscopic swallow evaluation. However, there was no difference in PEG removal in the pretreatment and post-treatment groups.[72]

In addition to swallowing exercises, patients may alter their diet to allow for smoother transit of the bolus or decreased aspiration of food contents. Diet alterations include thickening of liquids and changing the consistency of solids to include only soft foods. One randomized controlled trial demonstrated that there was no difference in the incidence of pneumonia, malnutrition, dehydration, and death between patients receiving daily speech therapy and patients who underwent a single therapy session. In this study, patients were instructed on compensatory swallowing techniques and dietary recommendations, which they performed independently.[73]

INTEGRATIVE TREATMENT APPROACHES AND OUTCOMES

Data regarding integrative treatments of swallowing disorders are limited; however, some studies have investigated acupuncture and Chinese herbal medicines in the treatment of dysphagia. A Cochrane review on acupuncture and post-stroke treatment of dysphagia identified one randomized controlled trial comparing Western medical treatment with and without adjunctive acupuncture.[74] In this trial, acupuncture patients were treated at acupoints RN 23, ST 9 (bilateral), GB 20 (bilateral), and DU 16. Patients were then evaluated for recovery defined as return of normal feeding. Results show no statistical difference in recovery of swallowing function in the 2 groups; however, there was an increase in percentage of patients who had marked improvement in swallowing in the acupuncture group, as defined by normal feeding with occasional bucking.[75] Conclusions from this Cochrane review state that more studies are required before any conclusions are made.[74]

Acupuncture has also been described in the treatment of dysphagia in patients with cancer. A retrospective review by Lu investigated acupuncture as a treatment of dysphagia in 10 patients with oral cavity or oropharyngeal squamous cell carcinoma undergoing chemoradiation.[76] Acupuncture sites varied according to patient complaints and whether the patient was currently undergoing radiation therapy, but included

- ST36
- SP6
- LI2
- LI11
- GV20
- Shenmen/ear
- Sanjiao/ear
- ST7
- ST6
- ST5
- CV23
- GB20
- Yintang

Results demonstrated that 9 of 10 patients reported some degree of improvement in swallowing function, xerostomia, fatigue, and pain. In addition, 6 of 7 patients with PEG tube at the start of acupuncture had their feeding tube removed. As a result of this study, the author is currently conducting a randomized controlled trial comparing acupuncture plus Western medicine to sham acupuncture plus Western medicine in this patient population.[77] Similarly, a randomized controlled trial comparing acupuncture to sham acupuncture in patients undergoing radiation therapy for nasopharyngeal carcinoma demonstrated that symptoms of xerostomia decreased and quality–of-life measures increased in the acupuncture group.[78] Acupoints used in this study were

- Ren 24
- LU 7
- K 6
- Shenmen
- Point Zero
- (SG 20)
- Larynx

Neuromuscular electrical stimulation (NMES) has also been studied in patients with head and neck cancer and dysphagia after surgery or radiation therapy. In a randomized controlled trial comparing NMES of the anterior neck musculature and swallow therapy to sham stimulation plus swallow therapy, a statistically significant improvement was noted in the functional dysphagia score in the NMES group.[79]

Furthermore, 3 separate randomized controlled trials by Iwasaki have investigated the traditional Chinese medicine Banxia Houpo Tang (BHT) in patients with dysphagia secondary to dementia, Parkinson, and stroke. BHT was found to improve the cough reflex and the latency of response of the swallow reflex. It was also found to decrease both the occurrence of pneumonia and mortality from aspiration pneumonia.[80–82] Because these studies have not been validated at other institutions further investigation is warranted.

MULTIMODAL APPROACHES AND OUTCOMES

The management of swallowing disorders involves comprehensive evaluation, including treatment plans and integrated approaches. Individual therapies, whether conservative, medical, or surgical have proved successful. However, multimodal approaches to treatment, which may include nontraditional therapies, will likely enhance management of this challenging disorder. Nearly every study that incorporates integrative medicine treatments of dysphagia investigates the integrative treatment in addition to Western medical treatments.[75,76,79] Because the use of integrative therapies alone has not been well studied, incorporation of these treatments into patient care should always be accompanied by medical or surgical treatments. **Fig. 2** proposes an algorithm for the integrative approach to managing swallowing disorders.

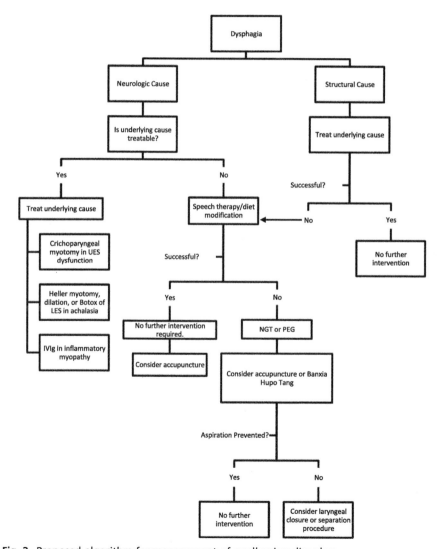

Fig. 2. Proposed algorithm for management of swallowing disorders.

REFERENCES

1. Cook IJ. Oropharyngeal dysphagia. Gastroenterol Clin North Am 2009;38: 411–31.
2. Tibbling L, Gustafsson B. Dysphagia and its consequences in the elderly. Dysphagia 1991;6:200–2.
3. Logemann JA. Upper digestive tract anatomy and physiology. In: Bailey BJ, Johnson JT, Newlands SD, editors. Head & neck surgery–otolaryngology. Philadelphia: Lippincott Williams & Wilkins; 2006. p. 685–92.
4. Kahrilas PJ, Lin S, Logemann JA, et al. Deglutitive tongue action: volume accommodation and bolus propulsion. Gastroenterology 1993;104:152–62.
5. Serra-Prat M, Palomera M, Gomez C, et al. Oropharyngeal dysphagia as a risk factor for malnutrition and lower respiratory tract infection in independently living older persons: a population-based prospective study. Age Ageing 2012;41: 376–81.
6. Caporali R, Caccialanza R, Bonino C, et al. Disease-related malnutrition in outpatients with systemic sclerosis. Clin Nutr 2012;31(5):666–71.
7. Barer DH. The natural history and functional consequences of dysphagia after hemispheric stroke. J Neurol Neurosurg Psychiatr 1989;52:236–41.
8. Gresham SL. Clinical assessment and management of swallowing difficulties after stroke. Med J Aust 1990;153:397–9.
9. Schmidt J, Holas M, Halvorson K, et al. Videofluoroscopic evidence of aspiration predicts pneumonia and death but not dehydration following stroke. Dysphagia 1994;9:7–11.
10. Brunnstrom HR, Englund EM. Cause of death in patients with dementia disorders. Eur J Neurol 2009;16:488–92.
11. Muller J, Wenning GK, Verny M, et al. Progression of dysarthria and dysphagia in postmortem-confirmed parkinsonian disorders. Arch Neurol 2001;58:259–64.
12. Ali GN, Wallace KL, Schwartz R, et al. Mechanisms of oral-pharyngeal dysphagia in patients with Parkinson's disease. Gastroenterology 1996;110:383–92.
13. Tandan R, Bradley WG. Amyotrophic lateral sclerosis: part 1. Clinical features, pathology, and ethical issues in management. Ann Neurol 1985;18:271–80.
14. Dalakas MC. Polymyositis, dermatomyositis and inclusion-body myositis. N Engl J Med 1991;325:1487–98.
15. Van Ruiswyk J, Cunningham C, Cerletty J. Obstructive manifestations of thyroid lymphoma. Arch Intern Med 1989;149:1575–7.
16. Hirano M, Kuroiwa Y, Tanaka S, et al. Dysphagia following various degrees of surgical resection for oral cancer. Ann Otol Rhinol Laryngol 1992;101:138–41.
17. O'Connell DA, Rieger J, Harris JR, et al. Swallowing function in patients with base of tongue cancers treated with primary surgery and reconstructed with a modified radial forearm free flap. Arch Otolaryngol Head Neck Surg 2008; 134:857–64.
18. Archontaki M, Athanasiou A, Stavrianos SD, et al. Functional results of speech and swallowing after oral microvascular free flap reconstruction. Eur Arch Otorhinolaryngol 2010;267:1771–7.
19. Uwiera T, Seikaly H, Rieger J, et al. Functional outcomes after hemiglossectomy and reconstruction with a bilobed radial forearm free flap. J Otolaryngol 2004; 33:356–9.
20. Nguyen NP, Sallah S, Karlsson U, et al. Combined chemotherapy and radiation therapy for head and neck malignancies: quality of life issues. Cancer 2002;94: 1131–41.

21. List MA, Mumby P, Haraf D, et al. Performance and quality of life outcome in patients completing concomitant chemoradiotherapy protocols for head and neck cancer. Qual Life Res 1997;6:274–84.

22. Huguenin P, Glanzmann C, Taussky D, et al. Hyperfractionated radiotherapy and simultaneous cisplatin for stage-III and -IV carcinomas of the head and neck. Long-term results including functional outcome. Strahlenther Onkol 1998;174:397–402.

23. Schrader M, Schipper J, Jahnke K, et al. Hyperfractionated accelerated simultaneous radiochemotherapy in advanced hypopharyngeal carcinomas. Survival rate, retained function quality of life in a phase II study. HNO 1998;46:140–5 [in German].

24. El-Deiry M, Funk GF, Nalwa S, et al. Long-term quality of life for surgical and nonsurgical treatment of head and neck cancer. Arch Otolaryngol Head Neck Surg 2005;131:879–85.

25. Siktberg LL, Bantz DL. Management of children with swallowing disorders. J Pediatr Health Care 1999;13:223–9.

26. Miller CK. Updates on pediatric feeding and swallowing problems. Curr Opin Otolaryngol Head Neck Surg 2009;17:194–9.

27. Mizuno K, Nishida Y, Taki M, et al. Infants with bronchopulmonary dysplasia suckle with weak pressures to maintain breathing during feeding. Pediatrics 2007;120:e1035–42.

28. Messina S, Pane M, De Rose P, et al. Feeding problems and malnutrition in spinal muscular atrophy type II. Neuromuscul Disord 2008;18:389–93.

29. Thompson DM. Abnormal sensorimotor integrative function of the larynx in congenital laryngomalacia: a new theory of etiology. Laryngoscope 2007;117: 1–33.

30. Franciosi JP, Liacouras CA. Eosinophilic esophagitis. Immunol Allergy Clin North Am 2009;29:19–27, viii.

31. Carr S, Watson W. Eosinophilic esophagitis. Allergy Asthma Clin Immunol 2011; 7(Suppl 1):S8.

32. Menezes C, Melo A. Does levodopa improve swallowing dysfunction in Parkinson's disease patients? J Clin Pharm Ther 2009;34:673–6.

33. Dalakas MC. High-dose intravenous immunoglobulin in inflammatory myopathies: experience based on controlled clinical trials. Neurol Sci 2003;24(Suppl 4): S256–9.

34. Walter MC, Lochmuller H, Toepfer M, et al. High-dose immunoglobulin therapy in sporadic inclusion body myositis: a double-blind, placebo-controlled study. J Neurol 2000;247:22–8.

35. Kiely PD, Heron CW, Bruckner FE. Presentation and management of idiopathic inflammatory muscle disease: four case reports and commentary from a series of 78 patients. Rheumatology (Oxford) 2003;42:575–82.

36. Battersby NJ, Bonney GK, Subar D, et al. Outcomes following oesophageal stent insertion for palliation of malignant strictures: a large single centre series. J Surg Oncol 2012;105:60–5.

37. Storr M, Allescher HD, Rosch T, et al. Treatment of symptomatic diffuse esophageal spasm by endoscopic injections of botulinum toxin: a prospective study with long-term follow-up. Gastrointest Endosc 2001;54:754–9.

38. Orlando RC, Bozymski EM. Clinical and manometric effects of nitroglycerin in diffuse esophageal spasm. N Engl J Med 1973;289:23–5.

39. Triadafilopoulos G, Tsang HP. Olfactory stimuli provoke diffuse esophageal spasm: reversal by ipratropium bromide. Am J Gastroenterol 1996;91:2224–7.

40. Clouse RE, Lustman PJ, Eckert TC, et al. Low-dose trazodone for symptomatic patients with esophageal contraction abnormalities. A double-blind, placebo-controlled trial. Gastroenterology 1987;92:1027–36.

41. Drenth JP, Bos LP, Engels LG. Efficacy of diltiazem in the treatment of diffuse oesophageal spasm. Aliment Pharmacol Ther 1990;4:411–6.

42. Annese V, D'Onofrio V, Andriulli A. Botulinum toxin in long-term therapy for achalasia. Ann Intern Med 1998;128:696.

43. Martinek J, Siroky M, Plottova Z, et al. Treatment of patients with achalasia with botulinum toxin: a multicenter prospective cohort study. Dis Esophagus 2003; 16:204–9.

44. Allen J, White CJ, Leonard R, et al. Effect of cricopharyngeus muscle surgery on the pharynx. Laryngoscope 2010;120:1498–503.

45. Robbins J, Gensler G, Hind J, et al. Comparison of 2 interventions for liquid aspiration on pneumonia incidence: a randomized trial. Ann Intern Med 2008; 148:509–18.

46. Sheppard JJ, Fletcher KR. Evidence-based interventions for breast and bottle feeding in the neonatal intensive care unit. Semin Speech Lang 2007;28: 204–12.

47. Baeten C, Hoefnagels J. Feeding via nasogastric tube or percutaneous endoscopic gastrostomy. A comparison. Scand J Gastroenterol Suppl 1992;194: 95–8.

48. Norton B, Homer-Ward M, Donnelly MT, et al. A randomised prospective comparison of percutaneous endoscopic gastrostomy and nasogastric tube feeding after acute dysphagic stroke. BMJ 1996;312:13–6.

49. Park RH, Allison MC, Lang J, et al. Randomised comparison of percutaneous endoscopic gastrostomy and nasogastric tube feeding in patients with persisting neurological dysphagia. BMJ 1992;304:1406–9.

50. Hamidon BB, Abdullah SA, Zawawi MF, et al. A prospective comparison of percutaneous endoscopic gastrostomy and nasogastric tube feeding in patients with acute dysphagic stroke. Med J Malaysia 2006;61:59–66.

51. Dennis MS, Lewis SC, Warlow C. Effect of timing and method of enteral tube feeding for dysphagic stroke patients (FOOD): a multicentre randomised controlled trial. Lancet 2005;365:764–72.

52. Saetti R, Silvestrini M, Peracchia A, et al. Endoscopic stapler-assisted Zenker's diverticulotomy: which is the best operative facility? Head Neck 2006;28: 1084–9.

53. Veenker E, Cohen JI. Current trends in management of Zenker diverticulum. Curr Opin Otolaryngol Head Neck Surg 2003;11:160–5.

54. Smith SR, Genden EM, Urken ML. Endoscopic stapling technique for the treatment of Zenker diverticulum vs standard open-neck technique: a direct comparison and charge analysis. Arch Otolaryngol Head Neck Surg 2002;128:141–4.

55. Cook RD, Huang PC, Richstmeier WJ, et al. Endoscopic staple-assisted esophagodiverticulostomy: an excellent treatment of choice for Zenker's diverticulum. Laryngoscope 2000;110:2020–5.

56. Payne WS, King RM. Pharyngoesophageal (Zenker's) diverticulum. Surg Clin North Am 1983;63:815–24.

57. Stoeckli SJ, Schmid S. Endoscopic stapler-assisted diverticuloesophagostomy for Zenker's diverticulum: patient satisfaction and subjective relief of symptoms. Surgery 2002;131:158–62.

58. Bonafede JP, Lavertu P, Wood BG, et al. Surgical outcome in 87 patients with Zenker's diverticulum. Laryngoscope 1997;107:720–5.

59. Zaninotto G, Narne S, Costantini M, et al. Tailored approach to Zenker's diverticula. Surg Endosc 2003;17:129–33.
60. Kos MP, David EF, Mahieu HF. Endoscopic carbon dioxide laser Zenker's diverticulotomy revisited. Ann Otol Rhinol Laryngol 2009;118:512–8.
61. Verhaegen VJ, Feuth T, van den Hoogen FJ, et al. Endoscopic carbon dioxide laser diverticulostomy versus endoscopic staple-assisted diverticulostomy to treat Zenker's diverticulum. Head Neck 2011;33:154–9.
62. Poirier NC, Bonavina L, Taillefer R, et al. Cricopharyngeal myotomy for neurogenic oropharyngeal dysphagia. J Thorac Cardiovasc Surg 1997;113:233–40 [discussion: 240–1].
63. Taillefer R, Duranceau AC. Manometric and radionuclide assessment of pharyngeal emptying before and after cricopharyngeal myotomy in patients with oculopharyngeal muscular dystrophy. J Thorac Cardiovasc Surg 1988;95: 868–75.
64. Herbella FA, Tineli AC, Wilson JL Jr, et al. Surgical treatment of primary esophageal motility disorders. J Gastrointest Surg 2008;12:604–8.
65. Boeckxstaens GE, Annese V, des Varannes SB, et al. Pneumatic dilation versus laparoscopic Heller's myotomy for idiopathic achalasia. N Engl J Med 2011;364: 1807–16.
66. Hoppo T, Jobe BA. Is laparoscopic Heller myotomy superior to pneumatic dilation to treat achalasia? Semin Thorac Cardiovasc Surg 2011;23:178–80.
67. McLarty AJ, Deschamps C, Trastek VF, et al. Esophageal resection for cancer of the esophagus: long-term function and quality of life. Ann Thorac Surg 1997;63: 1568–72.
68. Aghajanzadeh M, Safarpour F, Koohsari MR, et al. Functional outcome of gastrointestinal tract and quality of life after esophageal reconstruction of esophagus cancer. Saudi J Gastroenterol 2009;15:24–8.
69. Watanabe K, Nakaya M, Miyano K, et al. Laryngotracheal separation procedure for elderly patients. Am J Otol 2011;32:156–8.
70. Cook SP. Candidate's thesis: laryngotracheal separation in neurologically impaired children: long-term results. Laryngoscope 2009;119:390–5.
71. Kulbersh BD, Rosenthal EL, McGrew BM, et al. Pretreatment, preoperative swallowing exercises may improve dysphagia quality of life. Laryngoscope 2006; 116:883–6.
72. Carroll WR, Locher JL, Canon CL, et al. Pretreatment swallowing exercises improve swallow function after chemoradiation. Laryngoscope 2008;118:39–43.
73. DePippo KL, Holas MA, Reding MJ, et al. Dysphagia therapy following stroke: a controlled trial. Neurology 1994;44:1655–60.
74. Xie Y, Wang L, He J, et al. Acupuncture for dysphagia in acute stroke. Cochrane Database Syst Rev 2008;(3):CD006076.
75. Han J. An observation on the therapeutic effect of acupuncture for bulbar palsy after acute stroke. Henan Journal of Practical Nervous Disease 2004;7:81.
76. Lu W, Posner MR, Wayne P, et al. Acupuncture for dysphagia after chemoradiation therapy in head and neck cancer: a case series report. Integr Cancer Ther 2010;9:284–90.
77. Lu W, Wayne PM, Davis RB, et al. Acupuncture for dysphagia after chemoradiation in head and neck cancer: rationale and design of a randomized, sham-controlled trial. Contemp Clin Trials 2012;33(4):700–11.
78. Meng Z, Kay Garcia M, Hu C, et al. Sham-controlled, randomised, feasibility trial of acupuncture for prevention of radiation-induced xerostomia among patients with nasopharyngeal carcinoma. Eur J Cancer 2012;48(11):1692–9.

79. Ryu JS, Kang JY, Park JY, et al. The effect of electrical stimulation therapy on dysphagia following treatment for head and neck cancer. Oral Oncol 2009;45: 665–8.

80. Iwasaki K, Wang Q, Nakagawa T, et al. The traditional Chinese medicine banxia houpo tang improves swallowing reflex. Phytomedicine 1999;6:103–6.

81. Iwasaki K, Cyong JC, Kitada S, et al. A traditional Chinese herbal medicine, banxia houpo tang, improves cough reflex of patients with aspiration pneumonia. J Am Geriatr Soc 2002;50:1751–2.

82. Iwasaki K, Kato S, Monma Y, et al. A pilot study of banxia houpu tang, a traditional Chinese medicine, for reducing pneumonia risk in older adults with dementia. J Am Geriatr Soc 2007;55:2035–40.

Complementary and Integrative Treatments Facial Cosmetic Enhancement

James M. Hamilton, MD, Edmund A. Pribitkin, MD*

KEYWORDS

- Complementary and integrative medicine • Alternative medicine • CAM • CIM
- Facial cosmetic surgery • Aesthetic surgery • Herbal medicine • Phytomedicine

KEY POINTS

- Complementary and integrative medicine is particularly common among patients undergoing facial cosmetic enhancement.
- Most patients undergoing facial aesthetic surgery who practice integrative therapies do so for their purported wound-healing, antimicrobial, and analgesic properties.
- Well-controlled scientific trials regarding the efficacy of integrative therapies are extremely limited.
- The existing evidence regarding the efficacy of these therapies is contradictory.
- The inherent properties of many of these products have been reported to put patients at risk of increased bleeding, excessive sedation, and dermatitis.
- Many of these products have the potential to interact with conventional pharmacologic therapies that patients may be prescribed.

OVERVIEW

Over the last decade, the US public has shown a steady and substantial use of complementary and alternative medicine (CAM), with 2007 estimates placing the overall prevalence of use at 38.3% of adults (83 million persons) and 11.8% of children (8.5 million children less than 18 years old).[1] This CAM includes herbal remedies, massage, self-help groups, folk remedies, chiropractic manipulation, relaxation techniques, megavitamins, and others.[2] In 2007, adults in the United States spent $33.9 billion out of pocket on visits to CAM practitioners and purchases of CAM products, classes, and materials. Annual visits to alternative practitioners have been estimated at $629 million, higher than that of primary care visits.[1]

Department of Otolaryngology-Head & Neck Surgery, Thomas Jefferson University, 925 Chestnut Street, Sixth Floor, Philadelphia, PA 19107, USA
* Corresponding author.
E-mail address: Edmund.Pribitkin@jefferson.edu

Otolaryngol Clin N Am 46 (2013) 461–483
http://dx.doi.org/10.1016/j.otc.2013.02.007
0030-6665/13/$ – see front matter © 2013 Elsevier Inc. All rights reserved.

The use of Complementary and Integrative Medicine (CIM) is common among patients undergoing surgery. Reports have estimated its prevalence at 22% to 60% among certain adult surgical populations.[3] In a 2000 study of patients presenting for preoperative clinic evaluation surveyed by Tsen and colleagues,[4] 22% of presurgical patients reported the use of herbal remedies and 51% used vitamins. Another study from 2000 by Kaye and colleagues[5] surveyed 1017 patients presenting for preanesthetic evaluation before outpatient surgery and found that 32% reported using herbal medications. In 2004, Norred[6] surveyed 500 Denver patients about integrative medicine use in the 2 weeks before surgery and found that 67% disclosed the use of all types of CIM; 27% consumed herbs, 39% used dietary supplements, 54% took vitamins, and 1% reported the use of homeopathics.[6] In another study, 57% of the 2186 patients undergoing elective surgery polled by Adusumilli and colleagues,[3] in 2004, responded positively on a survey to have used herbal medicine at some point in their lives.

CIM seems to be especially popular among patients who undergo cosmetic surgery. Heller and colleagues[7] compared the results of a survey regarding the use of herbal medication given to cosmetic surgery patients with the results of the same survey given to randomly chosen members of the general public. Fifty-five percent of the cosmetic surgery patients used herbal medications versus 24% of the general population.[7] A 2011 UK study of 100 elective plastic surgery patients found that 44% were taking a dietary supplement, of which 17% were taking an herbal or homeopathic remedy.[8] It has also been shown that the use of herbs, vitamins, and dietary supplements is more prevalent among white, educated, and wealthy individuals. Tsen and colleagues[4] also reported that female patients use herbs more frequently than male patients (23.6% vs 19.2%). This description characterizes most aesthetic surgery patients.[9]

The risk of unforeseen morbidity and mortality in the perioperative period may be increased in patients using CIM not only because of the physiologic alterations that can occur secondary to the intrinsic properties of these supplements but also because of the drug interactions made more likely by polypharmacy.[10] The main concerns of the plastic surgeon are cardiovascular effects, alteration of coagulations, sedative effects, and interaction with other medications.[11] Here, the authors review the most common modalities of CIM and their potential benefit to patients undergoing facial cosmetic enhancement procedures as well as the potential adverse reactions stemming from their use.

INTEGRATIVE TREATMENT APPROACHES AND OUTCOMES
Herbal, Homeopathic, and Dietary Supplements

The reported effects of herbal therapies and natural dietary supplements, used for generations as antiinflammatory, antimicrobial, and wound-healing treatment, have played an important role in medicine. Although a lack of standardization and paucity of well-controlled scientific trials has made it difficult to determine their efficacy, which many attribute to the lack of financial support for the study of nonpatentable natural treatments, proponents and users argue that the lack of double-blind randomized controlled trials (RCTs) does not exclude the possibility of a therapeutic effect.[12]

Herbal
Aloe Aloe (Aloe vera, Aloe barbadensis) is a cactuslike perennial plant belonging to the Lilaceae family that is native to southern Africa and commonly grown in tropical climates.[13] Popular in traditional Chinese and Ayurvedic medicine, it has been used for thousands of years to treat wounds, skin infections, burns, and numerous other dermatologic conditions.[14] More recently, aloe has been reported to

- Improve reepithelialization of surgical wounds
- Provide antiinflammatory effects
- Possibly increase dermal perfusion to decrease ischemia[12,15]

Aloe leaves produce 2 substances, a gel and a juice or latex. The gel, a mucilaginous tissue from which most commercial cosmetic and medicinal products are made, is obtained from the inner part of the leaf and has been used topically to treat wounds and burns. The latex or juice refers to a bitter yellow fluid extracted from the specialized areas of the inner leaf skin and is generally sold as a powder that has very potent laxative effects.[15] Fractionation of extracts and purification of compounds from aloe resulted in the identification of β-sitosterol, an angiogenic factor that may be beneficial to the healing process, because angiogenesis is integral to the repair mechanism.[16] In view of the widespread use of aloe vera, the paucity of controlled clinical trials is surprising.

A 2012 systematic review of the literature summarizing the available evidence of the effectiveness of aloe vera in patients with both chronic and acute wounds, including surgical incisions, examined 7 small RCTs, with a mean sample size of 50. All had a moderate to high risk of bias caused by poor methodology. Evidence on wound healing was contradictory, and the investigators of the review concluded that there is little high-level evidence to support the use of aloe vera topical agents or aloe-derived dressings in the treatment of acute and chronic wounds.[13] There are, however, several small studies, case reports, and animal series that have suggested that aloe vera may help with the wound-healing process. A 1995 study by Heggers and colleagues[17] examined the role of aloe in enhancing the healing process in acute wounds in mice. Wounds treated with 10% aloe vera 3 times a day for 14 days had a significantly shorter half-life and healed faster than the control group. Additionally, the healed wound was markedly stronger than the control.[17] A 1990 study by Fulton[18] documented the effects of 2 different dressings for wound-healing management on full-faced dermabrasion patients. Eighteen patients suffering from acne vulgaris completed the study. Their abraded faces were divided in half. One side was treated with a standard polyethylene oxide gel wound dressing, whereas the other side was treated with a polyethylene oxide dressing saturated with aloe vera. After 48 hours with the aloe vera dressing, intense vasoconstriction and a reduction in edema was noted; less exudate and crusting were evident by the fourth day. By the fifth day, reepithelialization was complete to 90% on the aloe side compared with 40% to 50% on the control side. Overall, wound healing was approximately 72 hours faster on the aloe side. A 1995 study by Philips and colleagues compared the effect of an aloe vera derivative gel dressing with conventional treatment using hydrogen peroxide and an antibiotic with traditional dressing on 49 patients who had recently undergone shave biopsy excision for suspected skin cancers. There was no difference in the proportion of participants with a completely healed wound at 14 days; 26 out of 26 (100%) were healed in the aloe vera group compared with 23 out of 23 (100%) in the conventional therapy group, suggesting the noninferiority of aloe vera to conventional therapy.[13]

Arnica Arnica *(Arnica montana)* is an herbal remedy of European and Native American lineage used extensively in folk medicine to treat ecchymosis and pain after traumatic injuries. Arnica has frequently been cited in the herbal literature for its reported ability to promote wound healing and prevent postoperative hematomas, and it is also known as

- Leopard's bane
- Wolf's bane
- Mountain tobacco

- Arniflora
- Fallherb
- Fleurs d'arnica
- Guldblomme
- Monkshood
- Mountain daisy
- Mountain snuff
- Prickherb
- Smokeherb
- Sneezewort
- Snuffplant
- Spanish flower heads
- St. John's strength flower
- Strengthwort
- Thunderwort
- Woundherb
- Wolf's eye[19,20]

The arnica that is used for medicinal purposes is an extract of dried flowers from the plant native to the meadows and mountainous regions of Europe and North America. Formulations of arnica are available as sprays for topical application, creams, gels, ointments, sublingual preparations, tablets, teas, and tinctures.[19] It has been approved by the German Commission E as a topical agent with effective analgesic, antibacterial, and antiinflammatory properties; however, the Food and Drug Administration has classified arnica as an unsafe herb.[21]

Marketed and sold as SinEcch by Alpine Pharmaceuticals (San Rafael, CA), arnica is used by many plastic surgeons to limit postoperative edema and ecchymosis.[22] Anecdotal evidence is that arnica at a higher dose speeds the healing of bruises, and topical arnica is recommended to patients after soft tissue augmentation, Botox injections, fat transfer, and liposuction.[23] Although highly diluted homeopathic preparations are considered safe and are widely used for the treatment of injuries, many clinical trials have been conducted and have not found a statistically significant efficacy for herbal or homeopathic forms of arnica over placebo. In Ernst and Pittler's 1998 meta-analysis of 8 studies, 6 of which demonstrated no benefits for the use of arnica, the investigators concluded that this herbal agent is no more beneficial than a placebo.[24] Likewise, a 2002 study of 19 patients with facial telangiectasias demonstrated no effect of topical arnica (concentrated at $1\times$) on the prevention or quickened healing of laser-induced bruising whether applied before or after laser treatment.[25] A 2000 randomized, placebo-controlled, double-blind study performed by Ramelet and colleagues[26] of 130 patients undergoing saphenous vein stripping demonstrated no statistically significant difference between patients receiving a sublingual dose of homeopathic arnica or indistinguishable placebo the night before and immediately after surgery with respect to postoperative hematomas.[26] Most recently, a 2009 prospective, placebo-controlled, double-blind study of 30 male patients undergoing blepharoplasty found neither a subjective nor an objective difference in decreased ecchymosis or improved ease of recovery between the administration of homeopathic arnica and placebo.[27]

Still, evidence of the efficacy of arnica has been reported. Although many studies have produced contradictory results, several studies suggest that arnica is at least as effective as the current treatment of select conditions. Kulick[28] presented a randomized, prospective, double-blind, placebo-controlled trial of arnica in a series of 29 patients undergoing liposuction at the 2002 American Society for Aesthetic Plastic

Surgery meeting. He demonstrated a statistically significant reduction in bruising and swelling in the arnica-treated group.[22] The results of a 2007 study of 48 patients undergoing primary rhinoplasty with osteotomy demonstrated no differences between patients receiving arnica and those receiving corticosteroids or placebo with respect to the extent and intensity of postoperative ecchymosis. However, patients who received arnica had significantly less edema during the early postoperative period, suggesting a beneficial effect of arnica on this postrhinoplasty consequence.[29] A 2005 randomized, double-blind, placebo-controlled study of bruising and skin color changes following rhytidectomy in 29 patients who were treated with either homeopathic arnica or placebo found no subjective differences between patients in the two treatment groups. However, patients in the arnica group did have a smaller area of ecchymosis than those receiving placebo. This difference was found to be statistically significant on postoperative day (POD) 1 and 7 but not on POD 5 and 10. Objectively, no significant difference in the degree of ecchymosis, as measured by the extent of color change, was found.[30]

Although the subtle benefit that has occasionally been reported to be induced by arnica seems very difficult to definitively and reproducibly demonstrate in the studies involving the relatively small numbers of individuals considered in most trials to date, no serious adverse effects have been reported with the use of homeopathic arnica. Under a physician's supervision, patients can probably safely take arnica that is available in preparations manufactured for the prevention of bruising and swelling.[2] Patients should be discouraged from using oral arnica in amounts greater than commonly found in foods or in homeopathic formulations because of reports of severe health risks, including coma, hypertension, renal toxicity, cardiotoxicity, muscle paralysis, and death.[12,20] Also, patients should be instructed not to apply arnica to abraded skin or open wounds and advised against prolonged topical use because of the potential for irritant or allergic contact dermatitis.[20,31]

Bromelain   Bromelain (Ananas comosus, Ananas sativus) is a protease enzyme mixture derived from the pineapple plant that has been used by native cultures as a digestive aid and as a remedy for skin disorders. It is also known as

- Ananase
- Anansase100
- Ananase Forte
- Bromelain-POS
- Traumanase
- Wobenzym[32]

It has been reported to have antiinflammatory, antiedematous, anticoagulant, and antimetastatic properties and has also been shown to enhance antibiotic activity.[33] Bromelain may be of particular interest in plastic surgery because of its apparent antiedematous, antiinflammatory, and anticoagulation properties, which may be beneficial in postoperative healing. There is also some evidence that suggests that it may be beneficial in pain reduction, wound healing, burn debridement, and ischemia reperfusion.[33] It seems to be most effective when taken orally.[33]

An early double-blind, controlled clinical trial in obstetric patients reported faster rates of reduction of edema and bruising after episiotomy in patients who received bromelain treatment compared with those who received placebo. None of the results were statistically significant, however.[34] In another double-blind, placebo-controlled study, bromelain was shown to reduce edema and ecchymoses by one-half to one-third fewer days in patients who experienced surgical (eg, rhinoplasty) or nonsurgical trauma to the face.[33] More recently, a 2003 study of wound healing in healthy adults found that an oral nutritional supplement containing bromelain, as well as other vitamins and minerals, including other proteases, decreased the soft tissue wound healing time when administered during the early phase of wound healing, although the extent to which bromelain was responsible more than the other components was not elucidated.[35]

Grape seed extract Grape seed extract (*Vitis vinifera, Vitis coignetiae*) has been used to treat venous insufficiency, inflammatory conditions, and promote wound healing in Europe. It is also known as

- Pine bark
- Pinus maritima
- Grape complex
- Grape seed
- Grape seed oil
- Grape skin extract
- Muskat
- ActiVin
- Endotelon
- Grape seed standardized extract
- Leucoselect-phytosome
- Masquelier's Original OPCs
- Pycnogenol

It has been established as a potent antioxidant because of its constituent oligomeric proanthocyanidins and thought to exhibit a wide range of biologic, pharmacologic, chemoprotective, and antioxidant activity. Additionally, proanthocyanidins are thought to have the capacity to stabilize collagen and elastin, thereby improving the elasticity, flexibility, and appearance of the skin.[23]

Motivated by encouraging results in vitro and in animal models, grape seed, its oil, and its extract have been increasingly used for strengthening vessels and preventing bruising.[12] The extract has been reported to increase wound contraction and closure speed in mice, vascular endothelial growth factor (VEGF) and tenascin levels in the wound edge, and connective tissue deposition. A 2001 in vitro study by Khanna and colleagues[36] reported evidence showing that grape seed proanthocyanidin extract (containing resveratrol) facilitates oxidant-induced VEGF expression in keratinocytes. VEGF induces the migration and proliferation of endothelial cells and enhances vascular permeability consistent with the purported ability to promote angiogenesis. Angiogenesis plays a central role in wound healing.[36]

A 2002 study by Khanna and colleagues[37] examined the effect of topical grape seed proanthocyanidin extract (GSPE) on the healing of full-thickness excisional wounds in the mouse model. GSPE treatment was associated with a more well-defined hyperproliferative epithelial region, higher cell density, enhanced deposition of connective tissue, and improved histologic architecture in treated wounds compared with control wounds in the same animal. GSPE treatment also increased VEGF and tenascin expression in the wound edge tissue, which are markers in granulation tissue often used as indicators of cutaneous wound repair.[37]

A 2010 study by Nayak and colleagues[38] of the wound-healing activity in mice of a finely ground grape-skin powder derived from the Cabernet Sauvignon variety demonstrated that animals in the treatment group exhibited significant increases in the rate of wound contraction (100% by day 13 when compared with control [82.1%] and standard treatment with mupirocin [93.0%]) and an increased rate of epithelialization. Similarly, a 2004 study by Blazsó and colleagues[39] demonstrated that regular topical application of Pycnogenol, a patented nutrient supplement extracted from the bark of European coastal pine *Pinus maritime* that consists of flavonoids, catechins, procyanidins, and phenolic acids (which are the same constituents found in grape seed, although it is not the same supplement),[40] accelerated wound healing and reduced scar formation in rats. Gels of increasing concentration (1%, 2%, and 5%) were applied to wounds inflicted on the backs of the animals with a 100°C branding iron. The 1% gel significantly shortened the wound healing time by 1.6 days, the 2% gel reduced the time by 2.7 days, and the 5% gel by 5.3 days. Pycnogenol also reduced the diameter of the scars remaining following complete scab loss in a concentration-dependent manner.[39]

Ginkgo Ginkgo *(Ginkgo biloba)* is one of the top 10 best-selling herbs in the United States and the most widely sold phytomedicine in Europe.[31,41] It is also known as

- Maidenhair tree
- Duckfoot tree
- Fossil tree
- Yin xing
- Ich, ginnan
- Japanese silver apricot
- ArginMax
- BioGinkgo
- Gincosan
- Ginexin Remind
- Gingopret
- Ginkai
- Ginkgo Go
- Ginkgo Phytosome
- Ginkgo Powder
- Herbal vX
- Seredrin
- Tanakan

Ginkgo is widely used to treat a variety of conditions:

- Dementia
- Memory impairment
- Peripheral vascular disease
- Erectile dysfunction
- Premenstrual syndrome
- Macular degeneration
- Tinnitus
- Vertigo[42]

The known physiologic effects of ginkgo are congruent with a vascular mechanism of action.[43] Gingko has been researched among methods being devised to reduce tissue damage caused by ischemia in major surgical reconstructions that require extensive flap use.[44] The effects of ginkgo biloba extract on cellular membranes are scavenging oxygenated free radicals produced during arachidonic acid metabolism. Free oxygen radicals have been accused of causing cellular injury both during the course of ischemia and at the time when these total ischemic tissues are reperfused.[45]

A 1997 study of the effects of oral ginkgo biloba extract on flap viability in rats re-ported significantly lower rates of skin necrosis and levels of free radical scavenging biochemical enzymes malonyldialdehyde (MDA), superoxide dismutaste, and gluta-thione peroxidase, measures of free radical activity, in biopsy specimens. On electron microscope investigation, the treated group had more normal tissue structures compared with high levels of degeneration and loss of the dermal-epidermal junction in the control group. These results suggest that ginkgo biloba extract may be beneficial in modulating the no-reflow phenomena and subsequent tissue injury and may help to improve tissue salvage.[45] Another 1997 study of the effects of oral *Ginkgo biloba* on skin flaps in the rat model reported that biopsies of the flap site in ginkgo-treated groups had significantly lower MDA levels than control samples after 120 minutes of ischemia, indicating that ginkgo may decrease free radical activity and a possible benefit in modulating the no-reflow phenomenon and subsequent reperfusion injury, and may help to improve tissue salvage.[46] A 1998 study by Bekerecioğlu and col-leagues[47] examined the effect of *Ginkgo biloba* on caudal-based dorsal rat flaps. The investigators reported that the group that was administered ginkgo intraperitone-ally for 6 days beginning 24 hours after surgery demonstrated a significantly reduced area of flap necrosis after 10 days compared with the control.[45] A 2010 study by Sambuy and colleagues[44] analyzed the effect of *Ginkgo biloba* on the survival of fascio-cutaneous flaps in rats. They reported a statistically significant reduction in the area of necrosis of the total surface flap in the group administered ginkgo for 7 days starting 24 hours postoperatively and a reduction approaching statistical significance ($P = .053$) in the group administered ginkgo for 7 days beginning immediately after sur-gery.[44] These results suggest that the reduction in necrotic areas of the flaps by free radical scavengers, such as *Ginkgo biloba*, indicates that the extract may have an in-direct role in the survival of these flaps[47] and may be useful in salvaging some parts of distally necrotic flaps. Further research is warranted to determine if ginkgo might be advantageous in human patients.

Other herbs There are several less widely used herbs that have been associated with effects that may be beneficial to patients undergoing cosmetic enhancement proce-dures, including the following:

- Chamomile
- Marigold
- Honey
- Turmeric
- Cocoa

The wound-healing properties of these herbs have been explored in limited studies. Animal studies demonstrated that aqueous chamomile (*Matricaria recutita*) increased the rate of wound contraction and wound strength in addition to its antioxidant activ-ity.[48,49] Marigold (*Calendula officinalis*) is recommended as a topical preparation for the treatment of wounds, ulcers, burns, boils, rashes, chapped hands, herpes zoster, and varicose veins.[15] In animals, surgical wounds displayed faster reepithelialization and fibroblasts increased proliferation and migration.[12] In vitro and in vivo studies of honey have demonstrated not only its effectiveness against many human pathogens, including methicillin-resistant *Staphylococcus aureus* but also its ability to retain a proper amount of moisture in the wound and aid in the formulation of granulation tis-sue and reepithelialization, significant deodorization, and angiogenic activity.[16] Several in vitro studies of curcumin, the yellow-colored primary active constituent derived from the spice turmeric, have shown protective effects on keratinocytes and fibroblasts, cells involved in wound healing.[50,51] One human study also reported significantly reduced pain, fatigue, and the use of supplementary analgesics in postoperative patients.[52] External application of cocoa has been reported to have a variety of benefits, including soothing burns, disinfecting wounds, and acting as a moisturizer for the skin. Additionally, one study showed that consumption of flavanol-rich cocoa increased microcirculation in the skin, which may be important to the wound-healing process.[16]

Dietary supplements

Like herbal therapy, dietary supplements and topical applications containing one or more ingredients purported to exert a pharmaceutical therapeutic benefit but not necessarily a biologic therapeutic benefit, defined as *cosmeceuticals*, are used and promoted as improving outcomes in cosmetic surgery.[53]

Retinoids Derivatives of vitamin A, collectively known as retinoids, are used in topical preparations and have been studied extensively for the treatment of photodamage and acne.[54] Within cosmeceutical formulations, various derivatives of vitamin A can be found, including the following:

- Retinol
- Retinaldehyde
- Retinyl esters
- The oxoretinoids[55]

Retinoids are also known to have positive effects on wound healing. They have been shown to increase epidermal water content, epidermal hyperplasia, and cell renewal while enhancing collagen synthesis.[56] In a small 1995 study of 4 elderly men with extensively photodamaged skin, Popp and colleagues[57] reported that treatment with a topical retinoid significantly and dramatically accelerated wound healing. Examination of wounds inflicted with a punch biopsy revealed that the wound areas treated with the retinoid were 35% to 37% smaller on days 1 and 4 and 47% to 50% smaller on days 6, 8, and 11 compared with the controls. Also, reepithelialization occurred more rapidly both clinically and histologically.[57]

The use of topical retinoids is often recommended before laser resurfacing procedures because of the beneficial effects in accelerating wound healing, enhancing collagen production, and activating fibroblasts.[54] A 2004 study of 16 women undergoing nonablative laser remodeling treatment of the neckline and forehead reported that patients treated with a daily topical application of 0.05% retinaldehyde immediately after the first laser treatment and up to 3 months after the fifth treatment showed a statistically significant increase in dermal thickness compared with controls.[58] A survey of 339 dermatologists and plastic surgeons revealed that 80% of respondents recommended preoperative treatment with topical retinoids before laser resurfacing procedures.[59]

Vitamin C Vitamin C (L-ascorbic acid) is a naturally occurring antioxidant normally found in human skin that functions as a free radical scavenger.[54] Vitamin C–containing cosmeceuticals have been shown to promote collagen synthesis, improve fine rhytides, and decrease hyperpigmentation.[54] Vitamin C is often recommended to improve wound healing. Two intervention studies from the same research group aimed to evaluate the effect of vitamins (ascorbic acid and pantothenic acid) supplementation before and after tattoo resection on the healing of surgical wounds. In both studies, hydroxyproline in skin and scars decreased from day 8 to day 21, which was associated with an increase in fibroblasts. Also, rigidity and breaking energy of the scars were higher in a dose-dependent fashion, suggesting supplementation of ascorbic acid in combination with pantothenic acid before and after a planned surgery of the skin may partly improve the mechanical properties of scars.[60] Theoretical benefits to the use of topical vitamin C with laser resurfacing procedures include minimizing postprocedural inflammation and erythema and increasing new collagen formation.[54] A 1998 study by Alster and West[61] examined the effects of vitamin C in 21 patients who underwent carbon dioxide laser resurfacing followed by treatment of half of the face with topical ascorbic acid and half with petrolatum-based cream. Significantly reduced erythema was observed in skin treated with 10% L-ascorbic acid in aqueous formulation compared with placebo.[61]

Vitamin E Vitamin E (α-tocopherol) is a lipophilic antioxidant that occurs naturally in the skin and scavenges free radicals.[62] Topical vitamin E preparations have been marketed to assist in wound healing and in minimizing postsurgical scarring.[54] Data supporting these claims have been contradictory, however. Several studies have examined the effects of topical vitamin E on wound healing after laser resurfacing with conflicting results.[54] In a 1993 study by Simon and colleagues,[63] porcine skin was irradiated with various doses of argon and copper-vapor laser and evaluated for effects on healing time of pretreatment with topical or intramuscular vitamin E. Skin treated with vitamin E demonstrated significantly decreased wound healing time by approximately 1 week after exposures of intermediate duration.[63] A split-face study compared the effects of a topical formulation containing 4% tocopherol acetate among several other ingredients with petrolatum alone on wound healing after resurfacing with YAG laser. The investigators reported decreased time to reepithelialization, as well as decreased pain, erythema, and edema in the skin treated with the vitamin E–containing compound. As noted in a subsequent review article, however, the contribution of vitamin E is questionable because its effect was not isolated from the potential actions of the additional ingredients.[54,64]

Zinc Zinc is an essential trace element in the human body that plays key roles in each phase of wound healing and has antiinflammatory effects.[65] In the rat model, supplemental zinc administered orally to zinc-deficient patients in a 1970 study was found to increase the progression of wound healing,[66] and in a 1985 study, zinc applied topically for 12 days was beneficial in the treatment of full-thickness excisional wounds, regardless of the nutritional status of the rats.[67] A 1991 porcine study by Agren and colleagues[68] reported that topical zinc oxide enhanced reepithelialization of partial-thickness wounds in nutritionally balanced pigs. In human studies, a 1984 study of 37 geriatric patients with either venous or arterial leg ulcers showed statistically significant improvement in healing in nearly twice as many patients in the groups administered topical zinc, suggesting that healing of leg ulcers is improved after the addition of zinc oxide to the local regimen.[69] Whether zinc enhances wound healing in human beings is unclear for nondeficient individuals.

Acupuncture

Acupuncture is part of an age-old paradigm within traditional Chinese medicine (TIM), a holistic approach that addresses the entire body when treating a localized condition or anatomy.[70,71] Based on the concept of energy flow, or Qi, which is separated into yin and yang, the goal of TIM is to manipulate the balance of yin and yang along 12 basic channels that flow throughout the body to maximize health. Stimulation of special acupuncture points on the body surface with needles, heat, or pressure has been done in China for more than 2500 years to treat diseases and relieve pain.[72]

Within aesthetic plastic surgery, the use of acupuncture has been explored as a compliment or alternative to various procedures and also as an adjunct to conventional pharmacologic control of postoperative pain, nausea, and vomiting.

Facial rejuvenation
The goal of TIM in facial rejuvenation is to enhance facial muscle and skin tone to its optimum level without injections or surgery. Acupuncture has also been described as a compliment to improve results as a component of aesthetic surgery that is similar to physical therapy for orthopedic surgery.[71] Practitioners insert acupuncture needles into the face at different points along designated channels to attain tonification or sedation effects.[71] According to one California-based acupuncturist, many younger patients and established patients needing maintenance do not require major surgery and can benefit from a noninvasive approach. In a 2005 article, Barrett[71] outlined the major channels used in facial rejuvenation and the aspects of those channels that most strongly affect the face: tonification techniques are used in patients with flabby skin and poor muscle tone and to promote blood circulation, and sedation techniques are used to relax tense muscles and to reduce inflammation and acne. A single case of a 26-year-old woman seeking reduction in nasolabial fold prominence, facial edema, and poor muscle tone in her eyes and cheeks was presented. Over a 1-month period, the patient received 10 treatments with 2-Hz electroacupuncture needles inserted 1 to 2 mm at 0.5-in intervals for 20 minutes at approximately 5 mA "to strengthen local Qi and blood circulation while promoting collagen formation."[71] In the results, evaluated through the assessment of pretreatment and posttreatment photographs, the investigator reported a 50% shortening and 20% reduction in depth of the nasolabial fold, complete bilateral elimination of the lines above the eyes, and a 50% reduction of the depth and 20% reduction of the length of the lines under the eyes.[71]

Acupuncture analgesia
Acupuncture analgesia is a technique directed toward the relief of pain and regulation of the physiologic function of the human body by needling.[71] Relief of pain during surgery is conventionally provided by the administration of opioid drugs. Risks of undesirable side effects, such as nausea, vomiting, and decreased genitourinary and alimentary tract motility, can lead to delayed postoperative recovery. Therefore, the use of adjunct analgesics that provide opioid-sparing effects and decrease the incidence of opioid-related side effects has been explored.

There are increasing numbers of clinical trials evaluating the efficacy of acupuncture and related techniques as an adjuvant method for postoperative analgesia. Physiologically, acupuncture may inhibit gastric acid secretion and stimulate the release of endogenous endorphins, offering a potential explanation for therapeutic effects on nausea, vomiting, and pain.[72] The P6, or Neiguan acupuncture point over the median nerve on the volar aspect of the wrist, is thought to regulate these symptoms.[70] A 2008 meta-analysis evaluating the efficacy of acupuncture and related techniques as adjunct analgesics for acute postoperative pain management included 15 studies encompassing a wide range of interventions and types of surgery (not cosmetic). The investigators found that acupuncture and related techniques are effective adjuncts for postoperative pain management as demonstrated by a significant reduction of postoperative pain scores and opioid consumption.[73] A 2009 RCT by Larson and colleagues targeted patients undergoing cosmetic and reconstructive face, breast, and body-contouring cosmetic procedures and examined the effect of electro-acustimulation versus placebo on postoperative nausea, vomiting, and pain. Statistically significant findings included that patients in the electro-acustimulation group reported lower nausea scores at 30 minutes and 120 minutes postoperatively. There was no difference in emetic events. A shorter time to discharge was noted in treated patients undergoing abdominal procedures and a decreased need for intravenous (IV) fentanyl in treated patients undergoing breast procedures. However, these differences were not demonstrated in patients undergoing facial procedures.[74]

A 2005 randomized, double-blind, sham-controlled study of 105 adults undergoing elective plastic surgery by White and colleagues examined the effect of timing of acustimulation when administered in combination with ondansetron for preventing postoperative emetic symptoms. Results demonstrated that acustimulation at the P6 acupoint for 30 minutes before and up to 72 hours after surgery resulted in 25% less postoperative nausea and vomiting (PONV) than with preoperative treatment alone and 13% less PONV than with only postoperative treatment.[70] A 2010 study of 90 patients by Sahmeddini and colleagues[72] to test whether electroacupuncture (EA) of specific points is superior to sham acupuncture for complementary analgesia after nasal septoplasty reported that perioperative EA is a suitable alternative to intravenous morphine (0.1 mg/kg) in reducing postoperative pain scores. The results suggested that the use of both EA and 0.1 mg/kg IV morphine given intraoperatively resulted in a similar postoperative pain score and postoperative analgesic requirement, which meant EA had a similar analgesic effect to morphine in this study.[75]

Mind-Body Medicine

Numerous prospective randomized studies have investigated the effectiveness of mind-body techniques used before and after surgery in improving surgery outcomes as measured by

- Decreased anxiety
- Decreased pain
- Reduced need for pain medication
- Shortened hospital stays

Published pain management guidelines also recognize the role of the mind-body technique in the management of postoperative pain.[72] Facial neuromuscular training with electromyogram (EMG) biofeedback is a mind-body medicine technique that has been well described.[76] The process of monitoring and feeding back information to patients is used to aid in training patients to alter some characteristic of that activity. Biofeedback EMG instruments are essentially general-purpose physiologic monitoring devices that are designed to provide ongoing information about a physiologic function that normally occurs involuntarily, such as heart rate, blood pressure, or, in this case, muscle tension levels as measured by EMG.[77] A 2004 study by Vaiman and colleagues[77] described the outcome of biofeedback training of nasal muscles in cases of nasal valve stenosis and collapse. Fifteen nonrandomized patients with clinically evident nasal valve collapse were treated with 9 to 12 months of surface and intranasal EMG biofeedback-assisted specific strategies for nasal muscle education and a home exercise program of specific nasal movements. Although all patients improved subjectively, 86.66% (13 out of 15) showed objective improvement obviating endonasal surgery.[77]

Hypnosis

Hypnosis involves the intentional induction, deepening, maintenance, and termination of a natural trance state for a specific purpose, usually to reduce suffering or promote the healing of patients.[77] The hypnotic phenomenon has been used since antiquity to assist healing.[78] It may be induced using relaxation, meditation techniques, guided imagery, deep breathing, or self-induced focus. Hildebrand and Anderson[78] described techniques that can be used in the practice setting of the plastic surgery including

- Mindful focus
- Focused breathing
- Body scan
- Progressive muscle relaxation
- Guided imagery[79]

The use of hypnosis techniques has been promoted for a variety of situations in the plastic surgery setting. They have been used to assist with the use of Botox, the use of dermal fillers, and the removal of sutures or staples. Hypnosis has also been used to lessen the severity of pain associated with surgery when used in combination with a local anesthetic. A 2002 study of 20 women randomized to standard care versus preoperative hypnosis for excisional breast biopsy by Montgomery and colleagues[80] found that brief (10 minute) hypnosis was effective in reducing postsurgery pain and distress both before and after surgery. Patients in the hypnosis group required less propofol, and reported less pain intensity, nausea and discomfort than the control group.[78] Hypnosis has also been reported to be as helpful as complementary or integrative therapy for treating warts. In a controlled study by Surman and colleagues,[81] 53% of the experimental group consisting of 17 experimental patients with bilateral common or flat warts had improvement of their warts 3 months after the first of 5 hypnotherapy sessions, whereas none of the control group had improvement.

Adverse Effects

Many patients have the misconception that because integrative treatments are natural there are no adverse effects. Although there is no clear evidence that the preoperative use of herbal supplements will cause harmful effects, there are many potential complications that the surgeon should know.[79,81] A 2002 survey of surgical patients revealed that patients admitted to taking herbal medication that had coagulation effects (40.5%), blood pressure effects (32.7%), cardiovascular effects (20%), sedative effects (16.7%), and effects on electrolytes or diuresis (8.9%); 22.8% of patients reported using herbs that are known to cause adverse effects when combined with prescription medications.[82] Of the direct pharmacologic effects, the putative risk of bleeding imparted by the use of various herbal medicines is of particular concern. Certain remedies can increase the risk of intrinsic bleeding, which can result in serious problems for plastic surgeons and their patients.[83,84] Some herbals inherently possess significant pharmacologic activity to antagonize normal platelet aggregation and coagulation mechanisms; others contain coumarins, and their plants are similar in structure to warfarin.[85]

Garlic

There is substantial evidence to implicate garlic as a potential cause of bleeding, and studies indicate it may inhibit platelet aggregation in a dose-dependent fashion. In vitro studies have shown reduction in adenosine diphosphate (ADP)–induced platelet aggregation, thromboxane reduction, CA+ mobilization, and inhibition of the synthesis of thromboxane B2.[86] In vivo human studies have documented garlic's effect on hemostatic parameters, such as ADP-induced platelet aggregation, thromboxane reduction, and clotting time.[85] Garlic has also been implicated as a cause of spontaneous bleeding in several case reports, including a spontaneous epidural hematoma in an elderly man, a hematoma after breast augmentation that required evacuation, and a hemorrhage after a transurethral prostate resection in a 72-year-old patient taking no medications other than garlic that required transfusion of 4 units of blood.[85,87,88] The potential for irreversible inhibition of platelet function may warrant patients to discontinue garlic use at least 7 days before surgery, especially if postoperative bleeding is a particular concern or other platelet inhibitors are given.[85,87,88]

Ginkgo

Ginkgo also inhibits thromboxane synthetase, which may increase surgical bleeding. These antiplatelet effects are dose dependent, long lasting, and rapidly established after oral intake.[89] Several anecdotal reports of bleeding complications attributed to Ginkgo biloba use illustrate ginkgo's potential inhibitory effect on platelet activating factor and consequently on platelet aggregation, including

- Spontaneous bilateral subdural hematomas
- Fatal intracerebral mass bleeding
- Spontaneous hyphema
- Postoperative bleeding following laparoscopic cholecystectomy[89]

Attempts to scientifically demonstrate an in vivo effect of ginkgo on platelet or coagulation function have fallen short, however.[2,90] Clinical trials with small numbers of patients have not demonstrated complications from bleeding.[91] In 44 clinical studies with a total of 9772 patients, the incidence of adverse effects was 0.5%.[91] Recently, a 2003 prospective, double-blind, randomized, and placebo-controlled study was carried out in 32 young, male, healthy volunteers. No significant effect on hemostasis, coagulation, platelet function, and fibrinolysis was observed. Likewise, in a 2004 study of 50 healthy male volunteers taking ginkgo, none of 29 platelet and coagulation parameters was abnormal.[92] A 2007 study of 10 healthy adult volunteers taking ginkgo at the manufacturer's recommended dose for 2 weeks also showed no significant changes in platelet count, prothrombin time (PT), partial thromboplastin time (PTT), or bleeding time.[92]

Asian ginseng

Asian ginseng (Panax ginseng), the most expensive and probably the most popular herb sold worldwide, has been valued in Chinese medicine for more than 2000 years for its invigorating, adaptogenic, and tonic properties.[92] Presently marketed in the United States to increase alertness and energy, Asian ginseng has also been shown to exhibit irreversible antiplatelet effects.[93] In rats, ginseng has been shown to inhibit platelet aggregation induced by thrombin or collagen; a 1989 study suggested that it may exhibit irreversible antiplatelet activity in humans by the inhibition of thromboxane formation.[94] However, a 2007 study of the effects of ginseng administered at the manufacturer's recommended dose showed no significant alteration in platelet count, PT, PTT, or bleeding time.[94] Case reports implicating ginseng as a cause of bleeding are limited to 2 reports from the 1980s of vaginal bleeding in postmenopausal women after using ginseng either topically or orally and menometrorrhagia in a 39-year-old woman using oral and topical ginseng, which abated 10 days after she stopped taking the ginseng.[95] Although the elimination half-life of ginseng is relatively short, its irreversible platelet inhibition suggests that use should be discontinued at least 7 days before surgery.[96,97]

Ginger

Ginger, a popular remedy for nausea, gastrointestinal bloating, dyspepsia, and arthritic inflammation, has been shown to decrease platelet aggregation in randomized controlled studies; concern has been raised that ginger may prolong bleeding time because of its inhibition of thromboxane synthetase.[2,86,98] A 2003 Australian study showed that compounds in ginger and their derivatives are more potent antiplatelet agents than aspirin in vitro.[2,86,98] Several trials have found evidence contradicting these reports, including 2 trials that failed to demonstrate any association of ginger with platelet aggregation, fibrinolytic activity, or fibrinogen levels.[98] Still, most recommendations are that ginger should not be taken in the perioperative period because of the increased risk of hematoma and prolonged bleeding, and patients should be advised to discontinue the use of ginger 2 to 3 weeks before surgery.[99,100]

Feverfew

Feverfew is an herb that has been used traditionally as an antipyretic but is most commonly used for migraine prevention. No cases of bleeding problems in patients using feverfew have been reported; however, an in vitro study showed that feverfew extract inhibited the deposition of platelets on collagen in a dose-dependent way.[101] Caution dictates that patients should be advised to discontinue feverfew use before surgery. Plastic surgeons should advise patients to taper, then discontinue feverfew completely no later than 2 to 3 weeks before surgery[101] because abrupt cessation of feverfew therapy may result in a syndrome characterized by nervousness, tension headaches, insomnia, stiffness, joint pain, and tiredness.[101]

Kava and valerian

Kava and valerian, 2 popular herbal medications often taken as anxiolytics or sleep aids, have been associated with excessive sedative effects. It has been suggested that kava, a pepper plant derivative, has a therapeutic potential in the symptomatic treatment of anxiety. Its active constituents, kavalactones, have a dose-dependent potentiating effect on gamma-aminobutyric acid (GABA) inhibitory neurotransmission.[102] Although most Western countries suspended kava sales in 2002 following reports of liver toxicity, it may still be obtained through traditional herbalists and online distributors.[102] Potential for abuse exists; however, investigations into addiction, tolerance, and acute withdrawal are lacking.[11] Additionally, heavy users of kava have experienced a characteristic reversible kava dermopathy after several months at high doses.[10] Symptoms include reddened eyes, scaly skin eruptions, and a yellowish discoloration of the skin and hair.[31] The potential for interaction with anesthetic agents warrants its discontinuation at least 24 hours before surgery.[10]

Valerian, widely available as an herbal sleep aid, also acts by mediating GABA neurotransmission. Valerian produces dose-dependent sedation and hypnosis. There is a 1998 case report in which valerian withdrawal seemed to mimic acute benzodiazepine withdrawal syndrome in a patient who presented with symptoms of delirium and cardiac complications following surgery that were relieved with the administration of benzodiazepines.[10,103] Because of this unknown incidence of withdrawal effects, patients should be advised to taper the dose over several weeks before surgery or continue taking valerian up until the day of surgery.[10,103] St. John's wort, an herb with clinically proven antidepressant effects that is also used as an integrative treatment of anxiety and sleep disorders, may also potentially prolong postoperative sedation in some patients. However, no controlled studies support these observations.[104]

Cutaneous reactions

Many cutaneous reactions to herbal preparations have been reported. Numerous herbal medicines may profoundly affect the skin and thereby adversely interact with the facial plastic surgeon's efforts to improve skin quality through resurfacing techniques.[104] Kava dermopathy has previously been mentioned. St. John's wort poses a risk of photosensitivity reaction. Animal studies have noted the development of blisters similar to burns on exposure to bright sunlight with heavy consumption, and 2 case reports detail photosensitivity reactions in humans associated with the ingestion of the herb.[105]

A young woman has been described with leukemia-related Sweet syndrome elicited by pathergy to topical arnica; however, the most common cutaneous adverse effect of herbal preparations is allergic contact dermatitis.[106] Certain medicinal plants of the carrot family (*Apiaceae*) contain furanocoumarins and can also cause a photodermatitis in humans from sensitization of the skin to UV light. Use of herbal medicines containing furanocoumarins should be avoided while undergoing cosmetic surgery, UV exposure, or in conjunction with other photosensitizing agents or dermal irritants.[31]

Phytoestrogens

Many facial plastic surgery patients who are perimenopausal or postmenopausal have turned to herbal remedies following adverse outcomes of hormone replacement therapy reported by the Women's Health Initiative.[31,107] More than 500 plant species contain phytoestrogens, naturally occurring substances functionally similar to estradiol, which may potentiate or antagonize estrogen effects. Among the more commonly used phytoestrogen-containing herbs are

- Dong quai (*Angelica sinensis*)
- Red clover (*Trifolium pratense*)
- Alfalfa (*Medicago sativa var italica*)
- Licorice (*Glycyrrhiza glabra*)
- Black cohosh (*Cimicifuga racemosa*)[31,107]

These compounds may contribute to changes in skin pigmentation following plastic surgery procedures such as dermabrasion, laser skin resurfacing, microdermabrasion, and scar revisions. In one case, postmenopausal bleeding was attribute to the estrogenlike effect of topical ginseng.[108] Moreover, use of some phytoestrogens in conjunction with estrogen replacement therapies may result in symptoms, such as nausea, bloating, hypotension, breast fullness or tenderness, migraine headaches, and edema.[108]

Pharmacokinetic and Pharmacodynamic Interactions

The interaction of herbal medications with allopathic medicines is complex. A growing body of scientific literature has highlighted the pharmacokinetic and pharmacodynamic interactions between herbal and prescription medicines.[109] Many of the harmful interactions stem from the cytochrome P450 (CYP) pathway used by many medications.[109] St. John's wort induces the CYP isoform 3A4 as well as the drug efflux transporter P-glycoprotein. Documented St. John's wort interactions include a diverse group of drugs including

- The immunosuppressants cyclosporine and tacrolimus
- The protease inhibitor indinavir
- The non-nucleoside reverse transcriptase inhibitor nevirapine
- The tricyclic antidepressant amitriptyline
- The 5- hydroxy-3-methylglutaryl-coenzyme A (HMG-CoA) reductase inhibitor simvastatin
- Calcium channel blockers
- Serotonin receptor agonists
- Oral contraceptives[110]

The CYP isoform C is also induced by St. John's wort and can decrease levels of warfarin and nonsteroidal antiinflammatory drugs (NSAIDs).[110] Steady use may, on the other hand, lower digoxin levels. Both aloe vera (taken internally) and cascara (*Rhamnus purshiana*) may potentiate cardiac glycosides as well as antiarrhythmic drugs.[111]

Several studies support the avoidance of garlic usage with coagulation inhibitors, including heparin, warfarin, aspirin, and NSAIDs. In particular, garlic has been reported to increase the international normalized ratio when used in combination with warfarin and may potentiate bleeding postoperatively.[111] Concomitant use of *Ginkgo biloba* with antiplatelets, anticoagulants, and NSAIDs should also be avoided. Case reports of a spontaneous hyphema when a patient who had been on aspirin therapy commenced taking ginkgo and another who experienced cerebral hemorrhage when he added ginkgo to a regimen that included warfarin highlight the dangers of these combinations. Ginseng has been reported to interact with monoamine oxidase inhibitors, resulting in tremulousness and mania; concomitant use should be avoided. Caution should also be used when ginseng is taken along with anticoagulation and antiinflammatory pharmaceuticals because the platelet inhibition is irreversible.[86] Because valerian and kava can cause sedation, patients should be advised to avoid combining with benzodiazepines, barbiturates, and alcohol.[86] Furthermore, kava interacts with levodopa to potentiate Parkinsonian symptoms.[112]

SUMMARY

The growing popularity of CIM, including herbal and homeopathic supplements, in the last 2 decades has resulted in increased examination.[113] Natural compounds contain a wealth of interesting and possibly beneficial pharmaceutically active compounds.[86] A role for CIM therapies even as placebo use should not be discredited in aiding selected patients, especially as combined or complementary therapy.[12] A few RCTs have shown promising results in the use of herbal therapies for the treatment of cosmetic disorders. The addition of topical formulations to perioperative skincare regimens can serve to enhance the overall response of patients' skin to surgical procedures, such as skin resurfacing, and may allow for quicker healing, shorter recovery times, and fewer complications.[54]

Given the high rates of patient use, especially among plastic surgery patients; wide availability; potentially reduced costs; notable laboratory findings; and potential benefits, further study is recommended.[54] Well-controlled clinical trials may validate ancient remedies or yield valuable information about new and existing herbal medicines. A thorough review of the literature and the guidance of governmental research agencies when planning studies is likely to assist in gathering more reliable future evidence. Ideally, a medical professional with proper training in herbal medicine should supervise patients who take herbal supplements, but this is often impossible because the supplements are available over the counter and patients often research their proposed health benefits online via unregulated Web sites.[86] The side effects and potential complications warrant caution. Health care professionals have a responsibility to educate themselves and their patients about the risks and potential benefits of such supplements.[86] The limited evidence-based information about safety and efficacy, the absence of a standard regulatory mechanism for herbal medicine approval and surveillance, and improper patient assumptions are an evolving challenge.[10] Consideration may be given to these CIM therapies in the therapeutic armamentarium for selected patients undergoing cosmetic surgery, and open discussion with patients regarding possible risks and benefits is recommended for the best possible surgical outcomes.

REFERENCES

1. Anon. Search results: complementary alternative medicine barnes. Available at: http://www.cdc.gov/search.do?q=complementary+alternative+medicine+barnes&btnG.x=0&btnG.y=0&sort=date%3AD%3AL%3Ad1&oe=UTF-8&ie=UTF-8&ud=1&site=default_collection. Accessed October 6, 2012.

2. Broughton G, Crosby MA, Coleman J, et al. Use of herbal supplements and vitamins in plastic surgery: a practical review. Plast Reconstr Surg 2007; 119(3):48e–66e.
3. Adusumilli PS, Ben-Porat L, Pereira M, et al. The prevalence and predictors of herbal medicine use in surgical patients. J Am Coll Surg 2004;198(4):583–90.
4. Tsen LC, Segal S, Pothier M, et al. Alternative medicine use in presurgical patients. Anesthesiology 2000;93(1):148–51.
5. Kaye A, Clarke R, Sabar R, et al. Herbal medicines: current trends in anesthesiology practice—a hospital survey. J Clin Anesth 2000;12(6):468–71.
6. Norred CL. Complementary and alternative medicine use by surgical patients. AORN J 2002;76(6):1013–21.
7. Heller J, Gabbay JS, Ghadjar K, et al. Top-10 list of herbal and supplemental medicines used by cosmetic patients: what the plastic surgeon needs to know. Plast Reconstr Surg 2006;117(2):436–45.
8. Collins D, Oakey S, Ramakrishnan V. Perioperative use of herbal, complementary, and over the counter medicines in plastic surgery patients. Eplasty 2011;11. Available at: http://www.ncbi.nlm.nih.gov.proxy1.lib.tju.edu:2048/pubmed/21625528. Accessed October 2, 2012.
9. Schlessinger J, Schlessinger D, Schlessinger B. Prospective demographic study of cosmetic surgery patients. J Clin Aesthet Dermatol 2010;3(11):30–5.
10. Ang-Lee MK, Moss J, Yuan CS. Herbal medicines and perioperative care. JAMA 2001;286(2):208–16.
11. Rowe DJ, Baker AC. Perioperative risks and benefits of herbal supplements in aesthetic surgery. Aesthet Surg J 2009;29(2):150–7.
12. Reddy KK, Grossman L, Rogers GS. Common complementary and alternative therapies with potential use in dermatologic surgery: risks and benefits. J Am Acad Dermatol 2011. Available at: http://www.ncbi.nlm.nih.gov/pubmed/21890235. Accessed August 23, 2012.
13. Dat AD, Poon F, Pham KB, et al. Aloe vera for treating acute and chronic wounds. In: Cochrane database of systematic reviews. John Wiley & Sons, Ltd; 1996. Available at: http://onlinelibrary.wiley.com.proxy1.lib.tju.edu/doi/10.1002/14651858.CD008762.pub2/abstract. Accessed October 12, 2012.
14. Anon. Aloe (Aloe vera). In: Natural Standard: the authority on integrative medicine. Cambridge (MA): Natural Standard; 2012 [cited 25 October 2012]. Available at: http://www.naturalstandard.com. Subscription required to view. Accessed on October 25th, 2012.
15. Bedi MK, Shenefelt PD. Herbal therapy in dermatology. Arch Dermatol 2002; 138(2):232–42.
16. Davis SC, Perez R. Cosmeceuticals and natural products: wound healing. Clin Dermatol 2009;27(5):502–6.
17. Heggers JP, Kucukcelebi A, Stabenau CJ, et al. Wound healing effects of aloe gel and other topical antibacterial agents on rat skin. Phytother Res 1995;9(6):455–7.
18. Fulton JE Jr. The stimulation of postdermabrasion wound healing with stabilized aloe vera gel-polyethylene oxide dressing. J Dermatol Surg Oncol 1990;16(5):460–7.
19. Anon. Arnica (Arnica chamissonis, Arnica cordifolia, Arnica fulgens, Arnica latifolia, Arnica montana, Arnica sororia). In: Natural standard: the authority on integrative medicine. Cambridge (MA): Natural Standard; 2012 [cited 5 October 2012]. Available at: http://www.naturalstandard.com. Subscription required to view. Accessed on October 5th, 2012.

20. Dinman S. Arnica. Plast Surg Nurs 2007;27(1):52–3.
21. Widrig R, Suter A, Saller R, et al. Choosing between NSAID and arnica for topical treatment of hand osteoarthritis in a randomised, double-blind study. Rheumatol Int 2007;27(6):585–91.
22. Lawrence WT. Arnica. Plast Reconstr Surg 2003;112(4):1164–6.
23. Baumann LS. Less-known botanical cosmeceuticals. Dermatol Ther 2007;20(5): 330–42.
24. Ernst E, Pittler MH. Efficacy of homeopathic arnica: a systematic review of placebo-controlled clinical trials. Arch Surg 1998;133(11):1187–90.
25. Alonso D, Lazarus MC, Baumann L. Effects of topical arnica gel on post-laser treatment bruises. Dermatol Surg 2002;28(8):686–8.
26. Ramelet AA, Buchheim G, Lorenz P, et al. Homoeopathic arnica in postoperative haematomas: a double-blind study. Dermatology 2000;201(4):347–8.
27. Kotlus BS, Heringer DM, Dryden RM. Evaluation of homeopathic Arnica montana for ecchymosis after upper blepharoplasty: a placebo-controlled, randomized, double-blind study. Ophthal Plast Reconstr Surg 2010;26(6):395–7.
28. Reported at the Research and Innovative Technology Scientific Session of the American Society of Aesthetic Plastic Surgery (ASAPS) meeting in Las Vegas, April 29, 2002. Presented by Dr. Michael Kulick of San Francisco. Printed in the Abstract Book of the ASAPS Conference, p. 17–18: Arnica Montana, Role in Reducing Bruising and Swelling: Fact or Fiction?
29. Totonchi A, Guyuron B. A randomized, controlled comparison between arnica and steroids in the management of postrhinoplasty ecchymosis and edema. Plast Reconstr Surg 2007;120(1):271–4.
30. Seeley BM, Denton AB, Ahn MS, et al. Effect of homeopathic Arnica montana on bruising in face-lifts: results of a randomized, double-blind, placebo-controlled clinical trial. Arch Facial Plast Surg 2006;8(1):54–9. Accessed on October 5th, 2012.
31. deAzevedo Pribitkin E. Herbal medicine and surgery. Semin Integr Med 2005; 3(1):17–23.
32. Anon. Bromelain (Ananas comosus, Ananas sativus). In: Natural Standard: the authority on integrative medicine. Cambridge (MA): Natural Standard; 2012 [cited 5 October 2012]. Available at: http://www.naturalstandard.com. Subscription required to view.
33. Orsini RA. Bromelain. Plast Reconstr Surg 2006;118(7):1640–4.
34. Howat RC, Lewis GD. The effect of bromelain therapy on episiotomy wounds–a double blind controlled clinical trial. J Obstet Gynaecol Br Commonw 1972; 79(10):951–3.
35. Brown SA, Coimbra M, Coberly DM, et al. Oral nutritional supplementation accelerates skin wound healing: a randomized, placebo-controlled, double-arm, crossover study. Plast Reconstr Surg 2004;114(1):237–44.
36. Khanna S, Roy S, Bagchi D, et al. Upregulation of oxidant-induced VEGF expression in cultured keratinocytes by a grape seed proanthocyanidin extract. Free Radic Biol Med 2001;31(1):38–42.
37. Khanna S, Venojarvi M, Roy S, et al. Dermal wound healing properties of redox-active grape seed proanthocyanidins. Free Radic Biol Med 2002;33(8):1089–96.
38. Nayak BS, Ramdath DD, Marshall JR, et al. Wound-healing activity of the skin of the common grape (Vitis vinifera) variant, cabernet sauvignon. Phytother Res 2010;24(8):1151–7.
39. Blazsó G, Gábor M, Schönlau F, et al. Pycnogenol accelerates wound healing and reduces scar formation. Phytother Res 2004;18(7):579–81. Accessed on October 5th, 2012.

40. Anon. Grape seed (Vitis vinifera, Vitis coignetiae). In: Natural Standard: the authority on integrative medicine. Cambridge (MA): Natural Standard; 2012 [cited 15 October 2012]. Available at: http://www.naturalstandard.com. Subscription required to view.
41. Anon. Ginkgo (Ginkgo biloba). In: Natural Standard: the authority on integrative medicine. Cambridge (MA): Natural Standard; 2008 [cited 5 October 2012]. Available at: http://www.naturalstandard.com. Subscription required to view.
42. Stanger MJ, Thompson LA, Young AJ, et al. Anticoagulant activity of select dietary supplements. Nutr Rev 2012;70(2):107–17.
43. Blumenthal M, Busse WR, Goldberg A, et al, editors. Complete German Commission E monographs; therapeutic guide to herbal medicines. Austin (TX): American Botanical Council; Boston: Integrative Medicine Communications; 1998. [Kelin S, Risler RS, trans].
44. Sambuy MT, da Costa AC, Cohen C, et al. Effect of Ginkgo biloba extract (GbE-761) on the survival of fasciocutaneous flaps in rats. Phytother Res 2012;26(2): 299–302.
45. Çeliköz B, Aydin A, Kubar A, et al. The effects of Gingko biloba extract and deferoxamine on flap viability. Eur J Plast Surg 1997;20(4):197–201.
46. Deveci M, Dibirdik I, Çeliköz B, et al. Alpha-tocopherol and Ginkgo biloba treatment protects lipid peroxidation during ischemic period in rat groin island skin flaps. Eur J Plast Surg 1997;20(3):141–4.
47. Bekerecioğlu M, Tercan M, Ozyazgan I. The effect of Gingko biloba extract (Egb 761) as a free radical scavenger on the survival of skin flaps in rats. A comparative study. Scand J Plast Reconstr Surg Hand Surg 1998;32(2):135–9.
48. Nayak BS, Raju SS, Rao AV. Wound healing activity of Matricaria recutita L. extract. J Wound Care 2007;16(7):298–302.
49. McKay DL, Blumberg JB. A Review of the bioactivity and potential health benefits of chamomile tea (Matricaria recutita L.). Phytother Res 2006;20(7):519–30.
50. Phan TT, See P, Lee ST, et al. Protective effects of curcumin against oxidative damage on skin cells in vitro: its implication for wound healing. J Trauma 2001;51(5): 927–31.
51. Madhyastha R, Madhyastha H, Nakajima Y, et al. Curcumin facilitates fibrinolysis and cellular migration during wound healing by modulating urokinase plasminogen activator expression. Pathophysiol Haemost Thromb 2010;37(2–4):59–66.
52. Agarwal KA, Tripathi CD, Agarwal BB, et al. Efficacy of turmeric (curcumin) in pain and postoperative fatigue after laparoscopic cholecystectomy: a double-blind, randomized placebo-controlled study. Surg Endosc 2011;25(12):3805–10.
53. Brody HJ. Relevance of cosmeceuticals to the dermatologic surgeon. Dermatol Surg 2005;31:796–9.
54. Lupo M, Jacob L. Cosmeceuticals used in conjunction with laser resurfacing. Semin Cutan Med Surg 2011;30(3):156–62.
55. Zussman J, Ahdout J, Kim J. Vitamins and photoaging: do scientific data support their use? J Am Acad Dermatol 2010;63(3):507–25.
56. Choi CM, Berson DS. Cosmeceuticals. Semin Cutan Med Surg 2006;25(3): 163–8.
57. Popp C, Kligman AM, Stoudemayer TJ. Pretreatment of photoaged forearm skin with topical tretinoin accelerates healing of full-thickness wounds. Br J Dermatol 1995;132(1):46–53.
58. Mordon S, Lagarde JM, Vienne MP, et al. Ultrasound imaging demonstration of the improvement of non-ablative laser remodeling by concomitant daily topical application of 0.05% retinaldehyde. J Cosmet Laser Ther 2004;6(1):5–9.

59. Duke D, Grevelink JM. Care before and after laser skin resurfacing. A survey and review of the literature. Dermatol Surg 1998;24(2):201–6.
60. Ellinger S, Stehle P. Efficacy of vitamin supplementation in situations with wound healing disorders: results from clinical intervention studies. Curr Opin Clin Nutr Metab Care 2009;12(6):588–95.
61. Alster TS, West TB. Effect of topical vitamin C on postoperative carbon dioxide laser resurfacing erythema. Dermatol Surg 1998;24(3):331–4.
62. Huang CK, Miller TA. The truth about over-the-counter topical anti-aging products a comprehensive review. Aesthet Surg J 2007;27(4):402–12.
63. Simon GA, Schmid P, Reifenrath WG, et al. Wound healing after laser injury to skin–the effect of occlusion and vitamin E. J Pharm Sci 1994;83(8):1101–6.
64. McDaniel DH, Ash K, Lord J, et al. Accelerated laser resurfacing wound healing using a triad of topical antioxidants. Dermatol Surg 1998;24(6):661–4.
65. Lansdown AB, Mirastschijski U, Stubbs N, et al. Zinc in wound healing: theoretical, experimental, and clinical aspects. Wound Repair Regen 2007;15(1): 2–16.
66. Sandstead HH, Lanier VC, Shephard GH, et al. Zinc and wound healing effects of zinc deficiency and zinc supplementation. Am J Clin Nutr 1970; 23(5):514–9.
67. Hallmans G, Lasek J. The effect of topical zinc absorption from wounds on growth and the wound healing process in zinc-deficient rats. Scand J Plast Reconstr Surg 1985;19(2):119–25.
68. Agren MS, Chvapil M, Franzén L. Enhancement of re-epithelialization with topical zinc oxide in porcine partial-thickness wounds. J Surg Res 1991;50(2):101–5.
69. Strömberg HE, Ågren MS. Topical zinc oxide treatment improves arterial and venous leg ulcers. Br J Dermatol 1984;111(4):461–8.
70. Larson JD, Gutowski KA, Marcus BC, et al. The effect of electroacustimulation on postoperative nausea, vomiting, and pain in outpatient plastic surgery patients: a prospective, randomized, blinded, clinical trial. Plast Reconstr Surg 2010;125(3): 989–94.
71. Barrett JB. Acupuncture and facial rejuvenation. Aesthet Surg J 2005;25(4): 419–24.
72. Sahmeddini MA, Farbood A, Ghafaripuor S. Electro-acupuncture for pain relief after nasal septoplasty: a randomized controlled study. J Altern Complement Med 2010;16(1):53–7.
73. Arnberger M, Stadelmann K, Alischer P, et al. Monitoring of neuromuscular blockade at the p6 acupuncture point reduces the incidence of postoperative nausea and vomiting. Anesthesiology 2007;107(6):903–8.
74. Sun Y, Gan TJ, Dubose JW, et al. Acupuncture and related techniques for postoperative pain: a systematic review of randomized controlled trials. Br J Anaesth 2008;101(2):151–60.
75. White PF, Hamza MA, Recart A, et al. Optimal timing of acustimulation for antiemetic prophylaxis as an adjunct to ondansetron in patients undergoing plastic surgery. Anesth Analg 2005;100(2):367–72.
76. Diaz M, Larsen B. Preparing for successful surgery: an implementation study. Perm J 2005;9(3):23–7.
77. Vaiman M, Shlamkovich N, Kessler A, et al. Biofeedback training of nasal muscles using internal and external surface electromyography of the nose. Am J Otol 2005;26(5):302–7.
78. Hildebrand LE, Anderson RC. Hypnosis and relaxation in the context of plastic surgery nursing. Plast Surg Nurs 2011;31(1):5–8.

79. Shenefelt PD. Applying hypnosis in dermatology. Dermatol Nurs 2003;15(6): 513–7, 538; [quiz: 518].

80. Montgomery GH, Bovbjerg DH, Schnur JB, et al. A randomized clinical trial of a brief hypnosis intervention to control side effects in breast surgery patients. J Natl Cancer Inst 2007;99(17):1304–12.

81. Surman OS, Gottlieb SK, Hackett TP, et al. Hypnosis in the treatment of warts. Arch Gen Psychiatry 1973;28(3):439–41.

82. Morris CA, Avorn J. Internet marketing of herbal products. JAMA 2003;290(11): 1505–9.

83. Norred CL. A follow-up survey of the use of complementary and alternative medicines by surgical patients. AANA J 2002;70(2):119–25.

84. Tessier DJ, Bash DS. A surgeon's guide to herbal supplements. J Surg Res 2003;114(1):30–6.

85. Beckert BW, Concannon MJ, Henry SL, et al. The effect of herbal medicines on platelet function: an in vivo experiment and review of the literature. Plast Reconstr Surg 2007;120(7):2044–50.

86. Wong WW, Gabriel A, Maxwell GP, et al. Bleeding risks of herbal, homeopathic, and dietary supplements: a hidden nightmare for plastic surgeons? Aesthet Surg J 2012;32(3):332–46.

87. Rose KD, Croissant PD, Parliament CF, et al. Spontaneous spinal epidural hematoma with associated platelet dysfunction from excessive garlic ingestion: a case report. Neurosurgery 1990;26(5):880–2.

88. German K, Kumar U, Blackford HN. Garlic and the risk of TURP bleeding. Br J Urol 1995;76(4):518.

89. Smith PF, Maclennan K, Darlington CL. The neuroprotective properties of the Ginkgo biloba leaf: a review of the possible relationship to platelet-activating factor (PAF). J Ethnopharmacol 1996;50(3):131–9.

90. Akiba S, Kawauchi T, Oka T, et al. Inhibitory effect of the leaf extract of Ginkgo biloba L. on oxidative stress-induced platelet aggregation. Biochem Mol Biol Int 1998;46(6):1243–8.

91. Fessenden JM, Wittenborn W, Clarke L. Gingko biloba: a case report of herbal medicine and bleeding postoperatively from a laparoscopic cholecystectomy. Am Surg 2001;67(1):33–5. Accessed on October 5th, 2012.

92. Koch E. Inhibition of platelet activating factor (PAF)-induced aggregation of human thrombocytes by ginkgolides: considerations on possible bleeding complications after oral intake of Ginkgo biloba extracts. Phytomedicine 2005;12(1–2):10–6.

93. Anon. Ginseng (American ginseng, Asian ginseng, Chinese ginseng, Korean red ginseng, Panax ginseng: Panax spp., including P. ginseng C.A.Mey. and P. quinquefolius L., excluding Eleutherococcus senticosus). In: Natural Standard: the authority on integrative medicine. Cambridge (MA): Natural Standard; 2012 [cited 5 October 2012]. Available at: http://www.naturalstandard.com. Subscription required to view.

94. Teng CM, Kuo SC, Ko FN, et al. Antiplatelet actions of panaxynol and ginsenosides isolated from ginseng. Biochim Biophys Acta 1989;990(3):315–20.

95. Kuo SC, Teng CM, Lee JC, et al. Antiplatelet components in Panex ginseng. Planta Med 2007;56(02):164–7.

96. Greenspan EM. Ginseng and vaginal bleeding. JAMA 1983;249(15):2018. Accessed on October 5th, 2012.

97. Kabalak AA, Soyal OB, Urfalioglu A, et al. Menometrorrhagia and tachyarrhythmia after using oral and topical ginseng. J Womens Health (Larchmt) 2004;13(7): 830–3.

98. Anon. Ginger (Zingiber officinale Roscoe). In: Natural Standard: the authority on integrative medicine. Cambridge (MA): Natural Standard; 2012 [cited 5 October 2012]. Available at: http://www.naturalstandard.com. Subscription required to view.

99. Nurtjahja-Tjendraputra E, Ammit AJ, Roufogalis BD, et al. Effective anti-platelet and COX-1 enzyme inhibitors from pungent constituents of ginger. Thromb Res 2003;111(4–5):259–65.

100. Bordia A, Verma SK, Srivastava KC. Effect of ginger (Zingiber officinale Rosc.) and fenugreek (Trigonella foenum-graecum L.) on blood lipids, blood sugar and platelet aggregation in patients with coronary artery disease. Prostaglandins Leukot Essent Fatty Acids 1997;56(5):379–84.

101. Lösche W, Mazurov AV, Heptinstall S, et al. An extract of feverfew inhibits inter-actions of human platelets with collagen substrates. Thromb Res 1987;48(5):511–8.

102. Pepping J. Kava: Piper methysticum. Am J Health Syst Pharm 1999;56(10):957–8, 960.

103. Garges HP, Varia I, Doraiswamy PM. Cardiac complications and delirium asso-ciated with valerian root withdrawal. JAMA 1998;280(18):1566–7.

104. Leak JA. Perioperative considerations in the management of the patient taking herbal medicines. Curr Opin Anaesthesiol 2000;13(3):321–5.

105. Pribitkin ED, Boger G. Herbal therapy: what every facial plastic surgeon must know. Arch Facial Plast Surg 2001;3(2):127–32.

106. Ernst E, Rand JI, Barnes J, et al. Adverse effects profile of the herbal antidepres-sant St. John's wort (Hypericum perforatum L.). Eur J Clin Pharmacol 1998;54(8):589–94.

107. Rossouw JE, Anderson GL, Prentice RL, et al. Risks and benefits of estrogen plus progestin in healthy postmenopausal women: principal results From the Women's Health Initiative randomized controlled trial. JAMA 2002;288(3):321–33.

108. Hopkins MP, Androff L, Benninghoff AS. Ginseng face cream and unexplained vaginal bleeding. Am J Obstet Gynecol 1988;159(5):1121–2.

109. Williamson EM. Drug interactions between herbal and prescription medicines. Drug Saf 2003;26(15):1075–92.

110. Markowitz JS, Donovan JL, DeVane CL, et al. Effect of St John's wort on drug metabolism by induction of cytochrome p450 3a4 enzyme. JAMA 2003;290(11):1500–4.

111. Izzo AA, Ernst E. Interactions between herbal medicines and prescribed drugs: a systematic review. Drugs 2001;61(15):2163–75.

112. Hodges PJ, Kam PC. The peri-operative implications of herbal medicines. Anaesthesia 2002;57(9):889–99.

113. Brumley C. Herbs and the perioperative patient. AORN J 2000;72(5):785–94, 796; [quiz: 798–804].

Complementary and Integrative Treatments Integrative Care Centers and Hospitals: One Center's Perspective

Michael D. Seidman, MD*, Gerard van Grinsven

KEYWORDS

- Complementary and integrative medicine • Henry Ford Health System
- Optimal health • Wellness and prevention

KEY POINTS

- Complementary and integrative medicine (CIM) is generally described as any practice that can be used for the prevention and treatment of diseases, but which is not taught widely in medical schools, generally available in hospitals, or usually covered by health insurance.
- The mission of the Center for Integrative Medicine and the Henry Ford Health System West Bloomfield (HFWB) Hospital is to provide an environment in which patients resolve all health challenges and achieve optimal health.
- The average health status of the US population is steadily declining, while the use of increasingly higher-cost technology and pharmaceuticals in conventional medicine is not producing better health.
- Ultimately, success requires multiple "champions" from the medical and administrative sides, strong support from the leaders in the system, and a clear vision and strategy that embraces the importance of integrative care for our patients.
- The most successful systems seem to have secured significant funding, in the range or $10 million or more.
- It is paramount that the health system partner with many nearby community groups to address social, economic, and educational issues affecting people in the communities it serves.

OVERVIEW

The development of integrative care centers and hospitals is worth pursuing, and frankly, is no longer an option, but a requirement. Our existing paradigm of "health care" is nothing more than "sick care." Providing a more holistic and preventive approach is challenging, but a change we must implement. The Centers for Disease

Division of Otologic/Neurotologic Surgery, Department of Otolaryngology-Head and Neck Surgery, Center for Integrative Medicine, Henry Ford Hospital, Henry Ford Health System, 6777 West Maple Road, West Bloomfield, MI 48322, USA
* Corresponding author.
E-mail address: mseidma1@hfhs.org

Otolaryngol Clin N Am 46 (2013) 485–497
http://dx.doi.org/10.1016/j.otc.2013.02.010
0030-6665/13/$ – see front matter © 2013 Elsevier Inc. All rights reserved.
oto.theclinics.com

Control and Prevention estimates that two-thirds to three-fourths of all medical disorders are preventable. In 2013, "sick care" spending is estimated to approach $2.7 trillion and make up approximately 18% of the gross domestic product. This is not sustainable. Since 1998 at the Henry Ford Health System (HFHS), we have been implementing wellness initiatives designed to target many health care issues, with the goal of preventing disease, improving outcomes, and reducing health care expenditures. Some of these strategies involve complementary and integrative medicine (CIM).

CIM, perhaps better known as complementary and alternative medicine (CAM), can be defined in a variety of ways. CIM is generally described as any practice that can be used for the prevention and treatment of diseases, but which is not taught widely in medical schools, generally available in hospitals, or usually covered by health insurance. There are many widely accepted therapies that fall under the guise of CIM. Many of these practices had their inception in Asia thousands of years ago, whereas others originated in Europe or America. **Box 1** provides a partial list of CIM therapies.

History

The origins of what we now consider conventional medicine started approximately 200 years ago. The roots of complementary and integrative therapies have been present since civilization began. There are references, for example, to the healing applications of aloe vera in the Bible. During the mid-twentieth century there was a rapid elimination of CIM, as it was often considered to be quackery or charlatanism and was not validated by double-blind, randomized, placebo-controlled studies. It is difficult, if not impossible, to randomize and placebo control every type of therapeutic intervention, but the lack of strong, evidence-based research does not necessarily mean that a therapy is ineffective.

Clearly many clinicians with strong science backgrounds, coupled with the increasing demand for evidence-based medicine, find the following quotes or care model heretical on some level, and perhaps feel that these methodologies were germane only in the era of leeches and prayer. The authors of this article wholeheartedly endorse the concept that was adroitly articulated by Rich Rosenfeld: "the best care is likely to emerge from a skillful blend of best evidence with caring, humility, and behavior that engenders a placebo response."[1] Additionally, and in many ways not too dissimilar, in 1694 Voltaire is credited with saying, "the art of medicine consists in amusing the patient while nature cures the disease."[2] Last, Thomas Adams (English clergyman,1618) said, "Prevention is so much better than healing because it saves the labor of being sick."[3] Although some might consider these comments visionary for the times, cynics will argue that there was nothing else available, so all we could do was hold the hands of our patients and pray for them. The power of the body to heal itself is grossly underused in medicine today; the best physicians understand this and find ways to facilitate this healing.

Modern trends

CIM therapies are continuing to penetrate conventional Western medical health care. In 1997, the number of CIM visits to alternative practitioners was 629 million (a growing trend), whereas there were 386 million visits to primary care physicians (a declining trend).[4] The US Department of Health and Human Services issued a report dated May 27, 2004, regarding "Complementary and Alternative Medicine Use Among Adults: United States, 2002."[5] It showed that 62% of adults had used some form of CIM in the preceding 12 months. Interestingly, they included prayer (specifically for health reasons); when prayer was excluded, that number dropped to 36%. CIM was most often used for:

Box 1
Common CIM therapies
Acupuncture
Alexander technique
Ayurveda
Biofeedback
Chiropractic
Energy healing
Feldenkrais technique
Folk remedies
Healing touch
Herbal supplements
Homeopathy
Hypnotherapy
Imagery
Magnet therapy
Massage therapy
Meditation
Megavitamin therapy
Naturopathy
Neuromuscular therapy
Prayer
Qigong
Reflexology
Reiki
Relaxation
Remote healing
Rolfing
Self-help groups
Spiritual healing by others
Tai chi
Therapeutic touch
Yoga

- Back pain
- Upper respiratory infections
- Neck problems
- Anxiety
- Depression

It is evident that there continues to be a significant increase in both use and acceptance of CIM therapies by Americans.

There are many reasons cited for considering CIM, including peoples' dissatisfaction with conventional medicine, which is perceived to be authoritative, expensive, ineffective, and too intent on managing disease rather than focusing on wellness and prevention of disease.[6] Other reasons include the following:

- Market forces
- The desire of patients to have a more active role in their medical care
- The impression that conventional medicine fails to satisfactorily treat chronic ailments, such as chronic headache, back pain, fibromyalgia, cancer, and tinnitus and vertigo, among many others.

Thus, there are many patients who are engaging in alternative strategies. It is becoming clear that many CIM users are not necessarily dissatisfied with conventional care, but that they are developing a more holistic approach to their health and they want more health care options.[4,6] A matter of concern to health providers is that, according to a report in the *Journal of the American Medical Association,* 70% of CIM users do not inform their physicians about their use.[4] This statistic is alarming, as some of the herbal and nutritional supplements can interfere with common medications, at times with potentially life-threatening effects. Nondisclosure also minimizes the ability of the conventional physician to participate in the total care of the patient.

It is becoming increasingly apparent that patients are interested in being treated by a physician who is at least open to considering CIM therapies, particularly when conventional therapies may be less effective. Currently, approximately 75% of medical schools are offering courses on alternative medicine. Physicians must learn about CIM. In the best circumstances, we should use expertise from a variety of practitioners, and collaborations between physicians and people who practice CIM should become routine. Although CIM was conceived thousands of years ago, it exists as "frontier territory." However, we remain convinced that in certain situations, it might be and should be just what the doctor ordered.

Blending Conventional Medicine with CIM

It is important for medical practitioners to very seriously consider the integration of conventional medicine with CIM. Not only is there an increase of public interest in complementary and integrative therapies, but there is also a growing awareness of the effectiveness of CIM therapies, both on the part of consumers as well as the scientific community.

Generally speaking, chronic health problems respond well to a holistic approach based on state-of-the-art conventional medicine combined with CIM modalities to address suboptimal nutrition, emotional imbalances, structural abnormalities, blocked energy flow, and unsupportive belief systems, among other problems. There are many chronic diseases that simply do not respond well to conventional therapeutic intervention. These include such conditions as the following:

- Tinnitus and vertigo
- Chronic back pain
- Arthritis
- Headache
- Fibromyalgia
- Cancer

It is becoming increasingly clear that the best practices involve providing patients with a wide array of potential healing options. It is difficult for even the most open-minded provider to be an expert in all therapies, or be aware of everything that is available, what the research supports, and where to refer people. Providers must be honest with patients, especially if they do not know about a treatment modality. A lack of knowledge about a CIM modality does not provide a license to speak in a disparaging way about the modality.

The HFHS Center for Integrative Medicine (**Fig. 1**) and Vita Wellness Center provide excellent examples of integration of conventional medicine and CIM. These centers were conceived as a state-of-the-art program to provide optimal care for chronic illness and to support health and wellness. They provide integrative care with a strong research-based orientation to ensure the safe and effective blending of conventional and complementary medicine. CIM practitioners address patients as a whole in mind, body, and spirit. CIM professionals attempt to mobilize and enhance the healing ability inherent in each person, and they recognize that they are in partnership with their patients; treatment is directed toward the unique goals and values of each individual. Practitioners at the Center enter treatment notes in the patients' electronic records. We have collected data for more than 10 years on more than 5000 patients who have visited the center and received more than 35,000 treatments, including the following:

- Acupuncture
- Chiropractic
- Massage
- St. John neuromuscular therapy
- Feldenkrais movement reeducation
- Hypnotherapy.

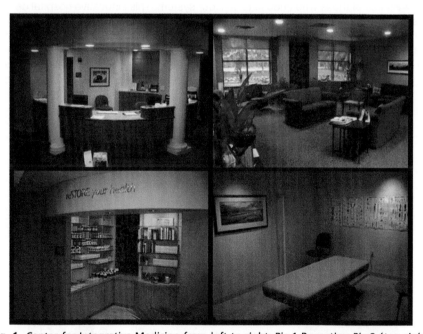

Fig. 1. Center for Integrative Medicine from left to right: Pic 1 Reception Pic 2 (*top right*) "Living Room" (where clients wait for their holistic provider), Pic 3 (*lower left*) Small storefront "reStore your Health" where we sell books and approved supplements and other tools to assist in improving health and wellness. Pic 4 (*lower right*) "Healing Room" there are 11 such rooms (note not called treatment or exam rooms, but HEALING ROOMS, to set the correct mindset).

Most patients treated at the center have failed all conventional medical options. In spite of this, our data show that pain levels in patients are reduced consistently by at least 50%, and some patients have eliminated their pain completely. Collecting data at centers is vital for identifying various alternative treatment strategies that are worthwhile.

In March 2009, HFHS opened a $370 million hospital based on the concept of health and wellness (**Figs. 2** and **3**). A critical part of the vision began with the very basic building blocks of food for our patients and employees. Henry Ford West Bloomfield (HFWB) Hospital does not use freezers or fryers, and serves organic and local food whenever possible. Every recipe is evaluated by a team of clinicians, ensuring that the meals are as healthy as possible. Because of these efforts, our patients and guests always enjoy fresh, delicious, and nutritious food. HFWB also offers a state-of-the-art greenhouse, which offers organic produce through hydroponics. The produce is used in our kitchens, and also used to educate community members about the importance of sustainable, healthy food sources. Additionally the Demonstration Kitchen, an educational facility located within the hospital, impacts patients and guests through cooking classes aimed at improving health.

The path to wellness at HFWB Hospital continues to the Vita Wellness center. Vita offers patients integrative therapy services in addition to conventional medical treatments. We offer mind-body therapies, acupuncture, chiropractic, traditional Chinese medicine, health coaching, and use of nutraceuticals, yoga studios, massage, and more within the same building. The health system built walking paths and an outdoor basketball court on our 160-acre property with the ultimate aim of improving the health and wellness of those who choose to visit our system. This innovative hospital design was greatly influenced by the president and CEO, Gerard van Grinsven. Gerard van Grinsven is a former executive in the hospitality industry, and led for the vision for distinction and innovation. This has led to further progress; through the direction of our in-house "think tank" of experts, we are creating a center of excellence based on wellness and prevention of disease. The model is supported by the CEO of our

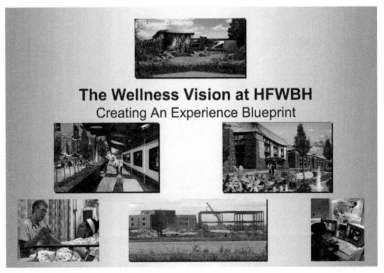

The Wellness Vision at HFWBH
Creating An Experience Blueprint

Fig. 2. Blueprint for Wellness Vision.

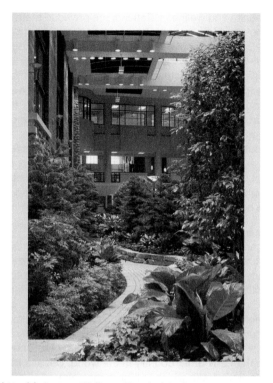

Fig. 3. Henry Ford Health System Wellness Hospital Atrium.

health system and other system leaders. We are driving a model that, when fully implemented, is predicted to significantly enhance the wellness of our patients, community,
and state, and when disseminated throughout the country will likely have
staggering positive effects on health care expenditures.

It is becoming clear that dramatic changes in our health care system are needed.
Health care costs are rising more rapidly than ever, and our country is being held hos-
tage by these high costs. Integrative medicine is one relatively inexpensive approach
that is helpful for many chronic, difficult-to- manage diseases. By incorporating the
best of conventional and complementary medicine, health care professionals can
work together to create an effective integrative health care system. Only in this way
may we succeed at producing the best health of our population at the lowest cost.

Mission and Vision

The mission of the Center for Integrative Medicine and the HFWB Hospital is to provide
an environment in which patients resolve all health challenges and achieve optimal
health.

> *"To administer medicine to diseases which have already developed and thereby
> suppress bodily chaos which has already occurred is comparable to the behavior
> of those who begin to dig a well after they had grown thirsty, or those who would
> begin to cast weapons after they have engaged in battle. Would these actions not
> be too late?" (The Yellow Emperor's Classic of Internal Medicine Circa 400 BC)*

HFWB Hospital and the Center for Integrative Medicine are the world's leader in pio-
neering unique, effective integrative care and wellness programs that propel patients

to achieve optimal health and wellness. Patients are provided state-of-the-art integrative care, combining the high-technology sophistication of conventional care with world-leading, novel, and innovative holistic approaches that, together, take health and healing beyond what has previously been possible.

Cutting-edge research supports the implementation of the most proven-effective healing and wellness programs. All patients and their families have access to wellness programs that support them in taking full control of their lives to achieve optimal health. The paradigm of long-term management and maintenance of chronic illnesses gives way to the eventual resolution of chronic disease.

As the clinical population of HFHS and the Center for Integrative Medicine grows out of our successes, a higher percentage of patient visits are to support achieving optimal health through participation in wellness programs. These programs are disseminated throughout health care to produce unprecedented cost savings and improvement of the health of the global population.

Health status in America

The cost of health care is increasing rapidly, which is having an adverse effect on our national economy, corporations, and individuals. Stress is a major contributor to the exacerbation of acute and chronic illness, maintenance of suboptimal health, loss of employee productivity and job satisfaction, and difficulties in interpersonal relationships. The average health status of the US population is steadily declining, whereas the use of increasingly higher-cost technology and pharmaceuticals in conventional medicine is not producing better health. The United States currently spends $2.7 trillion each year or 18% of gross domestic product on health care, more than $6000 per individual and more than any other country in the world. Despite these expenditures, our infant mortality is 6.37/1000, which is higher than almost all other developed nations. Our life expectancy is 78 years (45th overall), well behind Switzerland, Germany, Bosnia, and Jordan to name a few. Americans should have the best health status in the world; unfortunately, we are ranked 37th. As noted in the *Wall Street Journal* editorial of March 19, 2007, "The health system isn't healthy. There's no denying it. A system that was designed to make you feel better often just makes things worse."

Declining health status is likely to be the most significant event underlying the rising cost of health care. That, coupled with the escalating cost of pharmaceuticals and diagnostic testing, gives rise to a view of the future that is even bleaker than the present if nothing were to change. In spite of all the successes of conventional medicine, we have not delivered reliable ways of *resolving* chronic illness. The HFHS and the Center for Integrative Medicine has now proven in clinical trials for chronic back pain that complementary therapies are significantly more effective than the conventional care for resolving pain. Other research activities include completed clinical trials to evaluate the efficacy of complementary therapies to reduce or eliminate hot flashes in women with breast cancer, as well as migraine headaches.[7]

The excellent research activities are limited only by resources to fund more groundbreaking work. Our centers are seeking philanthropic partners to provide funding to obtain the evidence that is critical for accelerating the integration of proven-effective complementary therapies into mainstream medicine.

Background on Our Center for Integrative Medicine

In December of 2001, HFHS began helping people with chronic back pain, persistent headaches, uncontrolled allergies, digestive problems, and a long list of other conditions to find permanent relief through treatments such as chiropractic, acupuncture, St. John neuromuscular therapy, Feldenkrais, mind-body therapies, and nutritional counseling. HFHS operates the free-standing Center for Integrative Medicine, head-quartered in Novi, Michigan, which formally opened in June of 2002. The center represents one of the few that has a direct-care component in addition to research, and that is integrated with a nationally known medical center, such as HFHS.

Many of these therapies, which have been around for thousands of years, have been routinely rejected by mainstream Western medicine on the grounds of being unproven. Despite this resistance, our center sees nearly 1000 patients each month and more than 25% are referred to us from their physicians. Although this is exciting on the surface, we are usually seeing patients who have failed all forms of conventional options. Patients will benefit and health care costs will diminish when the paradigm of care provides patients concurrent access to complementary and conventional therapies; this is precisely what HFWB wellness hospital is providing. For example, the current paradigm for the patient with a cancer is to have a multidisciplinary conventional approach that includes the oncologist, the radiation therapist, and the surgeon. Our CIM philosophy supports the inclusion of the mind-body therapist, the acupuncturist, and the holistic nutritionist to the team to allow best practices from all vantage points to facilitate healing. This has yet to be implemented because of scant resources, but it is part of our vision and ultimate plan.

Current approaches
At HFHS, we employ practitioners that offer a variety of therapeutic approaches, both individual and combined, to support the total health and well-being of each person. Services offered include the following:

- Acupuncture
- Chiropractic
- Feldenkrais movement reeducation
- Herbal and nutritional counseling
- Holistic support for patients with cancer
- Health coaching
- Massage therapy
- Mind-body therapies (eg, hypnosis)
- Neuromuscular therapy.

The therapies are designed to compliment and integrate with conventional medicine for the treatment of many conditions including the following:

- Chronic pain (such as back, neck, hip, shoulder)
- Headaches (including migraines)
- Postural problems (scoliosis and "dowager's hump")
- Cancer
- Anxiety, depression, and stress
- Gynecologic and fertility problems
- Autoimmune diseases, such as rheumatoid arthritis
- Respiratory problems
- Wellness (smoking cessation, nutrition, weight management)
- Chronic fatigue
- Arthritis
- Digestive problems
- Vertigo and tinnitus
- Sports injuries
- Fibromyalgia
- Mobility problems
- Circulatory problems.

Our system offers these complementary therapies to patients both within and outside the HFHS, and works closely with Henry Ford specialties and centers, including the Josephine Ford Cancer Center, the Vattikuti Urology Institute, neurology, obstetrics and gynecology, otolaryngology, and orthopedics.

The HFHS Center for Wellness and the Center for Integrative Medicine research teams have already generated exciting research that has convinced the medical community and general public of the effectiveness of complementary therapies. A major example of the innovative, high-impact research conducted by Center for Integrative Medicine personnel is the recent successful group intervention program at Chrysler Corporation for employees with chronic back pain. Initial research has compared one-on-one conventional physical therapy to a hands-off group treatment approach with up to 48 Chrysler employees at a time. Although conventional physical therapy for people with chronic back pain provided a 5% resolution to zero pain, the group intervention produced a 55% resolution to zero pain (none of the control patients resolved to zero pain). The group intervention reduced the time of treating patients by more than 98% compared with typical one-on-one care. These remarkable results in resolving back pain at such high percentages using an efficient group intervention have never before been accomplished. Additional funding is paramount to validate this approach and apply it to other chronic conditions such as cancer, cardiovascular disease, diabetes, obesity, and others (Robert Levine, PhD, personal communication, 2012).

The Philosophy of CIM

The philosophy behind integrative medicine is that optimal health occurs when an individual has balance in mind, body, and spirit. When imbalances occur, they cause dysfunctions that can lead to organ and structural problems, as well as disease. Holistic practitioners recognize that people possess their own healing ability, so they work in partnership with patients to mobilize and enhance that ability in a way that takes into account each patient's unique background and make-up.

Before the 1600s, this holistic view of the individual was prevalent. René Descartes was the first to divide the human into separate and distinct entities. He proposed that the body could be treated for medical conditions independently, without considering other domains, such as mind or spirit. In **Fig. 4**, the left panel provides a pictorial of the holistic view. The right panel shows that the Western medical paradigm, or way of thinking, developed as an outgrowth of Descartes' philosophy. The predominant hypothesis of conventional medicine is that diseases are caused by dysfunctions within

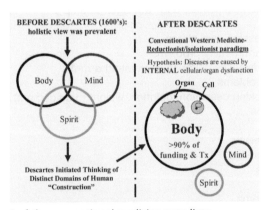

Fig. 4. Development of the conventional medicine paradigm.

cells. This reductionist, or isolationist philosophy has permeated Western medicine. Long-term use of expensive medicines that only manage symptoms rather than correct problems is why chronic diseases are so prevalent and very costly to treat. Thus, chronic conditions are managed, but not cured. Most funding for basic research and clinical trials is focused on discovering and reversing dysfunction at the cellular level. There is minimal funding for any other approaches, which has limited most patients' choices to conventional medicine options covered by health insurance.

Fig. 5 highlights one of the fundamental hypotheses in holistic medicine: that diseases are caused by imbalances of body, mind, and spirit. When these imbalances occur, they cause dysfunctions in cells that ultimately lead to organ problems and disease. If this hypothesis is correct, then cellular dysfunction would not be the primary cause of disease, and searching for the source of disease at the cellular level would be futile. Cellular and organ abnormalities would be a result of imbalances in body, mind, and spirit rather than the source of disease. Yet, holistic medicine is often rejected by mainstream medicine as unproven by scientific research, while minimal funds are available to provide appropriate evidence. Whether or not this hypothesis related to holistic medicine is true, complementary therapies that address the patient as a whole with potentially unique underlying causes of disease are effective, and often more effective than conventional medicine in addressing chronic disease, as we have proven with some of our clinical trial research at HFHS Center for Integrative Medicine.

Fortunately, there are key philanthropists that have the foresight to provide resources for gathering evidence showing the effectiveness of complementary therapies. An initial donation to HFHS allowed for the construction and opening of our first Center for Integrative Medicine. Philanthropy is the key resource that is catalyzing the transformation of conventional medicine to true integrative medicine that combines the best of both worlds to optimize patient care and promote wellness.

Growth of CIM

Despite this perceived conflict with conventional medicine, integrative therapies are popular with the general population. More than 60% of Americans use complementary health care services.[5] The American public spends more than $34 billion each year from personal resources on complementary therapies. It is also remarkable that there are nearly twice the number of visits to practitioners of complementary medicine than to primary care physicians in the United States, and the spread is growing.

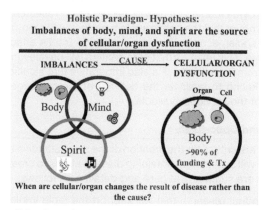

Fig. 5. A holistic medicine hypothesis.

There is limited insurance coverage for these therapies, in part because of the lack of evidence demonstrating their effectiveness in clinical trials. This is unfortunate, as access to these therapies is currently limited to those who can afford to allocate personal resources. Exacerbating the situation is that little research money is available, which limits the speed with which these therapies can be tested and made available to all people once validated.

How to Succeed in the Development of Integrative Care Centers and Health Systems

Succinctly put, success requires nothing short of a paradigm shift in the way we approach health care. It requires champions who are willing to put their careers at some risk and take chances. The path is challenging and will be met with both rewards and frustration. When we began our journey in 1998, we were charged with evaluating the possibility of bringing CIM to our health system; one that, like many, remains very conservative. The process began with a task force that included stakeholders from every discipline, including 2 lay individuals from the community. Surveys were sent out in multiple formats to our 23,000 employees to gain a pulse of the current sentiment regarding CIM. We asked not only the medical and nursing staff, but the administrators, allied health personnel, valet attendants, janitorial staff, and more. We asked simple questions, such as one gauging their awareness of acupuncture, chiropractic, homeopathy, naturopathy, vitamins and herbs, hypnotherapy, and so forth. Ratings were 1 to 5, with 1 being no knowledge and 5 being intimate understanding. The questions also asked (providers) if they would be open to recommending these services to their patients. Some providers were already "certified" as acupuncturists, and others were already suggesting alternative options to their patients. We also received some concerning responses; for instance, "If you even consider the quackery of homeopathy, I will quit." Over a period of several years, the team met weekly to create our vision and strategy to develop CIM within our health system. We had strong support from the CEO of our health system and from other system leaders, both on the medical and administrative sides. We also had high-level individuals within our system who set out to derail this venture and frankly continue to be less than supportive.

Ultimately, success requires multiple "champions" from the medical and administrative sides, strong support from the leaders in the system, and a clear vision and strategy that embraces the importance of integrative care for our patients. Additionally, and critically important, is extensive philanthropic resources to fuel the vision and the implementation. The most successful systems seem to have secured significant funding in the range of $10 million or more, and much of the funds are used to fuel an endowment to provide funding for new projects, "risky" research projects, and sustainability. It is paramount that the health system partner with many nearby community groups to address social, economic, and educational issues affecting people in the communities it serves. This ensures that care centers will be relevant to the population that would benefit from its services. It is also imperative that significant resources are earmarked for marketing to facilitate the delivery of the message and to make the community aware of the services available.

The Future Vision and Opportunity

The following goals are critical for the creation of the most effective and efficient health care. The paradigm will shift from maintaining disease states to creating optimal health and wellness. They are summarized here and detailed as follows.

- *Goal One:* Conduct research that will support the rapid implementation of integrative medicine. Cost savings will accumulate for the system and for insurance

Table 1			
Estimated funding requirements			
	Year 1, in Millions of Dollars	Year 2, in Millions of Dollars	Year 3, in Millions of Dollars
Research	1.0	0.5	0.5
Education	1.0	1.0	1.0
Centers for integrative medicine	1.0	1.0	1.0
Group interventions	1.0	1.0	1.0
Endowment	1.0	3.5	3.5
Total	5.0	4.5	4.5

Total investment needed over 3 years: $14M.

companies through more efficient patient care. Patients will find relief both from their ailments and for their financial resources; out-of-pocket expenses will decrease when therapies shorten illnesses and are covered under insurance plans.

- Goal Two: Educate medical practitioners on the ways in which alternative therapies can compliment conventional therapies, so that physicians refer their patients to the Center for Integrative Medicine when an integrative treatment can enhance their recovery. Education is fundamental to facilitate integration of complementary medicine therapies into conventional medicine.
- Goal Three: Open additional centers for integrative medicine to increase convenience and accessibility for patients around the region.
- Goal Four: Expand group interventions to address many conditions that can be managed in group settings. This model can be expanded to provide onsite services to major corporations.

Success depends on acquiring funds to cover the costs associated with these 4 goals (**Table 1**). Philanthropy will play a key role in the creation of an approach that incorporates the best of conventional and complementary patient care and will create a model that will be recognized and emulated internationally.

REFERENCES

1. Rosenfeld RM. Nature. Otolaryngol Head Neck Surg 2009;141(1):1–2.
2. Lock S, Last JM, Gunea G. The Oxford illustrated companion to medicine. 3rd edition. Oxford University Press; 2001. p. 698.
3. Adams T. The Happiness of the Church considered in contemplations upon Hebrews. SI Grisman; 1618. p. 146.
4. Eisenberg DM, Davis RB, Ettner SL, et al. Trends in Alternative Medicine Use in the United States, 1990-1997: results of a follow-up National Survey. JAMA 1998; 280(18):1569–75.
5. Barnes PM, Bloom B, Nahim RL. Complementary and alternative medicine use among adults and children: United States, 2007. Natl Health Stat Report 2008; 10(12):1–23.
6. Astin JA. Why patients use alternative medicine: results of a national study. JAMA 1998;279(19):1548–53.
7. Walker EM, Rodriguez AI, Kohn B, et al. Acupuncture versus venlafaxine for the management of vasomotor symptoms in patients with hormone receptor–positive breast cancer: a randomized controlled trial. Clin Oncol 2010;28(4):634–40.

Index

Note: Page numbers of article titles are in **boldface** type.

A

Acetyl L-carnitine, 283
Acupuncture, 267–268, 287–288
  in allergy, 304
  in balance disorders, 416–417
  in facial cosmetic enhancement, 470–472
  in facial pain, 376
  in obstructive sleep apnea, 386–387
  in rhinosinusitis, 353, 355
  in sore throat, 333
  in swallowing disorders, 454
  in tinnitus, 402–403
  in upper respiratory infection, 341
Adenotonsillar disease, and sore throat, integrative treatment approaches in, 331
    surgical treatment approaches in, 330–331
  complex and integrative treatments in, **329–334**
Aging, healthy, factors in, 280–281
  processes of, physiology and anatomy of, 278–281
Aging strategies, successful, 288
Allergic rhinitis, complementary and integrative medicine in, 301–304
Allergy, classification of, and symptoms of, 297
  complementary and integrative treatments in, **295–307**
  "hygiene hypothesis" and, 297
  medical treatment approaches in, and outcomes of, 297–301
  overview of, 295–296
  physiology of, 296–297
  reactions, 296–297
Aloe, in facial cosmetic enhancement, 462–463
Alpha lipoic acid, 282
Anesthetic agents, topical, in facial pain, 373
Anti-inflammatory agents, nonsteroidal, in upper respiratory infection, 338
Antibiotics, in upper respiratory infection, 336–337
Anticonvulsant drugs, in facial pain, 372–373
Antidepressants, in tinnitus, 397
Antihistamines, in allergy, 297–298
  in upper respiratory infection, 337–338
Antioxidants, for successful aging, 282–284
  in balance disorders, 415
  in voice disorders, 437–439
Arnica, in facial cosmetic enhancement, 463–465
Ayurveda, 265–266

Otolaryngol Clin N Am 46 (2013) 499–506
http://dx.doi.org/10.1016/S0030-6665(13)00060-1
0030-6665/13/$ – see front matter © 2013 Elsevier Inc. All rights reserved.

oto.theclinics.com

Moving?

Make sure your subscription moves with you!

To notify us of your new address, find your **Clinics Account Number** (located on your mailing label above your name), and contact customer service at:

Email: journalscustomerservice-usa@elsevier.com

800-654-2452 (subscribers in the U.S. & Canada)
314-447-8871 (subscribers outside of the U.S. & Canada)

Fax number: 314-447-8029

Elsevier Health Sciences Division
Subscription Customer Service
3251 Riverport Lane
Maryland Heights, MO 63043

*To ensure uninterrupted delivery of your subscription, please notify us at least 4 weeks in advance of move.

ELSEVIER